AF498879

Second Edition corrected and extended
Aze Shiatsu Editorial

Aze Shiatsu

Basic Treatment

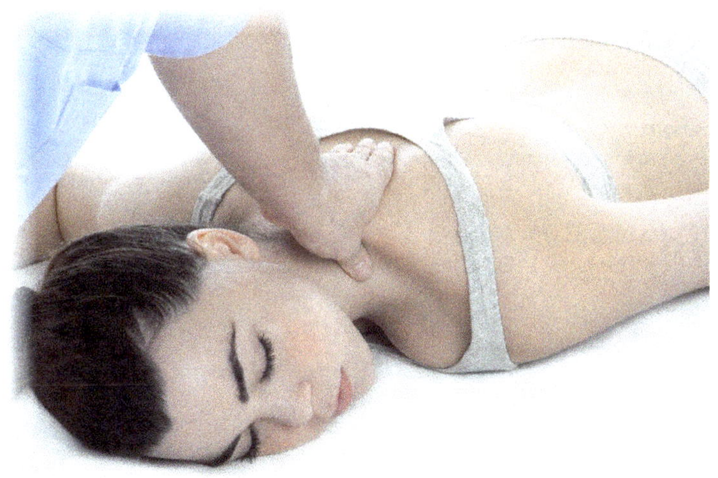

Shigeru Onoda

Supervisor: Dr. Hiroshi Ishizuka

© Aze Shiatsu Editorial 2022
Calle Juan Hurtado de Mendoza, 9 esc. B Apto 107, 28036, Madrid (España).
Tel.: +(34) 913 457 124 Fax.: +(34) 913 456 676
e-mail: centro@shiatsudo.com.

First edition: July 2011

Second Edition: March 2015

Third Edition: October 2022

Illustrations:
   María Torres Dos Ramos, Raquel García Fernández, Tatio Viana, Carmen Toro de Federico, Daigo Ohnuma.

Supervision of anatomical terminology:
   Dr. Hiroshi Ishizuka (Director of the Japan Shiatsu College).

Photography:
   Claudia Costanzo, Loukia Stathatou.

Legal Deposit: M-18621-2020
ISBN: 978-84-09-22107-3

Printed by: Amazon
Layout: María Torres
English translation: Briony Campbell

Index

CHAPTER 1. PRONE

Aze Shiatsu. Basic Treatment in Prone Decubitus 50

CHAPTER 2. SUPINE

Aze Shiatsu. Basic treatment in Supine Decubitus 144

Introduction

DUE to the many treatment sessions I perform everyday and my experience with hundreds of patients, I can assure you that Japanese and Western bodies are completely different; both anatomically and structurally.

Life expectancy has noticeably increased; however, let's not forget that the number of young victims who die

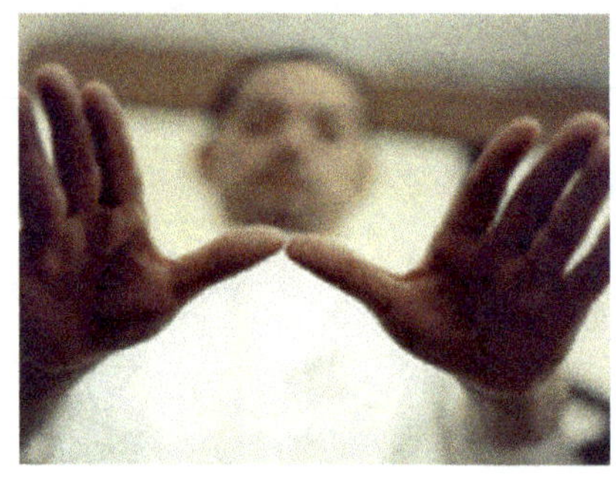

from diseases such as cancer has also increased. We will analyze this data more closely, as although rectal cancer has the highest incidence rate in Spain, it is stomach cancer in Japan; mainly because of the differences in food, and even for the length of the intestine, as this organ is longer in the Japanese.

Another fact to be reviewed, and which I find extremely curious, is that the Japanese do not possess the main enzymes that metabolize alcohol; although this may seem like a disadvantage to the naked eye, they have a much lower risk for developing alcoholic liver disease, presumably because of their sensitivity to alcohol poisoning.

The inclination of the sacrum in Westerners is very acute, so more than 20% suffer from herniated discs; in Japanese, however, this pathology is 2%.

During my years of treatment, I have also discovered that my patients have very fragile cervical vertebrae, I could almost say that they were like glass; that's why I always try to perform neck movements with great care and observe the reactions of all my patients.

Shiatsu is of Japanese origin; it was conceived to increase and improve the self-defenses of the Eastern body, so after many years of study with Westerners, I realized that my patients evolved very slowly when working with the Namikoshi style, the "bible" of shiatsu that I was involved with in Japan.

Over time, I decided to adapt it to the Western body by creating a system of techniques and variants of Namikoshi Shiatsu that gradually yielded its fruit, with quite noticeable improvements in all my patients.

I have worked on this book, the result of my years of study with patients, and I have called it Aze Shiatsu, which means "to look for the key points outside the meridians lines".

This book is the standard Aze Shiatsu theory and today it is the basis of the work of all my students.

Shigeru Onoda
Founder of Aze Shiatsu
Shiatsupractor

1. What is Shiatsu?

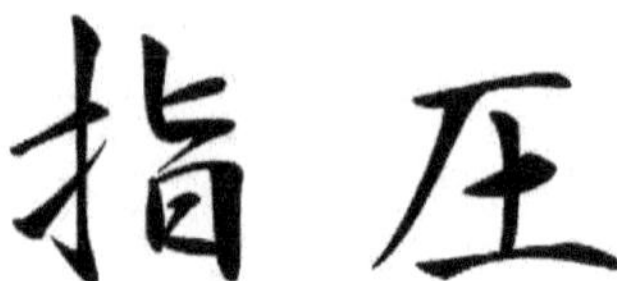

THE literal translation of the word Shiatsu is "finger pressure", but in Japan everyone understands what it really means. Shiatsu is a manual therapy originating in Japan, whose objective is to maintain and improve health. Japan's Ministry of Health defines Shiatsu as: "Treatment that, by applying pressure with the thumbs and palms of the hands on certain points, corrects irregularities, maintains and improves health, and contributes to alleviating certain diseases (discomfort, pain, stress, nervous disorders, etc.), thereby activating the human body's ability to self-heal. IT HAS NO SIDE EFFECTS".

Currently in Europe, along with Karate or Judo, Shiatsu treatment is well-known and there is no need to explain what it is. Its more than forty-year history gives it its own position within the world of manual therapies.

The primitive origin of Shiatsu goes back to our unconscious act of rubbing or pressing the body with the hands when we feel some kind of slackness, stiffness, numbness or pain. Instinctive actions like these to cure disorders predate medicine and history itself. The Japanese, when using the word TEATE, understand that it refers to any manual treatment.

TEATE literally means "touching with your hand". For them a manual therapy should balance the body, maintain its ability to defend itself and improve the patient's quality of life.

It was Tokujiro Namikoshi who developed the method of teaching and applying Shiatsu. Currently, to be a Shiatsu therapist you have to do three years of study (2,145 hours) in one of the schools authorized by the Japanese Ministry of Education. Upon completion, you get an academic degree that entitles you to take a state exam that, if passed, qualifies you as a Shiatsu therapist. There are several schools that train future Shiatsu professionals, but the Japan Shiatsu College, founded by Tokujiro Namikoshi, is the most recognized and prestigious.

It should additionally be noted that another of Namikoshi's objective was to promote this therapy outside Japan. Its line has spread worldwide and, in particular in Spain, the Japanese Shiatsu School, run by Shigeru Onoda, has been responsible for boosting knowledge of Shiatsu across Europe. The collaboration between the School and the Japan Shiatsu College is ongoing. Periodically a Japanese delegation attends different events that are organized to support the work of the School.

Technically, Shiatsu is based on the use of three different techniques:

1. Finger pressure.
2. Alignment of the spinal column.
3. Exercises to maintain and/or increase flexibility.

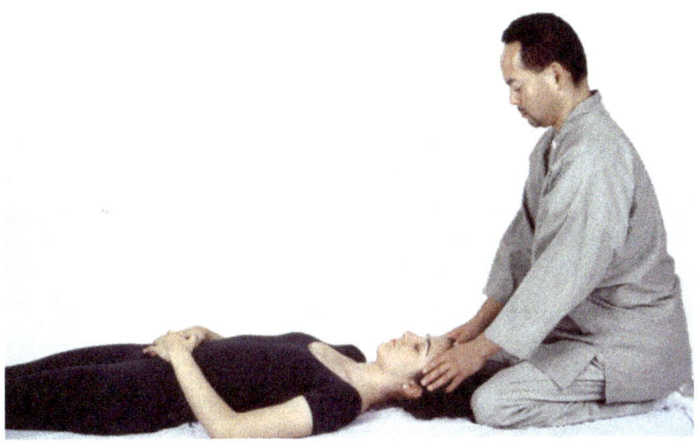

Therapist Shigeru Onoda, founder of Aze Shiatsu.

Currently, Shiatsu in Japan focuses on teaching the finger pressure technique. Aze Shiatsu takes up the other two techniques, and from its particular point of view elaborates a complete Shiatsu adapted to the Western body. It keeps the essence of therapy for maintaining health, but meets the needs posed by 21st Century society's lifestyle.

2. Tokujiro Namikoshi (1905-2000)

Founder of Shiatsu therapy

SHIATSU was created by the master Tokujiro Namikoshi in Japan.

Tokujiro was born in Kagawa Province on the southern island of Shi-koku, and when he was 7 years old his family moved to Hokkaido, the island to the far north of Japan. The sudden change from Shikoku's mild climate to Hokkaido's harsh cold, along with other problems, caused Tokujiro's mother to develop rheumatoid arthritis with severe joint pains. At that time, Rusutu village in Hokkaido was a place without doctors or any way to get medicines or injections. The only thing that the young Tokujiro could do for his mother was to try to relieve the pain; by rubbing, kneading, massaging or applying pressure to the painful areas. In his fight against his mother's pain, he found that the most effective way to relieve the pain was by applying pressure to the area with his fingers.

From that moment on, Tokujiro researched different types of pressure techniques on the area of pain, and so developed the Shiatsu technique. He made the decision to dedicate this therapy to helping people with health problems. He then moved to Tokyo. There he began his personal struggle

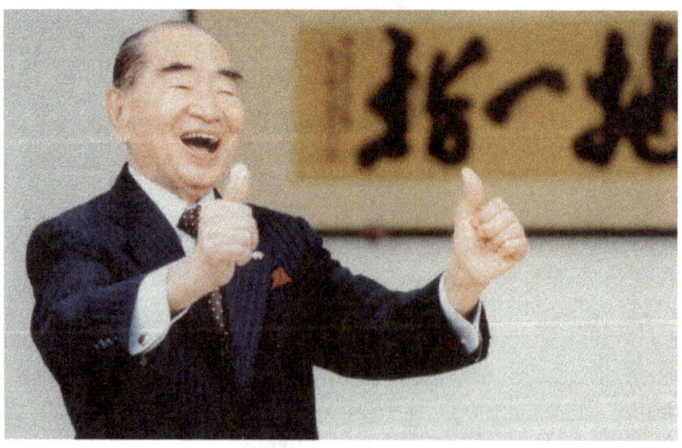

Tokujiro Namikoshi, Shiatsu legend.

to get Shiatsu recognised as a manual therapy by the Japanese authorities. In 1940 he founded Shiatsu's first school, the present-day Japan Shiatsu College.

At one time, he had a programme on Japanese television called "Three Minutes of Shiatsu". His charisma attracted people to become interested in Shiatsu, giving him many students and national popularity. Finally, in 1957, Shiatsu was recognized by Japan's Ministries of Health and Labour as a therapy per se.

After Tokujiro's death, his eldest son, Toru, led the Japan Shiatsu College. It is currently his youngest son, Kazutami, who is at the helm of the institution. Both maintain the premise that Tokujiro Namikoshi left as a testament: "To spread Shiatsu around the world". Many of his disciples are responsible for carrying out this task in every corner of the planet.

Shiatsu was known before Tokujiro, but with his dedication and commitment he managed to standardize a teaching and therapy method with his own organisation for approval by the health authorities of Japan. The essence of Shiatsu is summed up in the words of Master Tokujiro Namikoshi:

The heart of shiatsu is like a mother's love, pressure on the body stimulates the source of life.

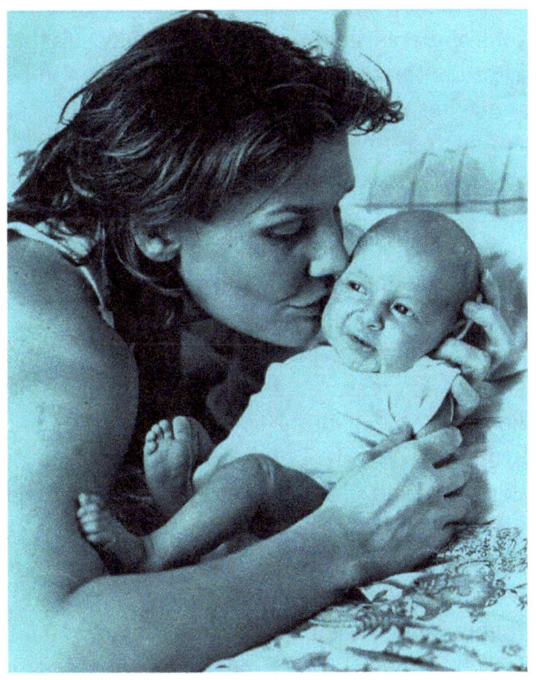

A mother's love.

3. What is Aze Shiatsu?

THE NEED TO CREATE
A STANDARD TREATMENT

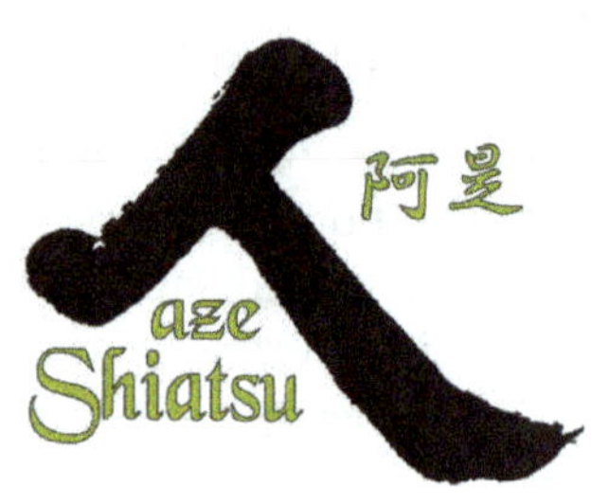

WHEN the Japanese hear the word Shiatsu, they associate it directly with problems of the back. This therapy has done a lot of good to this area and so this idea has remained in the collective subconscious. However, Shiatsu is not used exclusively to alleviate spinal problems; we have also proven, through many years of experience, that it can be used to treat numerous ailments.

Shiatsu professionals know that Shiatsu therapy can help to treat numerous ailments, although it is especially suitable for treating spinal problems. There is the popular saying: "Prevention is better than the cure". Its coherence lies in the nature of the body's self-defense system that has an innate ability to self-heal. It uses pain as an alarm signal to let us know that something isn't working properly, so that we can anticipate the problem in time. Each person has a different sensitivity and pain threshold; when it is passed, the alarm goes off and the body converts it into physical symptoms, receiving it as a message of pain (does the level of pain change depending on the person and the age?).

Over the years, poor posture, stress and tiredness weaken that innate resilience, increasing the pain threshold and making recovery slower.
For pain, the general tendency is to use medications that eliminate the symptoms quickly. But don't be confused; the cause is still there even if we don't feel pain. The mechanisms of pain and inflammation are what the body uses to self-heal. When an area is inflamed and we take an anti-inflammatory, what we are doing is interrupting the regeneration process that our own body puts into operation; let's say that the tissues are repaired, but not regenerated, which affects their quality and durability. Therefore, the pathology becomes chronic (macrophages cannot clean the area and pathogens remain).There are anatomical differences among the different races. For example, Asians and Europeans have a different constitution, especially in

the lumbar curvature, which makes a difference in how frequently they suffer from herniated discs; in the West it is around 20%, while in the East it is 2%.

But, unfortunately, even though there are cultural differences, lower back pain is universal and almost inevitable. In the world of manual therapies, there are different theories about pathologies and their origins. As the lumbar area is in the centre of the body, and the human being the only bipedal mammal, an affected lumbar area can be caused by problems both of the lower body (poorly cured sprains), and of the upper body (cervical whiplash).

From Shiatsu's point of view, the body must be seen as a whole in which all parts are interconnected, influencing each other, so it is risky to perform a treatment as an assembly of separate parts.

Since ancient times, man has received manual treatment to cure his ailments; besides, Chinese medicine says that "in the pursuit of balance in the body, there is an inviolable union between the mental and the physical". Which suggests that back pain may have emotional causes, among other reasons. An emotional state can create an ulcer, tachycardia or weaken any organ, liver irritation also influences the emotional state (there is a saying that says "being in a liver mood").

Our treatment does not focus on the ailment, although it does arise according to the symptoms and pain that the patient presents. The main goal is to balance the body and increase the defenses. The pursuit of such a balance should not be confused with the search to bring the body closer to a Greek ideal, but to find the patient's tendencies and understand the balance within its structure. From birth, each person's DNA determines each person's structural and postural tendency. That is why there are as many possibilities as many as there are people. It is, in short, a holistic and individual treatment.

It is the body itself, through the stimuli received (pressure), that balances and restores health, thereby keeping the body young, flexible and with high defenses to deal with any ailment.

With Shiatsu we work to correct the asymmetries, finding the pressure limit that the patient can tolerate to achieve their balance.
Why is there a need for standard European patient treatment?
As this technique was born in the East, the standard treatment has been developed from the experiences and needs of that community. As it spreads in the West, Shiatsu has to meet new needs; the difference between Asians and Westerners is not only structural but also cultural. In Japan, people are accustomed to deep pressure treatment that is bordering on pain. Their physical structure better supports this type of pressure; the Japanese are also used to receiving Shiatsu regularly and that's why the stimulus need to be increased. In addition, culturally there is the idea that a massage is only effective if the pressure is strong. However, western people require lighter pressure, without causing pain. The ideal of manual therapy is to stimulate as little as possible.
We are used to tolerating heavy and continuous tensions accumulating in our bodies without trying to correct them. Sooner or later the body starts to warn of overload in the form of pain or discomfort. We then go to the doctor or manual therapist for a remedy that gradually has to offer greater stimulation to get positive results. If we think about maintaining a good quality of life, the stimulation of the patient's body should always be minimal. It will only increase because of the aging process that reduces organ function so there needs to be greater stimulation.

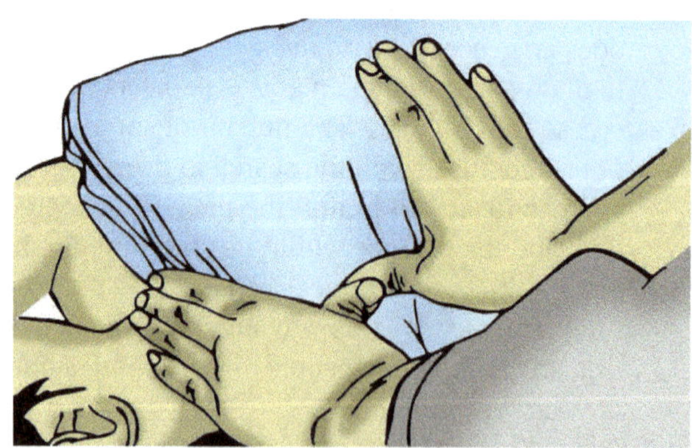

In general, a treatment is considered standard when, with a 60% effectiveness, it is able to achieve a substantial improvement in people. Normally the standard focuses on the lumbar region or back, which is considered the basis for all treatments, even beginners know how to adopt a specific treatment; if they do a standard treatment, the person gets better. It focuses on stimulating the body's self-defense and auto-immune system. From there comes the rest of the techniques. Metaphorically, standard treatment can be considered as the trunk of a tree and, the rest of the techniques are the branches.

In the case of the western tree, the key or first branch would be the specific treatment of the upper body and especially cervical pain, because it is the weak point of the vertebral structure. That's why Master Onoda's AZE style was created, based on his more than 30 years experience with Western patients. It is the birth of what can be considered an adaptation of the traditional Japanese method (Namikoshi) to a standard AZE style for the Western body and mind.

4. Key points, Aze points and Aze Shiatsu

Each Shiatsu work region consists of one or more lines and these in turn contain several points. Some of these points influence specific imbalances and must be treated in a special way, according to knowledge of Aze Shiatsu. References to these points continually appear in our Shiatsu style's literature. Let's define them briefly:

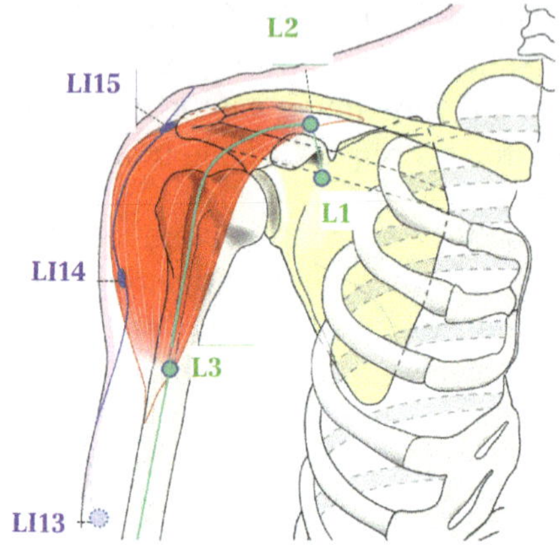

Key points: These are important points for treating some imbalances. Most are closely related to acupuncture points. Others are points of experience, effectively proven by working with Shiatsu, defined and localized after more than thirty years of work.

Aze Points: This is the Japanese way of naming ashi points, which are referred to by traditional Chinese medicine. Ashi points have no specific name or location; they are located in painful areas when imbalances exist.

Key points are always identified according to their traditional acupuncture location, but Aze Shiatsu's work requires searching for the nearby aze point. On many occasions they exactly agree, but in so many others, they do not.

It is important to distinguish between Acupuncture and Shiatsu. Both come from a common source and have the same goal, restoring the health and well-being of the patient, but the ways of diagnosis and treatment are different. Acupuncture is a technique that works directly on the energy that circulates through the body via the meridians and the points that form them. Between ten and thirty needles are normally used in each session. Shiatsu is a manual technique that works by correcting the structural imbalances that occur in the body for different reasons (postural, emotional, energetic, traumatic).

It works the whole body with the hands, the physical contact and its warmth being very important to the final result.

The way of working these points is also different in both techniques. Undoubtedly, you cannot compare the action of a needle inserted two or three centimeters deep for twenty minutes with the work of a thumb applying pressure three times for three seconds, which is the basic Shiatsu pressure. To make the pressure action effective, Aze Shiatsu proposes a simple technique to work on these important points. The therapist has to consider the region where the point is located as a wide area that must be bound by lines and these in turn with points that must be worked on gradually. It is about going from the broadest to the most specific: each point is located in a muscle area whose state irremissibly affects it. The muscle must be returned to its physiological state so that further work on the particular point is much more effective.

5. Characteristics of Shiatsu Treatment

1. Shiatsu is a complete treatment. Whenever work is done, the whole body is treated as well. When treatment is local, the effects are usually temporary and so, does not cure the real cause of the pain.

2. Shiatsu, as its etymology indicates, is a therapy in which only fingers are used, without resorting to any machinery or utensils. Neither fists nor elbows are used. It's because our fingers are endowed with more sensory receptors than the rest of the body and are very sensitive and able to feel the thickness of a thin paper.

3. Diagnosis and therapy are done at the same time in Shiatsu. By applying pressure to the patient's body, the therapist receives information about the skin, muscles, body temperature and so on, through the hands and fingers, and therefore knows what the best treatment is to perform.

4. Shiatsu is a way of treating the body by applying hand and finger pressure on the patient's body. This pressure is perpendicular and is modulated according to the response of the area being worked on, with the objective of stimulating not only the skin but also the muscles, the hormonal system and the central and peripheral nervous system.

5. Shiatsu has no side-effects since pressure is applied so as to produce pleasant sensations in the body. The pleasant pain threshold is never crossed, and the therapist should harmonize the pressure according to the area being treated.

6. Shiatsu can be applied to men, women and children of all ages and the objectives are to be determined in each case individually. With children, it is necessary to try to improve their constitution and strengthen the body. With adults, we should try to maintain and improve their general condition. Shiatsu is applied in pregnant women from the first to the last day of pregnancy; after childbirth, it speeds up the hip recovery process. With the elderly, it keeps the body flexible in order to prevent diseases.

7. Regularly receiving Shiatsu helps to detect possible changes and irregularities that can start showing up in the body. Therefore, it prevents the build-up of stress and toxins that can cause disease to appear. The goal of Shiatsu is to maintain and increase the body's self-defense capacity.

6. Physiological Functions of Shiatsu

Wₕₑₙ any part of our body hurts, we naturally move our hand to the painful area. This is an instinctive action humans are born with and does not need prior training; it is a natural way to relieve pain and is the origin of Shiatsu and other treatments. At the physiological level what happens is that positive ions accumulate in the inflammation causing the sensation of pain. By putting our hands laden with negative ions over the inflamed area, we neutralize the positive charge and the pain disappears. The Shiatsu therapist applies pressure on the areas of the patient's body where there is inadequate blood supply. When an area of the body does not receive the correct blood supply, we will observe the following on the skin of that area:

1. It has dull.
2. It is dry.
3. It lacks elasticity.
4. Hair appears to protect the area.

Applying pressure on these areas, which in general usually coincide with what we refer to as tsubos, improves circulation. To make a comparison, if the body were a railroad network, the tracks would be the lines connecting the pressure points and the stations would be the tsubos. These are usually found in greater numbers around the joints and near the muscle insertions. As sediments accumulate in river curves, tsubos accumulate around the joints and complicated structural areas of the human body. Tsubo in Japan has two meanings: "place of accumulated energy" and "bowl"; in this case, it's an energy deposit.

The therapist can, through his hands, perceive and get to know the patient's body condition and receive its vibrations even without speaking with him. The greater the therapist's experience, the more sensitive the information received from the patient's body is. Perception and experience allow the therapist to treat the right areas by creating communication through their hands.

The Shiatsu-shi (Shiatsu therapist in Japanese) uses their knowledge of Western medicine about the nervous system and viscero-cutaneous reflections. The peripheral nervous system is a part of the nervous system, considered to be an extension of the brain and spinal cord. It consists of sensitive nerves (centripetal fibres) that transmit the collected stimuli to the nerve centres; and motor nerves (centrifugal fibres) that carry the orders of these centres to different body structures, especially the muscles.

Through the centripetal fibres, the stimulus coming from an internal organ can cause reflective pain or other reactions that the nervous system channels to some areas of the body such as the shoulders, back, or abdomen. That would indicate that an exaggerated muscle contraction can be caused by organ disease. The distribution of nerves in the spinal cord is very orderly and the inert areas form segments around the body. These segments are called *dermatomes*.

Taking into account the location of pain and contracture areas we can know which organ or viscera is in bad condition. Knowing when an organ is affected by a viscero-cutaneous reflection is the key that opens the door to many Shiatsu treatments. This way we can help many people improve their organ function by applying pressure on the reflective areas. Depending on the patient's conditions, the therapist applies pressure on the affected areas of the body.

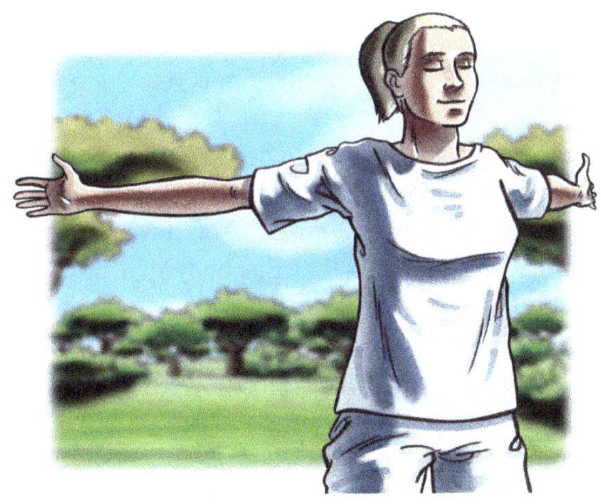

7. Effects of Shiatsu on the body

1. Makes the skin more flexible.
2. Improves the circulatory system.
3. Makes the muscle system more flexible.
4. Helps the digestive system to recover balance.
5. Eases the digestive system's functions.
6. Improves control of the endocrine system.
7. Regulates neural functions.

Stretches are an ideal complement after a Shiatsu session when the muscles received pressure from the hands. One of the fundamental points of Shiatsu is that it is always treats the whole body.

Patients usually tend to think that they should only be treated for the affected part of the body or the part that hurts them. In Shiatsu we know that a stomach disorder may be caused by the organs related to it functioning at a lower rate.

Therefore, we always work the whole body so that all organs function better and the body regains its natural harmony.

The human skeletal system is composed of 206 bones. Joints are where some bones bond with others so that the body can move freely. Without them we'd be like robots. Shiatsu helps the joints regain their natural synchronised movements.

The joints of the body are connected in such a way that if we lay a person of 100kg down on their back, a child of only a few years could, with the help of only his hand or a finger, push the lying person's big toe and move their whole body from the feet to the head. If a joint stops working and its movement is reduced, all joints related to it will be affected.

Let's imagine we twist an ankle; because of the pain, and to protect the affected joint, we use the other foot more by shifting our centre of gravity.

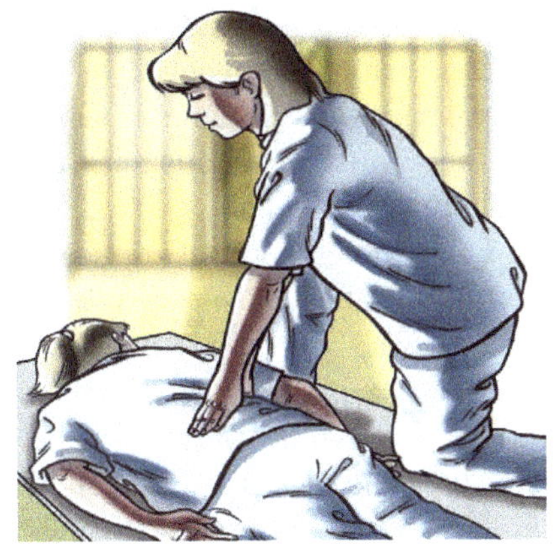

Such a change will undisputably affect all joints. Shiatsu works by regulating body imbalances from head to toe, treating each and every joint to regain their natural synchrony. This is another clear point of support for Shiatsu theory that advocates for treating the whole body and not just the affected area.

Shiatsu induces the patient to breath calmly and deeply from the abdomen, and balances the autonomic nervous system. When receiving shiatsu, the breathing deepens and if we breathe with the abdomen the whole body breathes.

Blood travels through the body from one end to the other, so by breathing deeply and abdominally the blood will circulate better, so we improve joint movements, the body's balance and our posture. With this type of breathing our mind moves into a meditative state, the body relaxes and stress is eliminated. The movement of the diaphragm up and down massages the gut, making it function better.

Shiatsu also plays an important role in rebalancing the body, correcting the alterations caused by the daily repetition of certain movements or exercises. Humans walk, act and stand upright on their feet, and often repeatedly perform movements and exercises daily, thereby putting more stress on some areas than others.

For example, we use one hand more than another, cross one leg over the other and so we take our centre of gravity always to the same side.

Tennis, golf and baseball are exaggerated examples of these tendencies. Shiatsu and a change of postural habits are paramount to fix these imbalances.

Shiatsu helps the patient reach the maximum limit of their body's self-healing capacity, something that every human being possesses. The body has the ability to always be in a good state of health. Instinctively, we reject what harms and accept what benefits.

Pain is an alarm signal that the body sends us to let us know we are hurt. People who have "anesthetized" this sensation do not know where their body's endurance limit is and often suffer from serious illnesses.

When animals get sick, they do not eat or drink, they only rest, making it possible for their body to heal thanks to their ability to self-heal. Instinct is what makes them act that way; it's only humans who do not rest when sick.

The best indicator of good health is that when we wake up in the morning, we feel rested and energized to start the new day. Humans must live according to their biorhythms and maintain a state of health which allows them to be sufficiently sensitive to receiving any signal that the body sends, and to be able to react promptly to any ailment. Our body changes daily, loses tone and health; it's normal and should happen.

Humans are born to end up dying, but we can enjoy life fully. If our measure of health were to drop to 50%, feel pain or have any symptoms of illness, the ideal would be to rest and receive Shiatsu to regain our usual level of health. Shiatsu's mission is to get the greatest number of people to enjoy their lives fully and be happy.

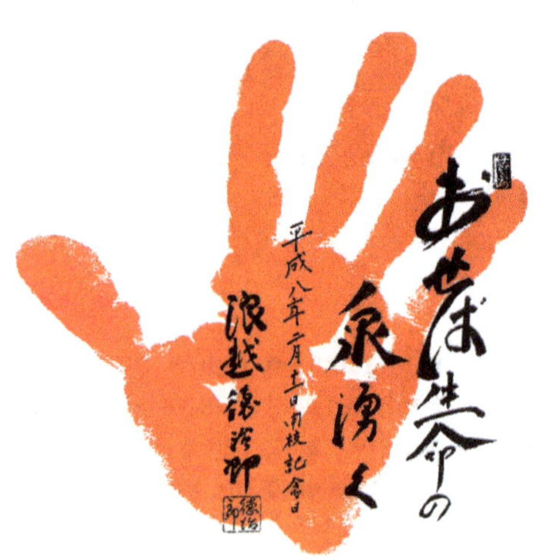

8. Pathologies that can be worked on with Shiatsu

1. Colds.
2. Senile dementia in older people (prevention).
3. ANS imbalance.
4. Insomnia.
5. Obesity.
6. Exhaustion.

Circulatory problems:

1. Hypertension.
2. Cerebral stroke (prevention and rehabilitation).
3. Diabetes (prevention and maintenance).
4. Hyperlipidemias.
5. Angina (prevention).
6. Arrhythmia.
7. Tachycardia.
8. Feeling of respiratory distress.
9. Stress.
10. Myocardial infarction (prevention).

Digestive system problems:

1. Balance the appetite.
2. Diarrhea.
3. Constipation.
4. Poor digestion.
5. Gases.

Skin problems:

1. Allergy.
2. Itchiness of the Skin.
3. Roughness of the skin.
4. Asthma (respiratory system problem).
5. Pollen allergy (respiratory system problem).

Problems with the genital tract:

1. Menstruation pain.
2. Irregular menstruation.
3. Menopause.
4. Myoma.
5. Symptoms during pregnancy.
6. Postpartum (hip) problems.

Leg problems:

1. Swollen feet.
2. Cramps.
3. Cold legs.
4. Heavy Legs.
5. Varicose veins.
6. Fluid retention.

Problems of the spinal column:

1. Cervicalgia.
2. Herniated disc.
3. Frozen shoulder (scapulahumeral periarthritis).
4. Lumbalgia.
5. Sciatica.
6. Scoliosis (rehabilitation and prevention).

9. Rules of Precaution

1. Hands should be clean at all times and nails cut to an adequate length.

2. Before beginning with a treatment, the therapist must breathe deeply to control his breathing and to mentally calm himself.

3. The basic principles of the therapy must be mastered.

4. Basic positions must be done properly. If positions are not carefully adapted, pressure will not be applied accurately.

5. Pressure points must be located exactly. From the beginning, pressure should have the right intensity, never too much.

6. When the patient suffers from a condition that prevents him from moving the body freely — shoulder pain, sprains, pregnancy, herniated intervertebral discs, whiplash syndrome, hemiplegia, etc.—, the therapist should be very careful to adapt patient's postures and regulate pressure intensity.

7. During therapy, the therapist must be sincerely and carefully concentrated on his work.

8. Therapeutic sessions last from thirty minutes to an hour depending on the patient's age, sex, condition and symptoms.

9. If need be, the patient should use the bathroom before the therapy starts. He should be mentally and physically relaxed. Of course, therapy can be interrupted if necessary.

10. Wait at least thirty minutes after meals before doing therapy; the patient's stomach should not be too empty or too full.

10. The correct way to apply pressure

THE thumb is the main tool of Shiatsu therapy. Applying Shiatsu pressure is done 90% of the time by the thumb; the remaining 10% is done with the palm of the hand.

Thumb penetration must always be perpendicular to the area where the pressure is being applied to; Therefore, pressure is applied with the thumb pad, while simultaneously inclining the body from the pelvic waist. With this movement the weight supported by the thumb can be up to 25 or 30 kilos (55 to 66 pounds). We must take care while applying pressure as, by adopting an incorrect thumb or body position, we could possibly cause some kind of damage or deformity of the thumbs.

The thumb must support weight on the first phalanx, which is the first joint linked to the metacarpal bone, and not the second. The thumb and the rest of the fingers must form a triangle to the area where pressure is applied.

RULES FOR APPLYING THUMB PRESSURE

1. Pressure applied to each point generally lasts for three seconds, with the exception being the individual points where pressure lasts for five seconds.
2. Pressure is repeated three times for each line, area or key point.
3. In the basic position, the Cross theory is applied for thumb over thumb pressure, meaning that the thumb which supports more weight is placed under the other one and is opposite to the foot resting on the ground.
4. When working on transverse lines, the thumb placed below will be the one closer and pointing to the line that is being treated.

5. There are several exceptions to the rules we have just seen, for improving pressure or getting a better hold on a specific area being treated, we use the thumb below of the hand which enables us to hold the area better.
6. In positions where the treated line is located centrally, right-handed people will place the right thumb under the left one, and left-handed people will place the left thumb under the right.

11. Characteristics of Pressure

1. Perpendicular: The pressure of the fingers must always be perpendicular to the body's surface where treating.
2. Constant pressure: Maintain the quality of the pressure throughout.
3. Concentration: Pressure must be highly concentrated on a specific point to enable the necessary penetration to relieve the pain or correct the condition.

Shiatsu Aze introduces four new concepts as an extension of the previous ones:

1. Direction.
2. Time.
3. Depth.
4. Relationship to patient.

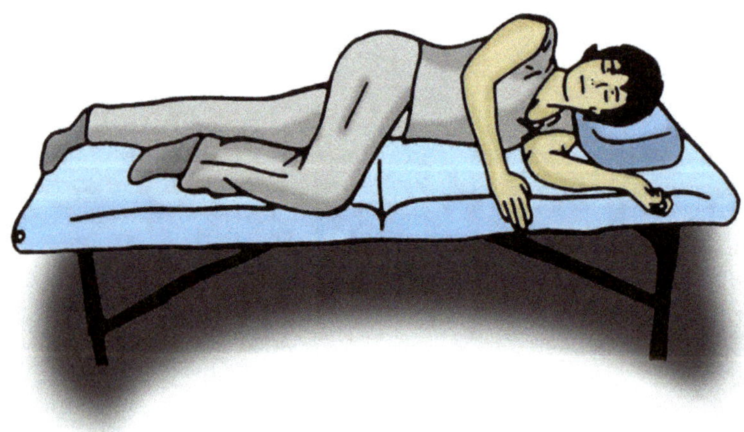

12. Conditions when Shiatsu should not be used

1. Infectious diseases.

2. If a patients suffers from the following pathologies: Pleurisy, peritonitis, appendicitis, pyelitis, pancreatitis, peptic ulcer, duodenal ulcer, liver cirrhosis, leukemia, stomach-ache, intestinal obstruction, cancer.

3. In the following special cases: High fever after a surgical operation, extreme physical weakness, infectious skin diseases.

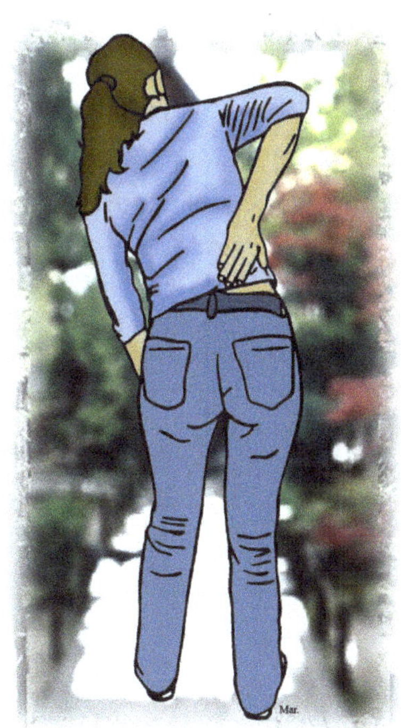

13. Autonomic nervous system reflections

T HERE are other reflections, but here are the two most important:

Reflections of the carotid area

Given the importance of Shiatsu on the anterior cervical area, the physiological functions of the carotid area must be understood meticulously. The carotid sinus is located at the point of the neck where the carotid artery branches in the direction of the head. The body carotid is located at this point, a distribution of nerve tissues connected to the vagus nerve, here called the sinus nerve. It is extremely sensitive to blood pressure and respiratory conditions.

Aschners phenomenon (oculo-cardiac phenomenon)

This reflection is especially important in relation to Shiatsu palm pressure applied on the eyes. A light and constant pressure on the eyes stimulates the trigeminal nerve extremities behind them. This, in turn, induces reflections in the central body of the vagus nerve, leading to a reduced pulse and decreased blood pressure.

14. Types of Pressure

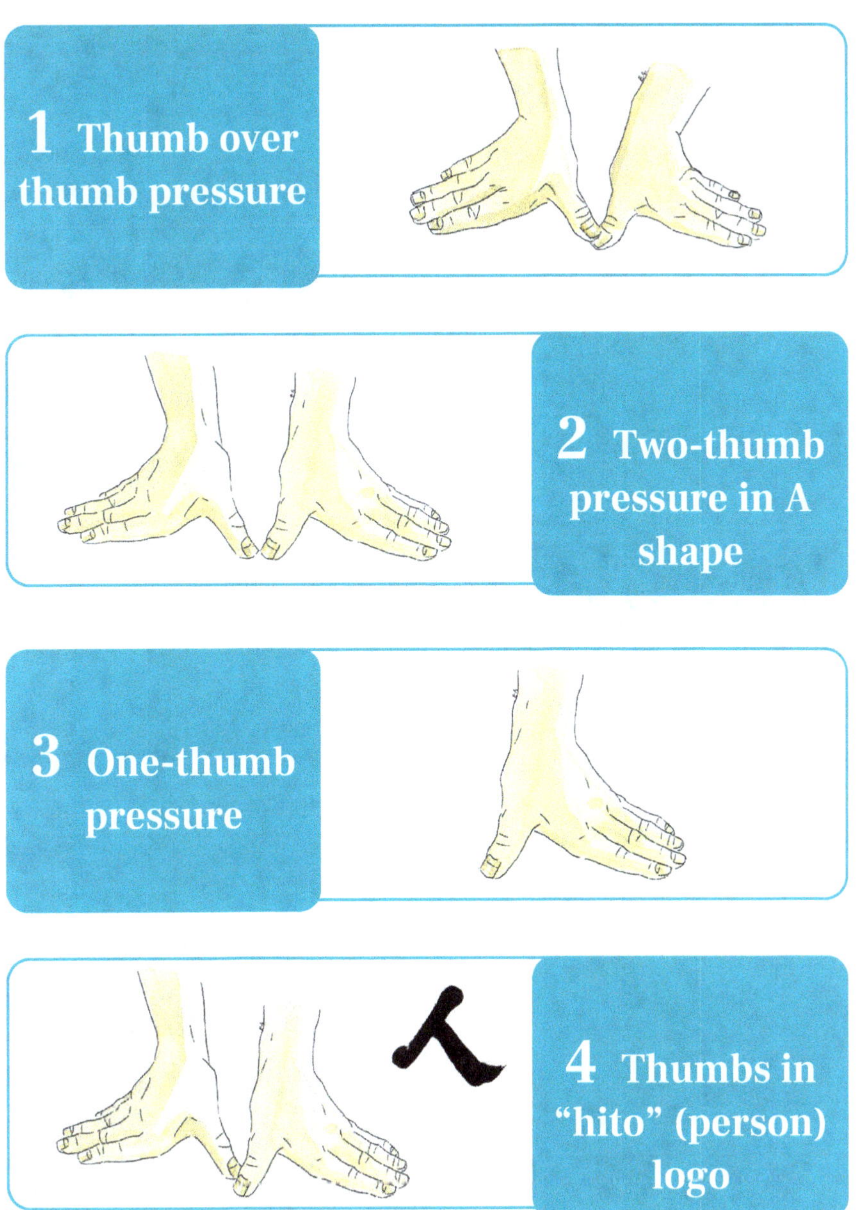

5 **Thumb and fingers pincer pressure.**

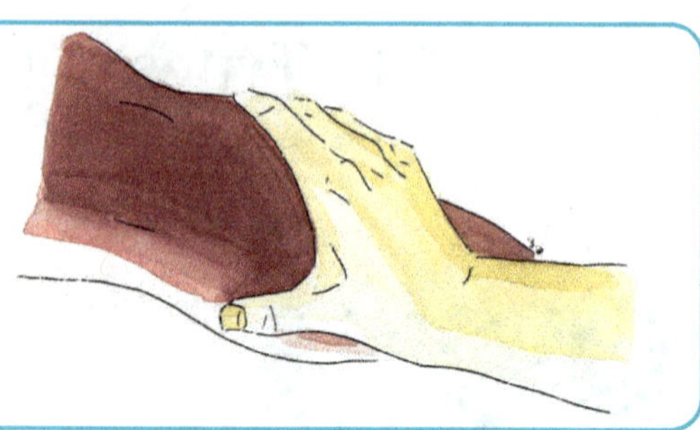

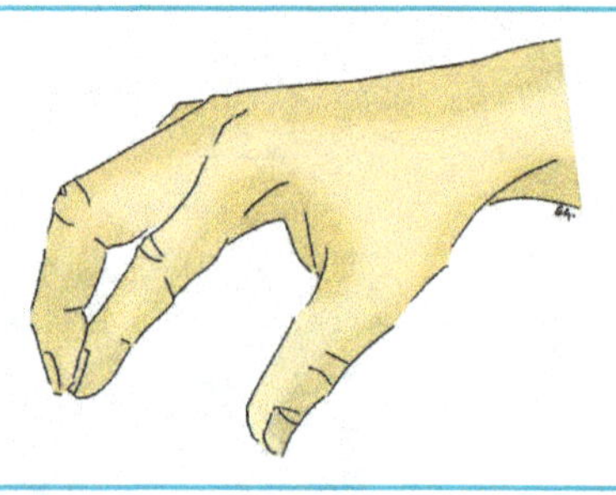

6 **Middle and index finger pressure**

7 **Hand palm pressure**

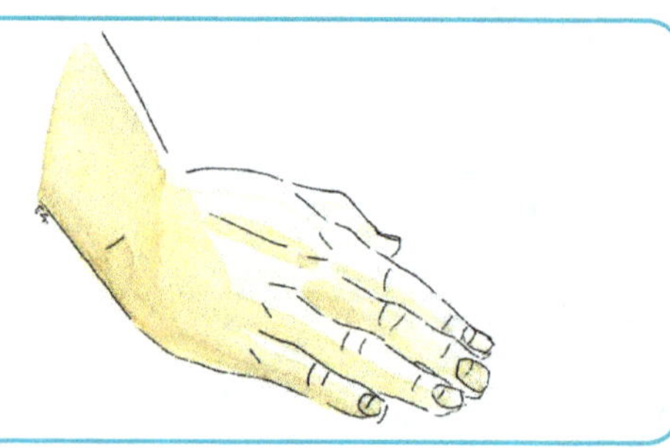

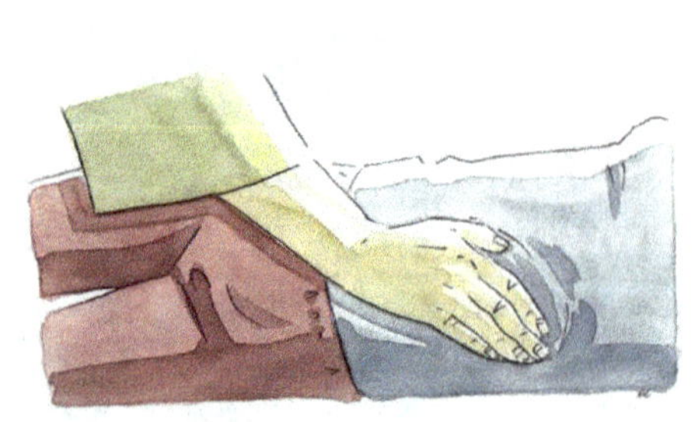

8 **Pressure with the heel of the hands (thenar and hypothenar pads)**

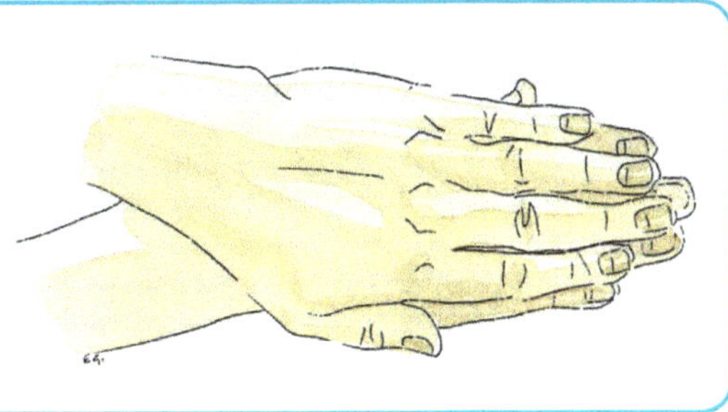

9 Two hand palm pressure

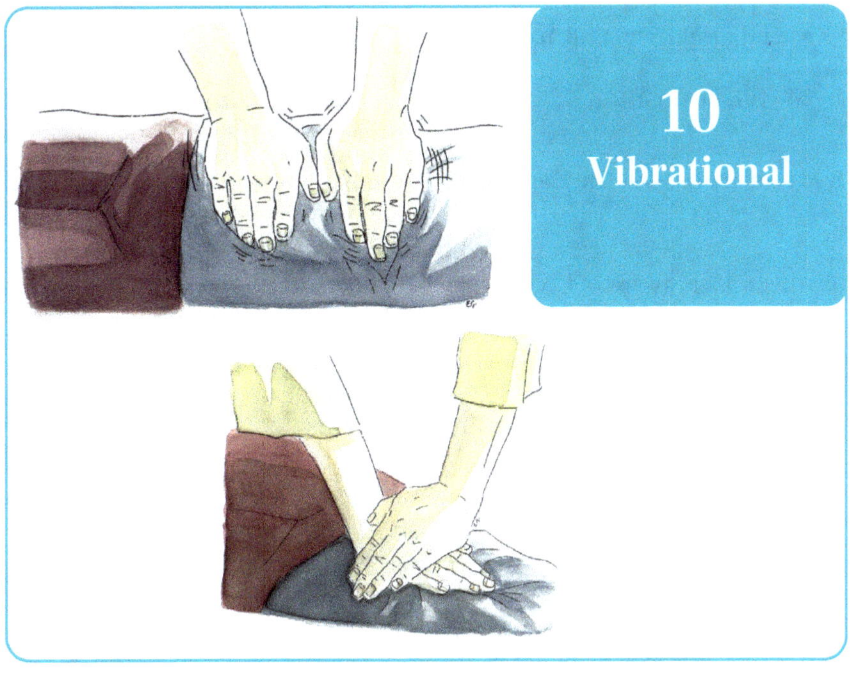

10 Vibrational

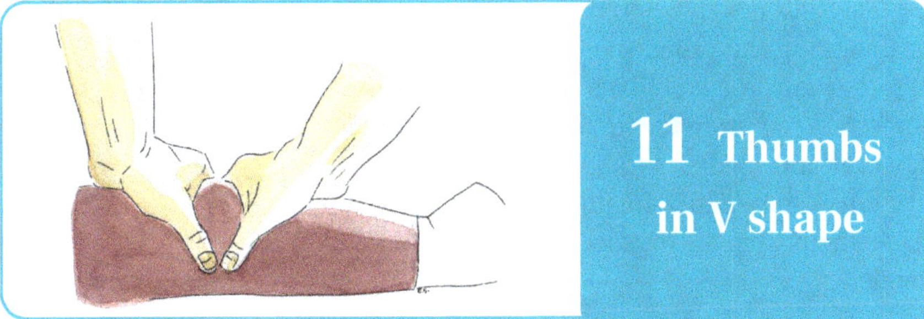

11 Thumbs in V shape

15. Therapist's Position

TYPES OF POSITION

Shiatsu therapists mainly use three basic positions to perform treatment:

1. Basic position.　　2. Seiza.　　3. Kneeling position.

Body awareness of the therapist's position

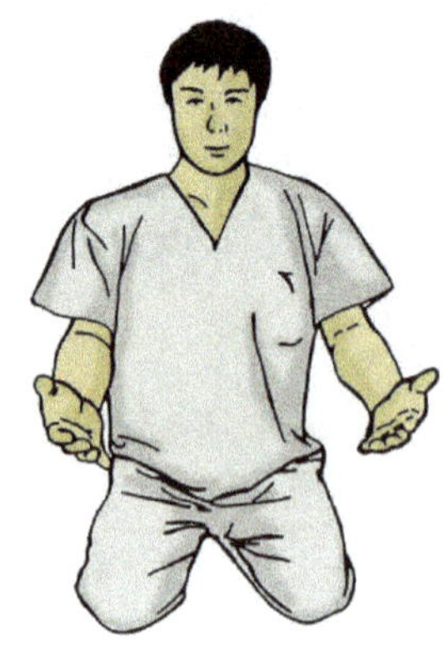

To work with Shiatsu it is very important that the therapist is aware of his own body. You need to know what your proper posture is to be balanced and administer better therapy.

The upper body should be completely relaxed. You must have your little fingers towards your trunk, this way the elbows stick to the body and relax the trapezoids. The position is therefore concentrated on the anterior part of the trunk, especially on the pectoralis major. A proper exercise is to make wide circles with the arms, gathering them up towards the hara, drawing in the little fingers.

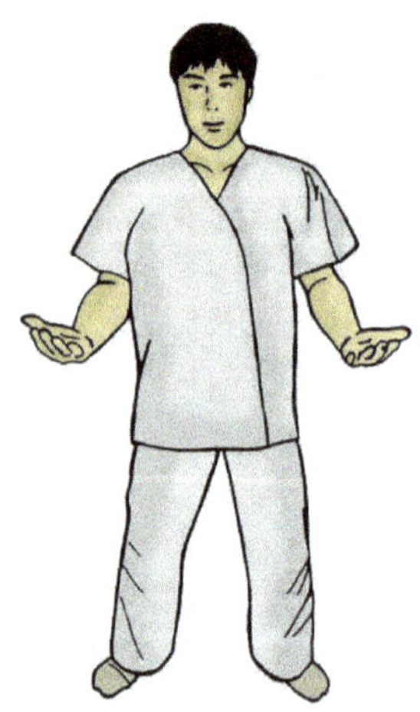

The lower body should be concentrated on maintaining the proper position. To do this the big toes must be well-fixed on the ground. The knees are therefore together and focused on the femoral and medial sural regions (the Spleen-Pancreas meridian), creating greater stability. Then the position is focused on the hara and the tanden.

This way of settling the body is good for both the standing position and the kneeling position (seiza).

The body and the pressure

The movement is generated from this position, and the pressure is performed through it. The weight of the body falls on the hands and therefore pressure is applied through them. Arm strength is not used.

The therapist's spinal column and hip should form a 90° angle, locking the hip area in order to avoid spinal problems.

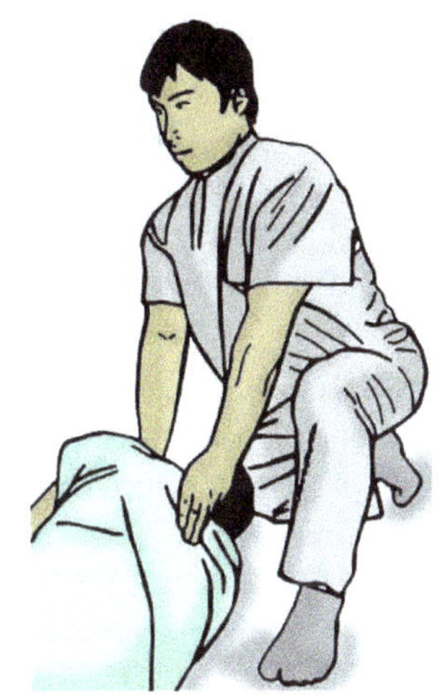

When working on a massage bed, the therapist should imagine the triangle formed by the big toes of both feet and the tanden to maintain the correct position; in addition to taking care of the triangle formed by the tanden, the perineum and the sacrum where the movement comes from to generate the pressure.

Breathing must be adapted to match the patient's rhythm. As the session progresses, the patient's breathing will become slower and deeper. The therapist should also concentrate on point MH8 of his hands. It is always necessary to leave a space between this point and the patient's body, as this is the place where energy is projected from the therapist to the patient. You must adjust the position of your hands to maintain this position.

1. How to work with the basic position

The basic position is the most commonly used in Shiatsu. It has three support points: the knee, the foot and the thumbs. The triangle they form should be as equilateral as possible. This way you can apply the appropriate pressure on the patient.

As we indicated at the beginning, it is essential to concentrate on supporting the big toe to keep the leg closed and maintain a good position that enables us to apply pressure correctly, making use of the hara and the tanden.

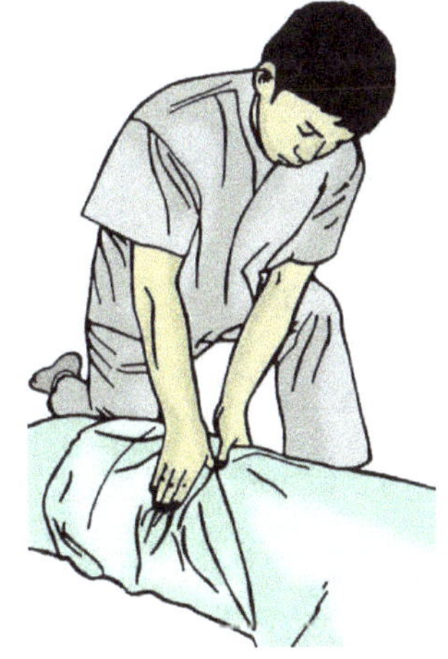

2. Seiza Position

The Seiza position is the traditional Japanese position. The back
is kept perfectly straight and is supported by resting the buttocks on
the heels. It is very important to
start the pressure from the hara
(tanden). As always it is the hara
that exerts the pressure, not the
arms or hands.

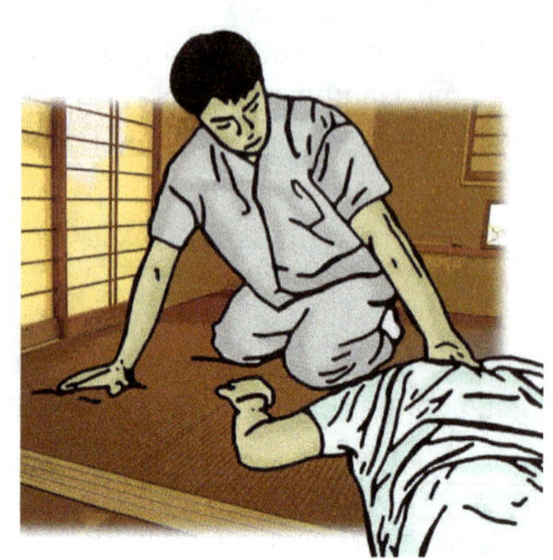

3. Kneeling position

In the kneeling position, the therapist rests
on his knees with his hips slightly raised. The
way to apply pressure is the same as in seiza,
but this position is somewhat more unstable.
The therapist should fix the top of both feet to
the ground to stabilize himself better.

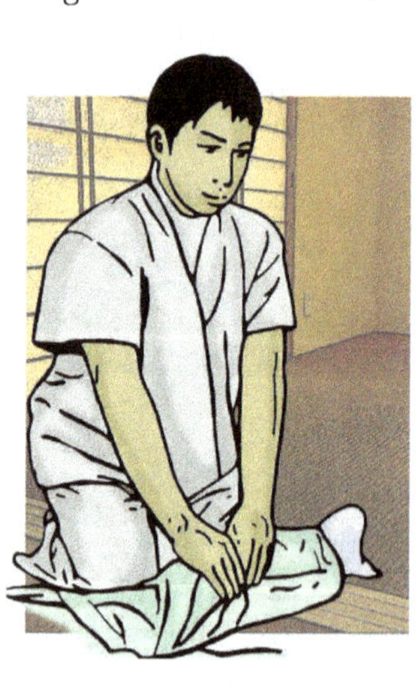

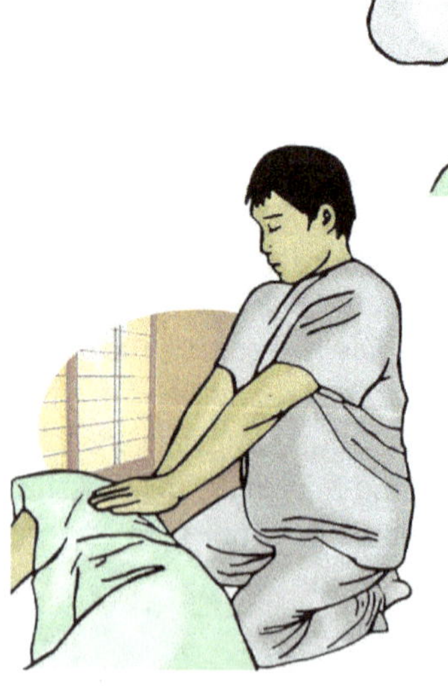

16. The spinal column and location of vertebrae

The spinal column is a flexible bone structure, whose function is to protect the spinal cord, support the skull, give mobility to the trunk and transmit force via the pelvis to the lower limbs. It is also called a dorsal spine or rachis and is composed of 33 or 34 small bones called vertebrae, whose posterior bumps (spinous process) can be felt when we touch the centre of the back. Between each vertebra are the intervertebral discs, formed by elastic cartilage with a gelatinous nucleus and a peripheral part composed of concentric layers of fibrous cartilage, whose function is to reduce the pressure the vertebrae are subjected to.

The spinal column consists of:

7 cervical vertebrae.
12 dorsal vertebrae.
5 lumbar vertebrae.
5 vertebrae joined to the sacrum.
4 vertebrae joined to the coccyx.

The first seven vertebrae, located in the neck, are the cervical ones, with the skull resting on the first one (atlas). Below the neck are the twelve dorsal vertebrae, which are attached to the ribs and finally the five lumbar vertebrae. All these vertebrae have mobility, while the sacrum and coccyx are fixed.

If we look laterally at the spinal column we will see that it is not straight, but has certain curvatures, two concave and two convex. The sacral and dorsal area are convex to the posterior part, while the lumbar and cervical areas are concave to the posterior area. The concave parts are called lordosis.

Due to the special importance we give to treating the back area in Shiatsu, which is related to regulating the autonomic nervous system, we can position the location of some vertebrae, having them as reference points, in more precise locations.

1. To locate the first dorsal vertebra we ask the patient to flex the head; this way we observe the large knotty vertebra that protrudes at the base of the neck and which corresponds to the seventh cervical vertebra or also called a prominent vertebra. There could be circumstances when we cannot distinguish between the seventh cervical vertebra and the first dorsal, because they form a large knotty surface. To be able to distinguish it, we ask the patient to make a slow rotation of the head so that we can check that the vertebra that rotates at the same time as the neck is the seventh cervical.

2. If we imagine the mamillary line in the chest, which reaches to the posterior part of the back, it would correspond to the intermediate point between the fifth and sixth dorsal vertebra.

3. If we draw an imaginary line between the inferior edges of the shoulder blades, it would roughly match the eighth dorsal vertebra.

4. The level of the navel corresponds to the point between the second and third lumbar vertebra in the back area.

5. Finally, if we draw an imaginary line that joins the iliac ridges, it corresponds to the fourth lumbar vertebra.

MULTIFIDUS AND ROTATOR MUSCLES

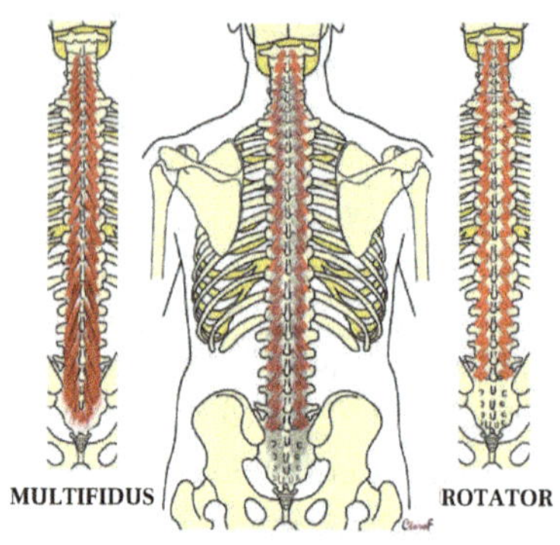

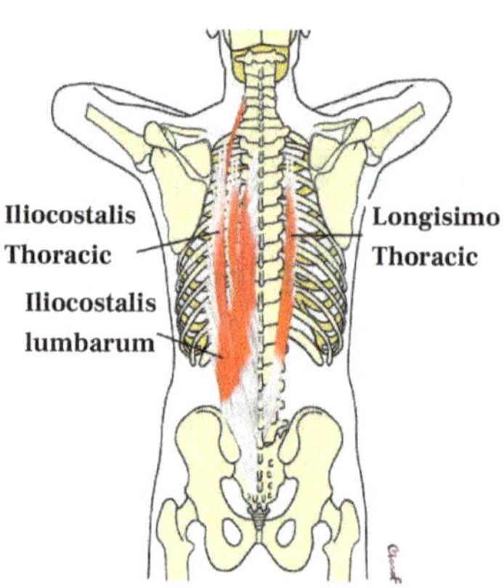

ILIOCOSTALIS THORACIC MUSCLE

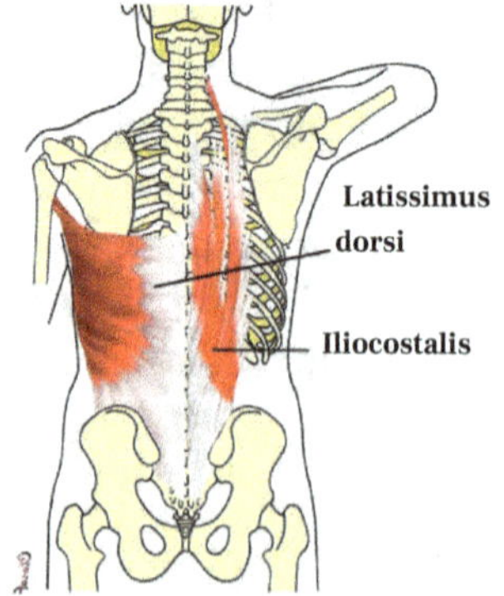

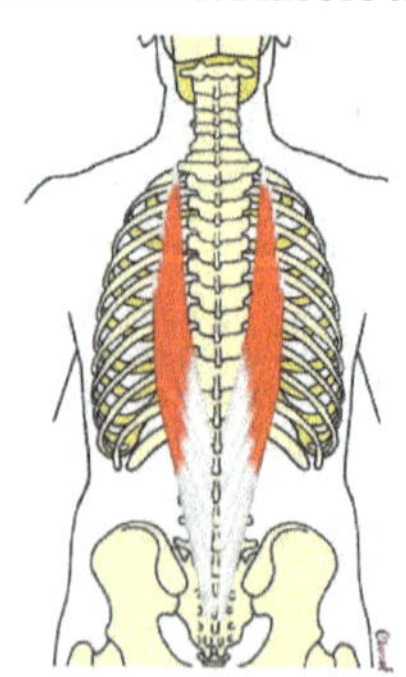

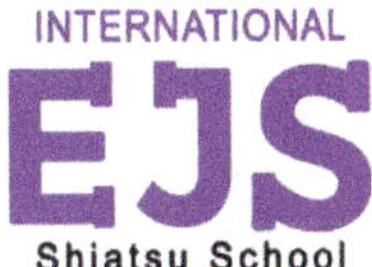

LOCATION OF VERTEBRAE

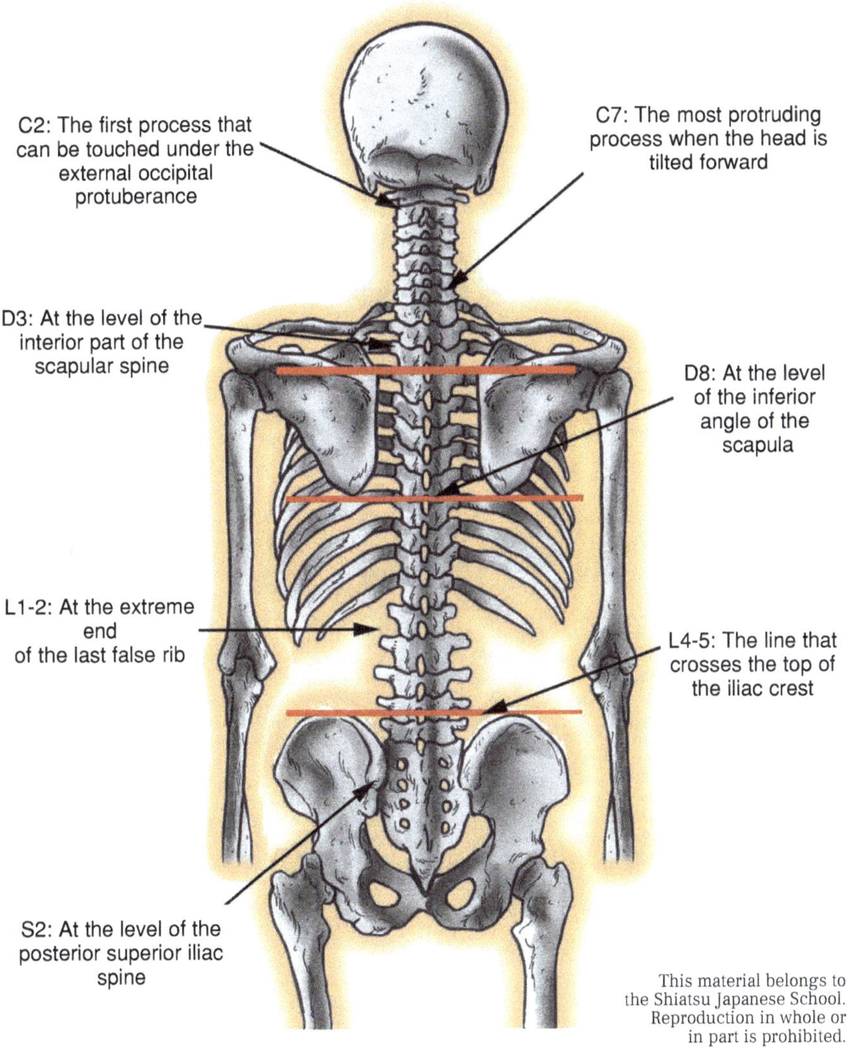

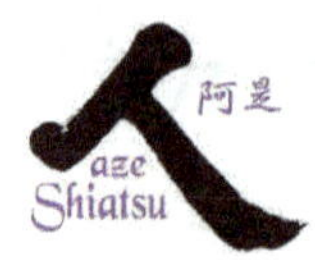

POINTS OF AZE SHIATSE BASIC STYLE
指圧療法基本圧点図

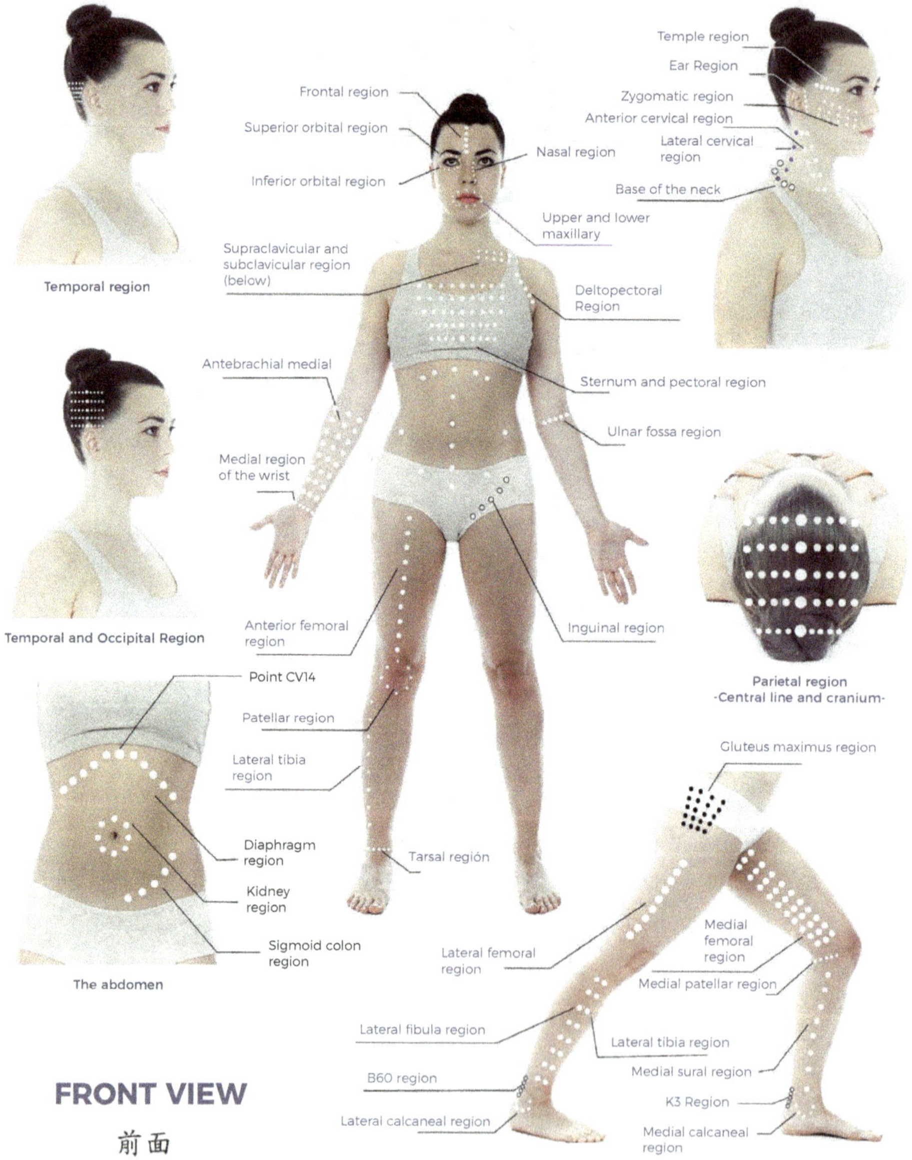

FRONT VIEW
前面

POINTS OF AZE SHIATSU BASIC STYLE
指圧療法基本圧点図

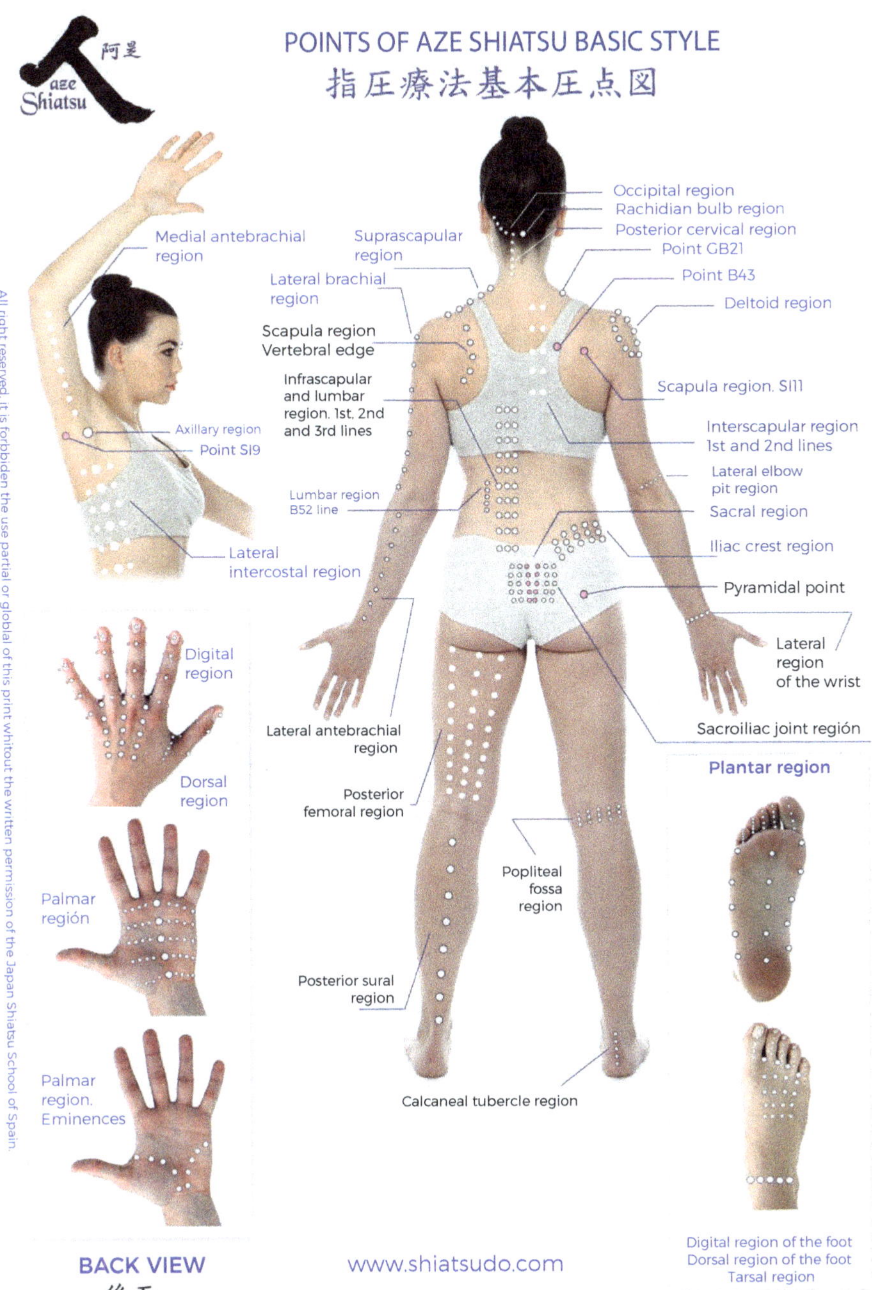

Aze Shiatsu

1. Basic treatment in Prone Decubitus

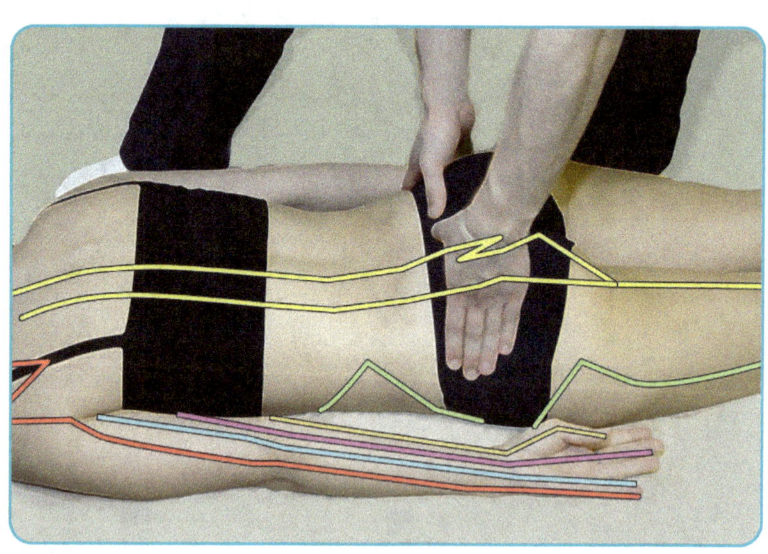

1. Preparing the back (I): Dorsal and lumbar

1.1. Cross-palm pressure.

1.2. Pressures with the eminences.

1.3. Stretching the spinal column.

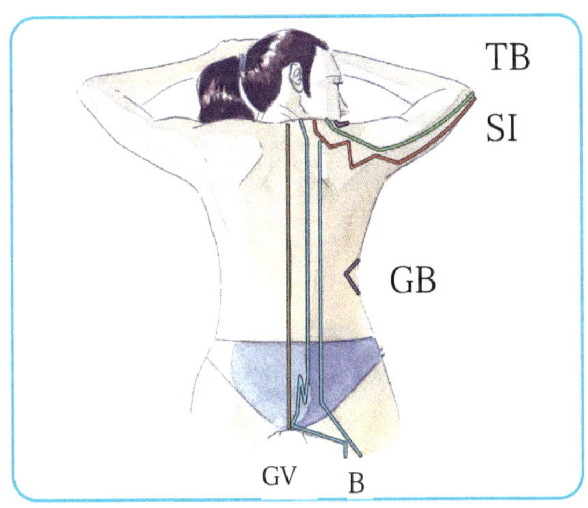

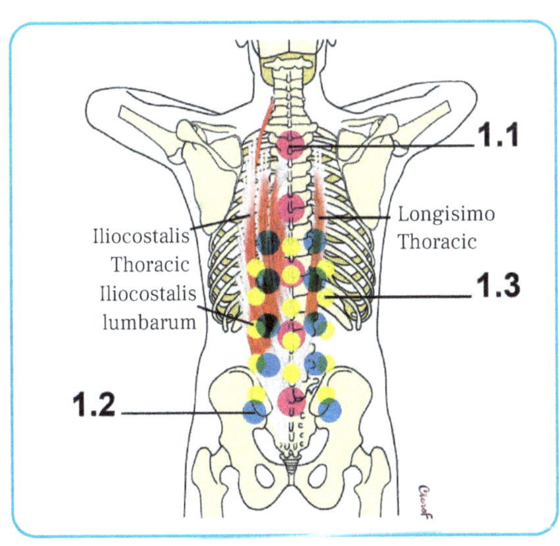

1.1. CROSS-PALM PRESSURE

PATIENT'S POSTURE: Prone. Head turned towards the therapist, shoulders in abduction and elbows bent.

THERAPIST'S POSITION: Basic, on the left side of the patient.

TYPE OF PRESSURE: Palm (palms crossed, right one below).

Nº. OF POINTS: Five zones.

DIRECTION OF THE LINE: From the interscapular zone to the sacrum region, along the spiny apophysis.

Three times for three seconds.

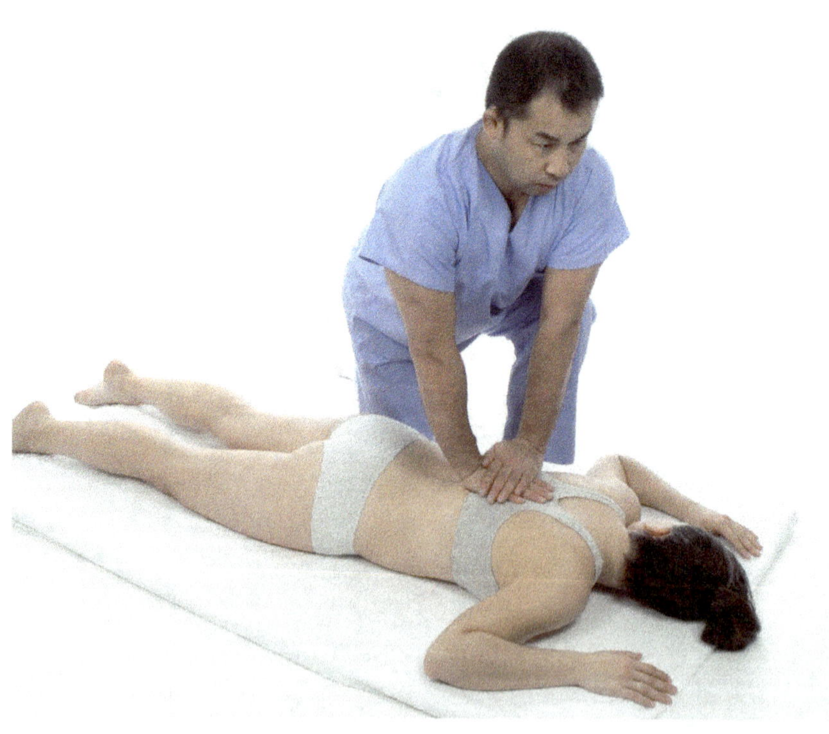

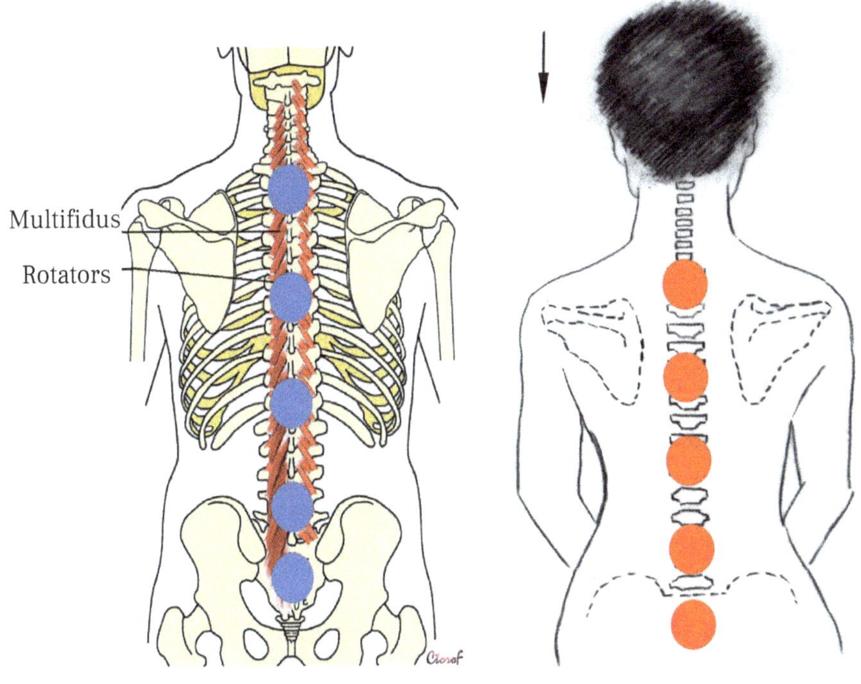

Multifidus
Rotators

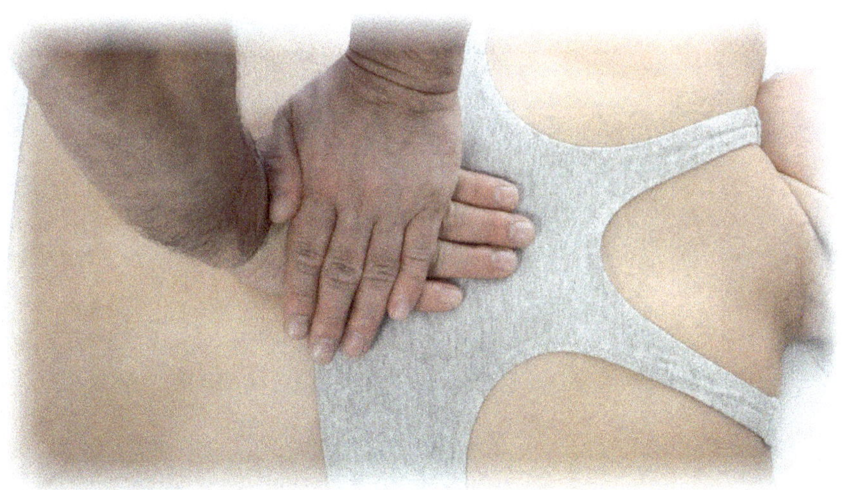

1.2. PRESSURE WITH THE EMINENCES

PATIENT'S POSTURE: Prone. Head turned towards the therapist, shoulders in abduction and elbows bent.

THERAPIST'S POSITION: Basic, on the left side of the patient.

TYPE OF PRESSURE: Hands in parallel, applying pressure with the heel of the hand, the spinal column is between the two hands, fingers facing out.

Nº. OF POINTS: Five zones.

DIRECTION OF THE LINE: From the inferior angle of the shoulder blade to the sacrum region, over the paravertebral muscles. The last pressure is applied on the sacrum and gluteus.

Several times attending to less flexible areas.

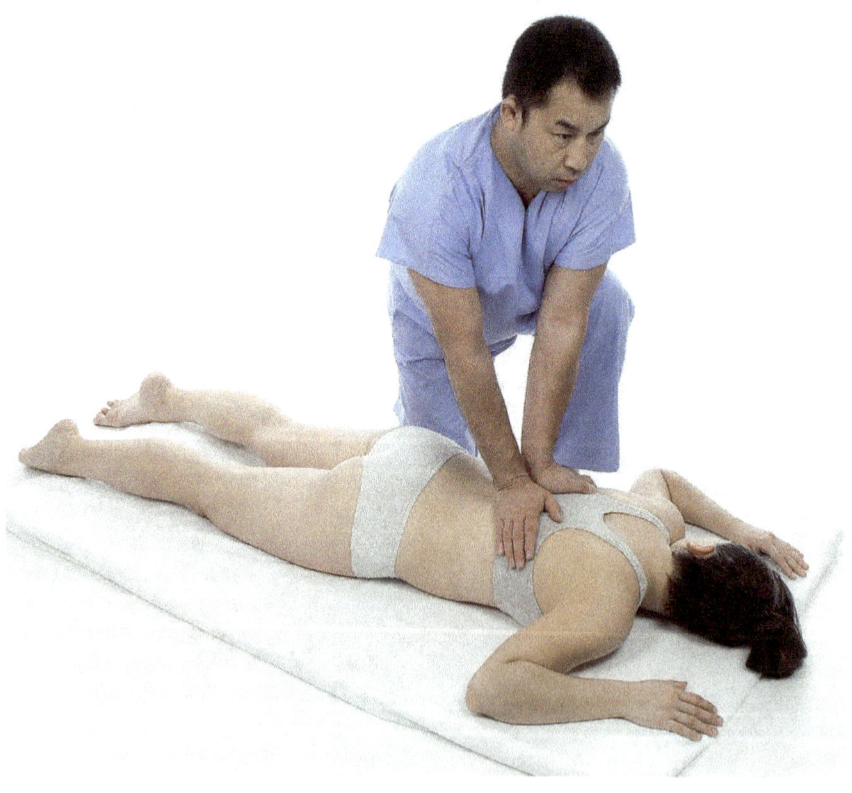

Iliocostalis
Thoracic
Iliocostalis
lumbarum
Longisimo
Thoracic

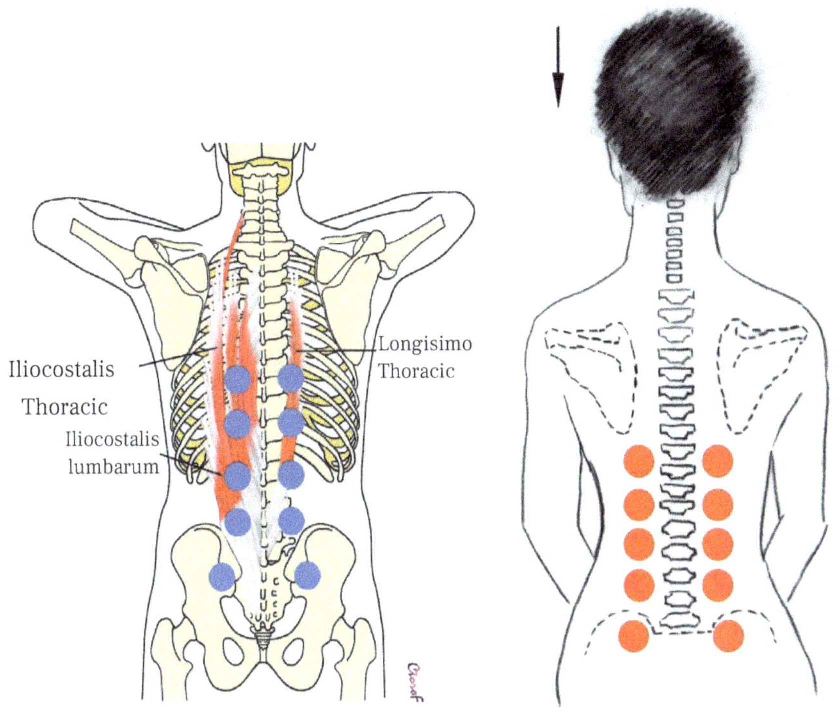

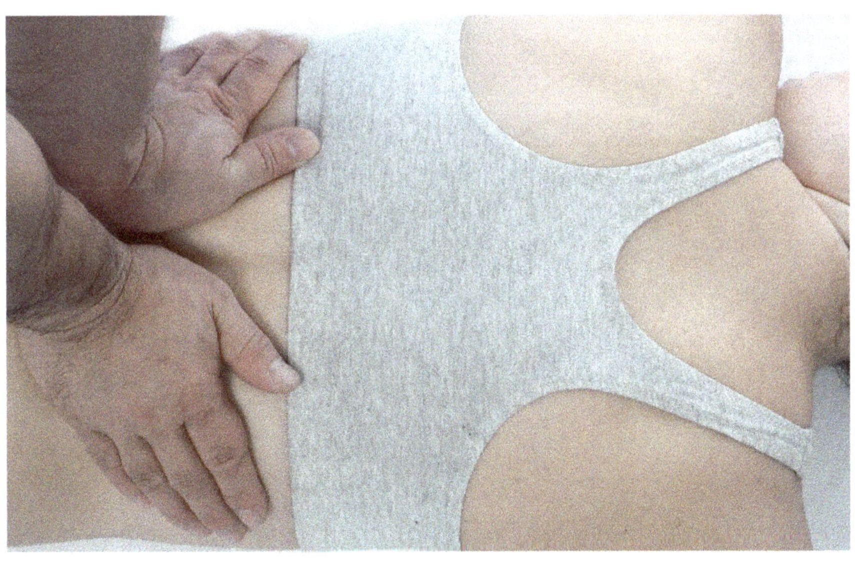

55

1.3. STRETCHING THE SPINAL COLUMN

PATIENT'S POSTURE: Prone. Head turned towards the therapist, shoulders in abduction and elbows bent.

THERAPIST'S POSITION: Kneeling.

TYPE OF PRESSURE: Palm pressure crossing the arms.

DIRECTION OF THE LINE: From the sacrum to the dorsal area (approx. D8). Block the sacrum with one hand without moving it until the work is complete. The other hand stretches the spinal column.

OBSERVATIONS: Three lines of work. A central along the spinous process, another two lines on each side of the spine, three fingers from the anterior and on the paravertebral musculature. The opposite iliac crest is blocked on the 2nd and 3rd lines. The number of pressures varies depending on how the patient's back functions. Slow and deep work.

**Five seconds and repeat depending on how much tension
the area has.**

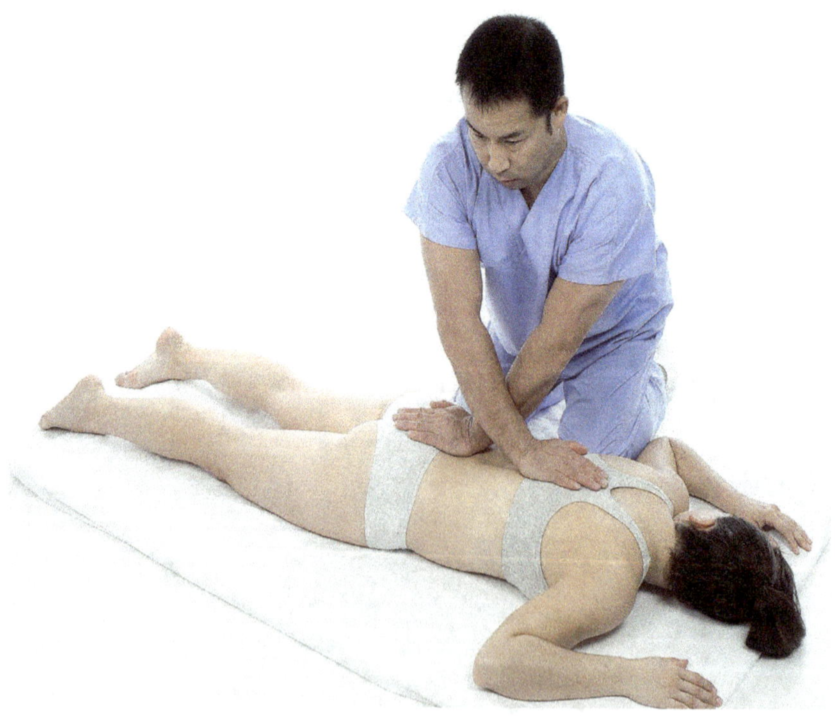

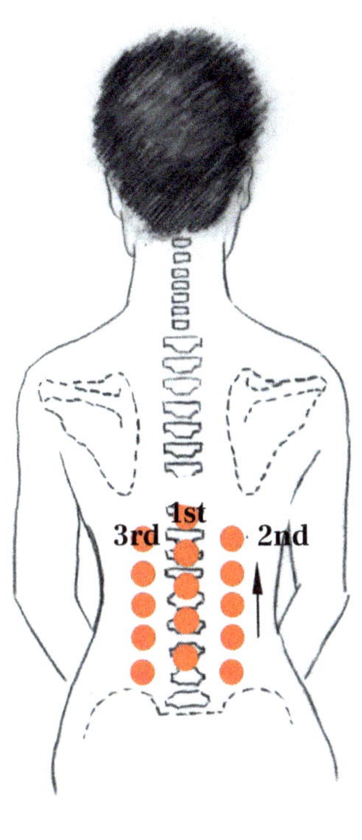

1st
3rd
2nd

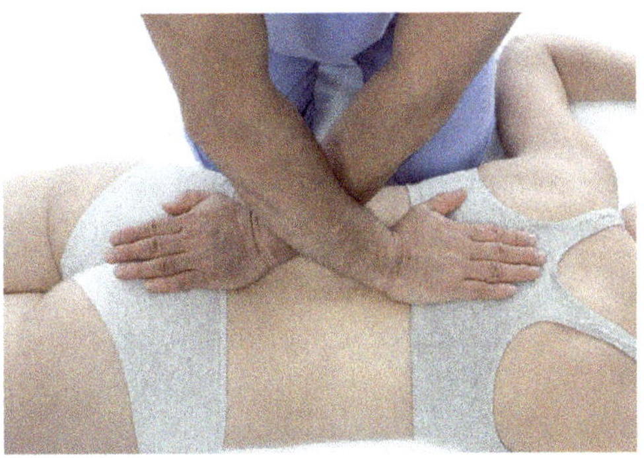

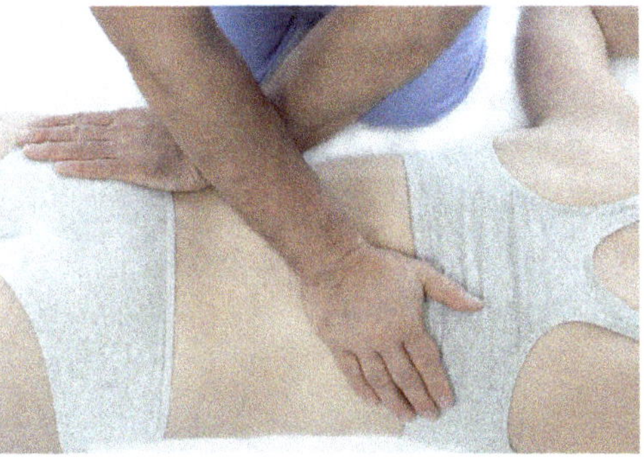

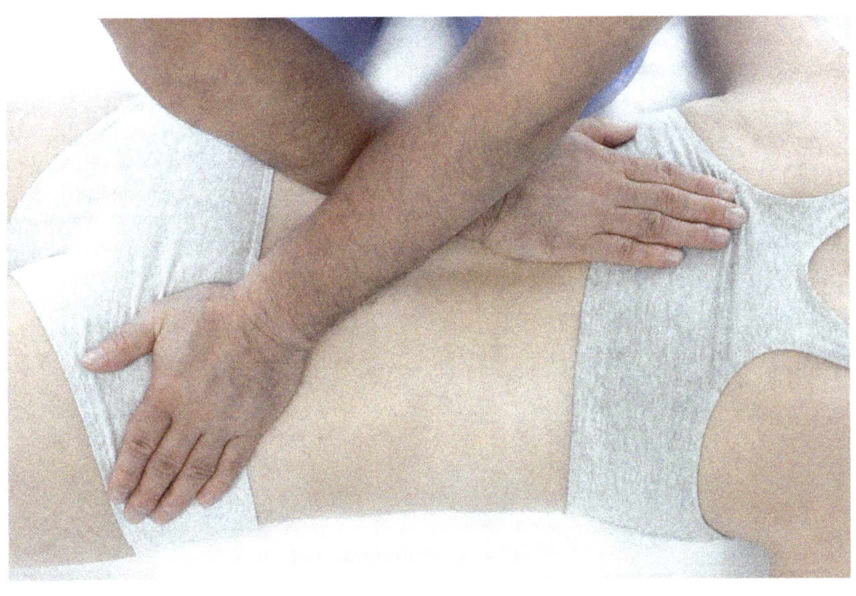

2. Preparing the back (II): Neck, shoulder and dorsal

2.1. Occipital Region. Traction.

2.2. Suprascapular point. Both sides.

2.3. Interscapular region. 1st and 2nd Lines. Both sides.

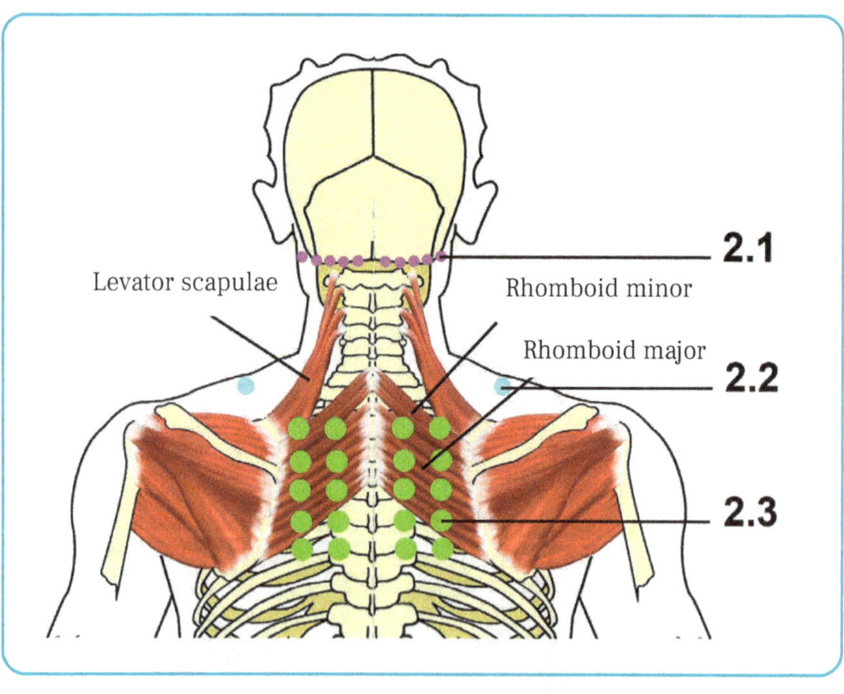

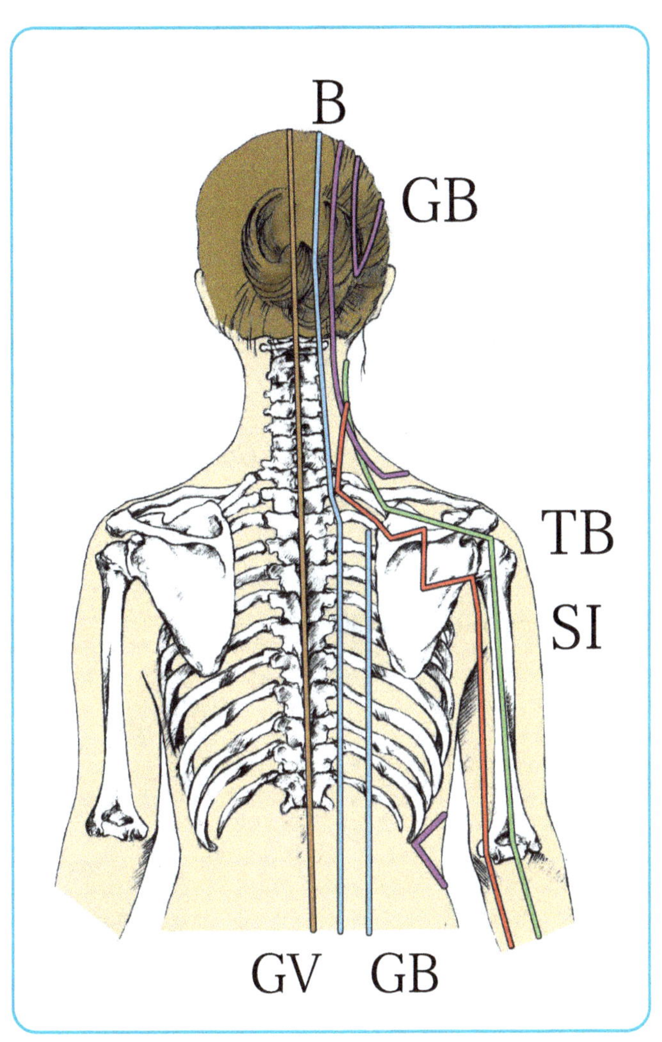

B
GB
TB
SI
GV
GB

2.1. OCCIPITAL REGION. TRACTION

PATIENT'S POSTURE: Prone. The forehead rests on a pillow, shoulders in abduction and elbows bent.

THERAPIST'S POSITION: Seiza facing the patient's head.

TYPE OF PRESSURE: Traction with the index, middle and ring finger-pads.

Nº. OF POINTS: Two five-point lines, worked simultaneously.

DIRECTION OF THE LINE: From the paravertebral musculature to the mastoid process, by the occipital rim.

OBSERVATIONS:The therapist concentrates his work in the tanden area with his elbows to his sides. Traction is performed by moving his body, without using the force of his arms.

The first point in this region corresponds to key point *B10 (Tenchuu)*, and the last point corresponds to key point *GB12 (Kankotsu)*.

It is a very important area because it is reflective of the state of many organ systems with symptoms such as headache, mental stress, tired eyesight, etc.

Three times for three seconds.

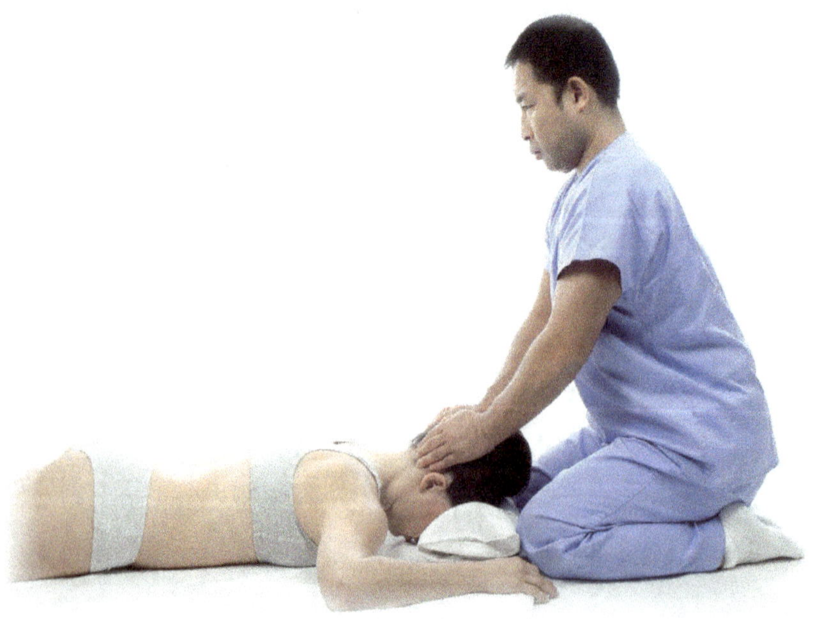

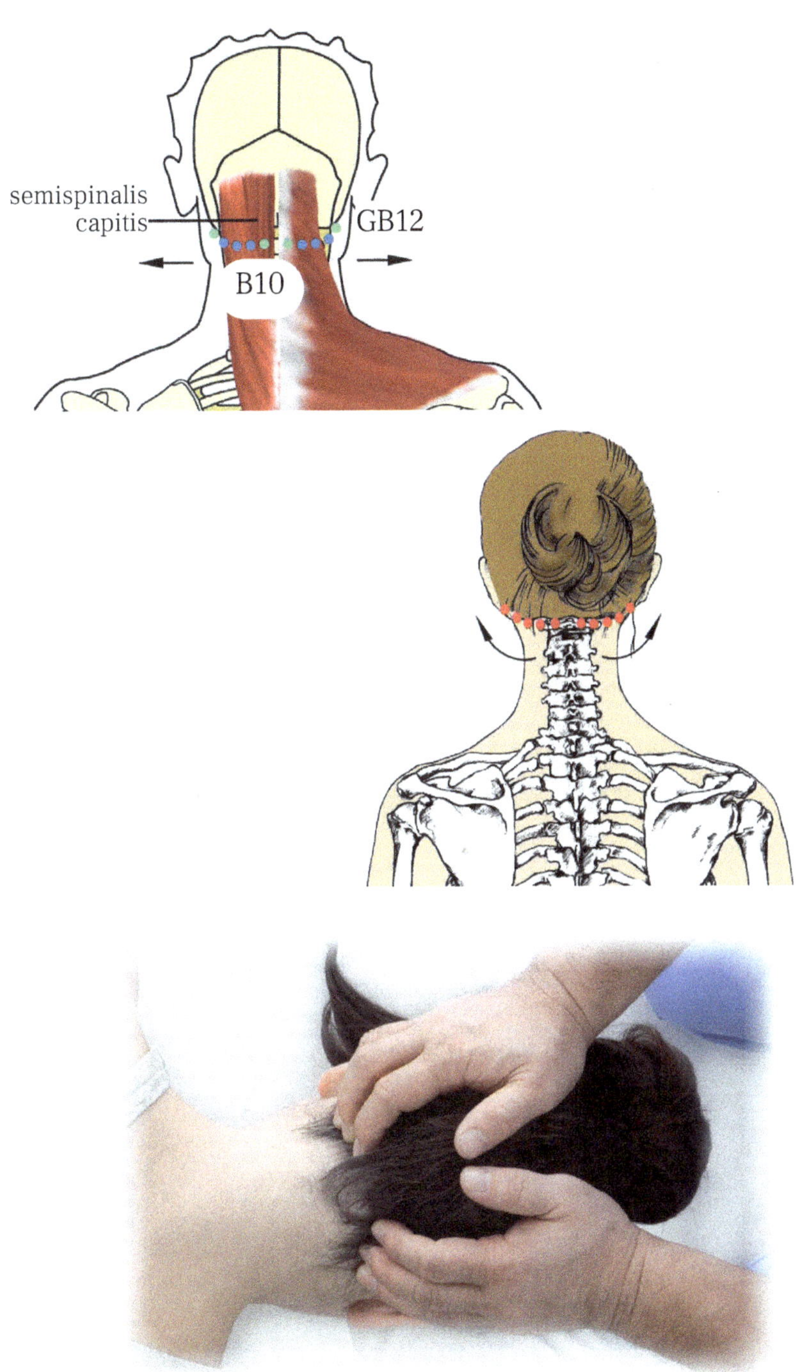

semispinalis
capitis
GB12
B10

2.2. SUPRASCAPULAR POINT. BOTH SIDES

PATIENT'S POSTURE: Prone. The forehead rests on a pillow, ahoulders in abduction and elbows bent.

THERAPIST'S POSITION: Seiza, above the patient's head.

TYPE OF PRESSURE: With both thumbs at the same time, arms slightly bent.

Nº. OF POINTS: 1/1. Worked simultaneously.

DIRECTION OF THE LINE: Applying Pressure towards the midline of the body at the D7 level.

OBSERVATIONS:This point coincides with the second in the suprascapular region, roughly at the location of key point *GB21 (Kensei)*.

Three times for five seconds.

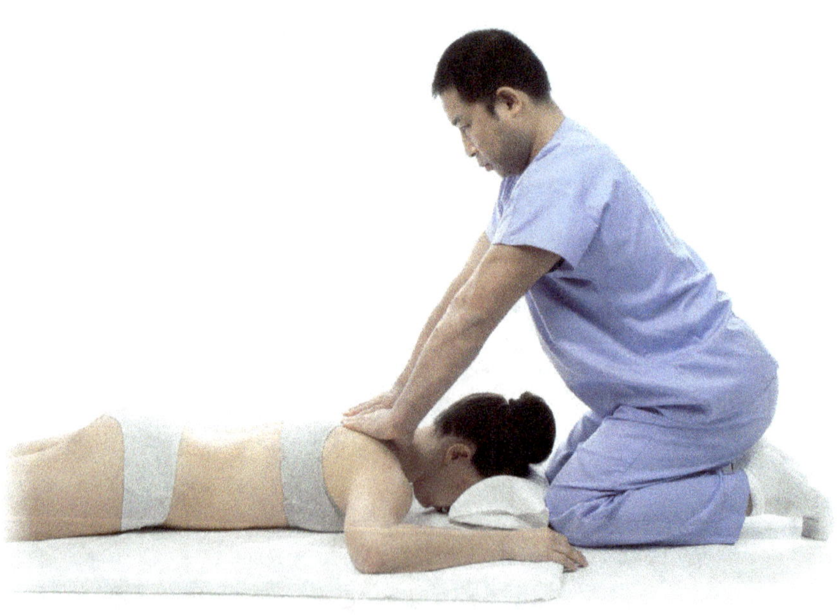

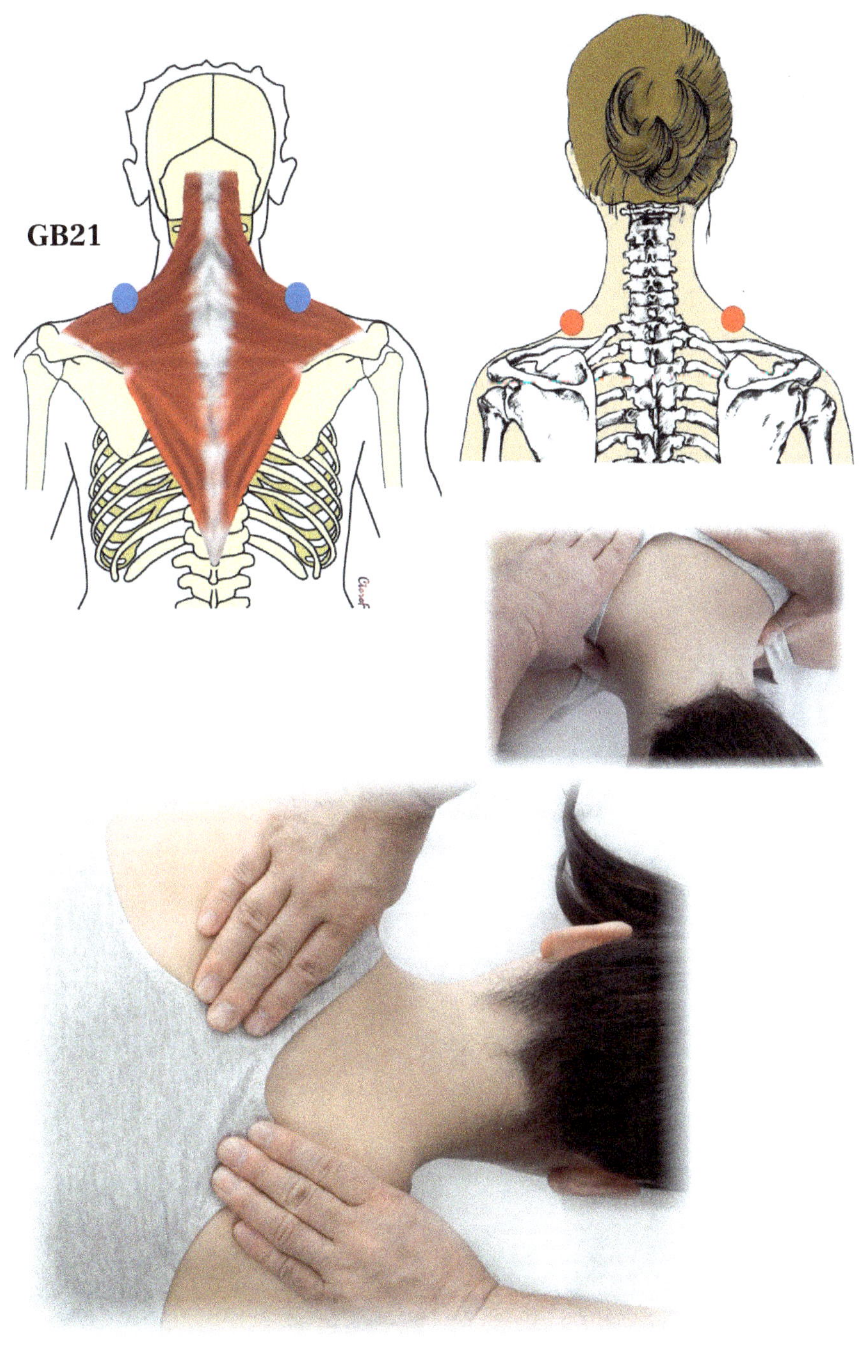

GB21

2.3. INTERSCAPULAR REGION 1st and 2nd Lines. Both sides.

PATIENT'S POSTURE: Prone. The forehead rests on a pillow, shoulders in abduction and elbows bent.

THERAPIST'S POSITION: Kneeling, above the patient's head.

TYPE OF PRESSURE: With both thumbs at the same time.

Nº. OF POINTS: Two five-point lines (1st line internal and 2nd external).

DIRECTION OF THE LINE: The 1st line is located on the internal edge of the paravertebral muscles. The first point is located at D1 running until D7/D8. The 2nd line runs parallel to the previous one by the lateral edge of the vertebral musculature. Repeat both lines alternately.

Three times for three seconds.

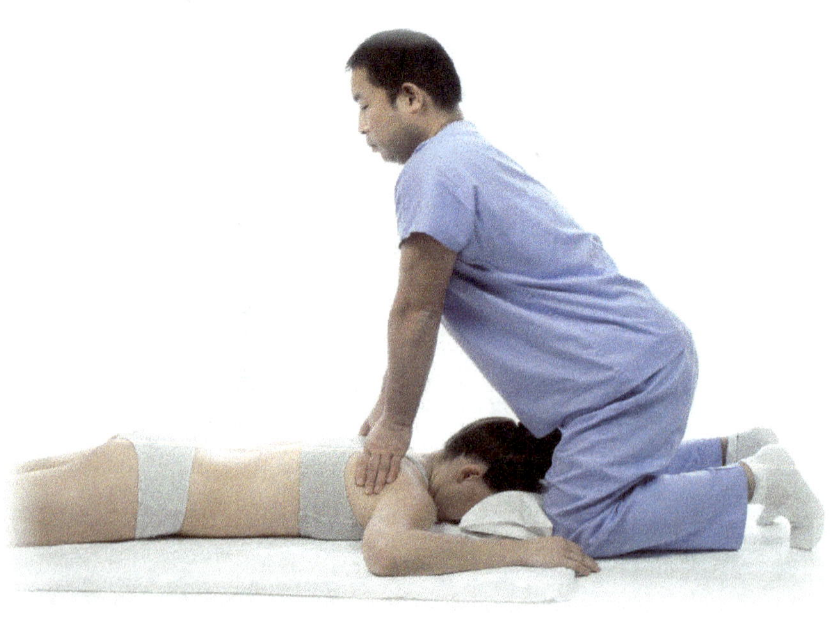

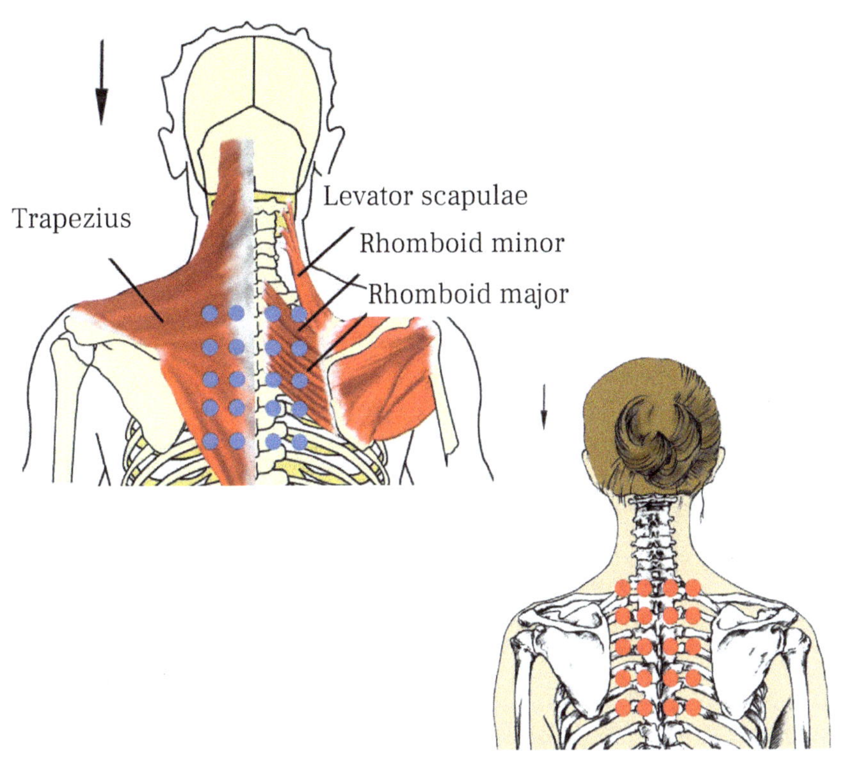

Trapezius
Levator scapulae
Rhomboid minor
Rhomboid major

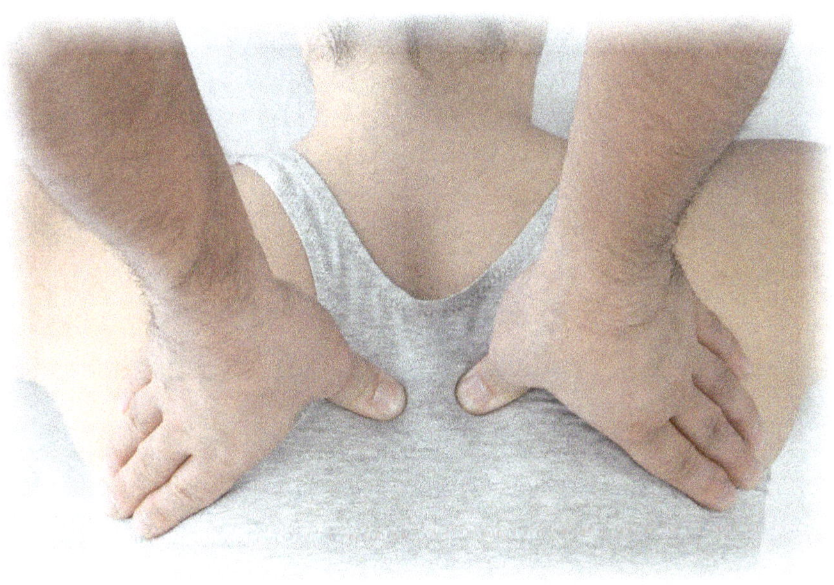

3. The neck

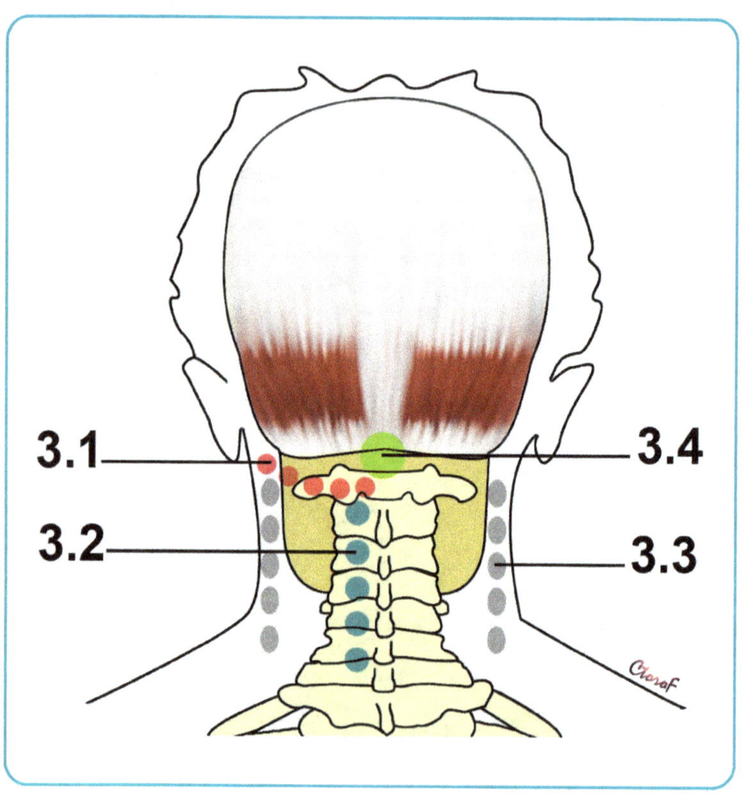

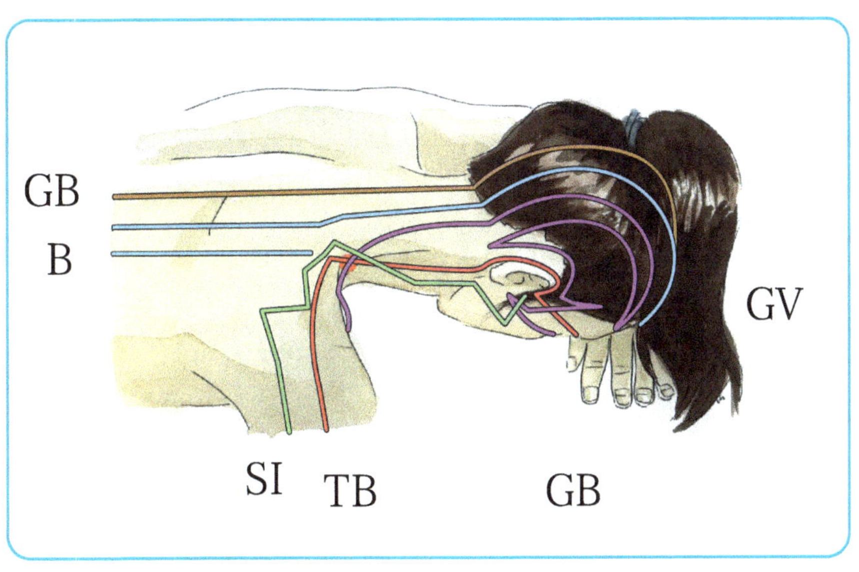

GB
B
SI
TB
GB
GV

3.1. OCCIPITAL REGION

PATIENT'S POSTURE: Prone, with the forehead resting on a pillow, shoulders in abduction and elbows bent.

THERAPIST'S POSITION: Basic, on the left side of the patient. Right knee at the level of the axillary region.

TYPE OF PRESSURE: Right thumb applies pressure and the left hand holds the top of the patient's head.

Nº. OF POINTS: One five-point line.

DIRECTION OF THE LINE: From mastoid tuberosity to the Rachidian bulb. Apply pressure towards the centre of the hand holding the head.

OBSERVATIONS:The hand holding the head adopts a 'bowl' form to avoid unpleasant contact with the patient. In addition, this position helps the therapist concentrate energy in the centre of his palm (key point *H8, Roukyuu*).

The last point in this region corresponds to key point *B10 (Tenchuu).*

Three times for three seconds.

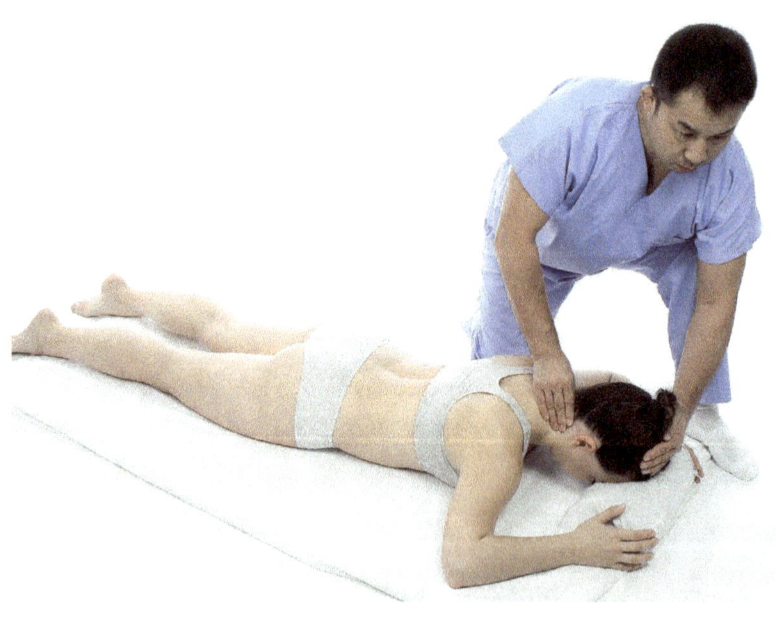

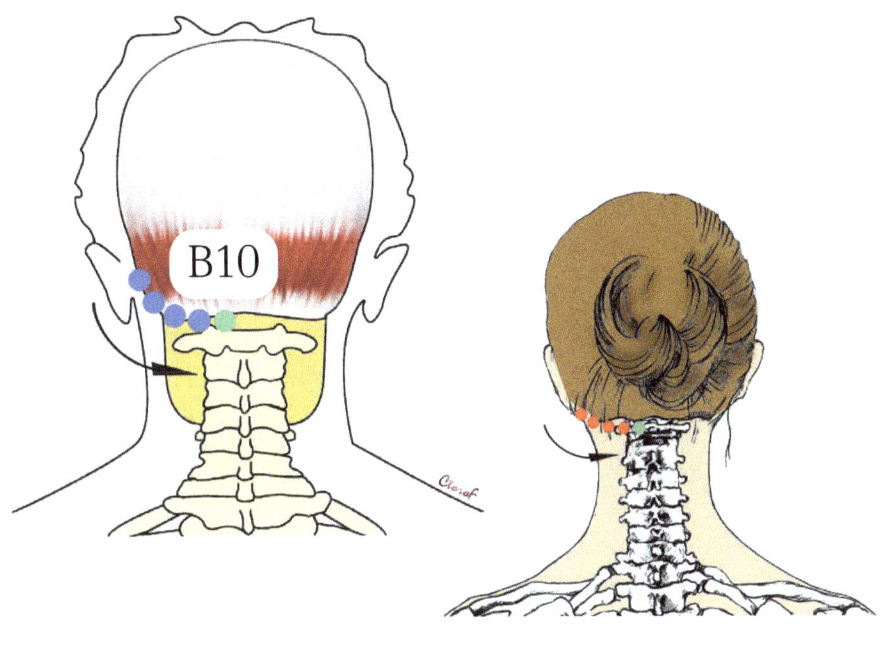
B10

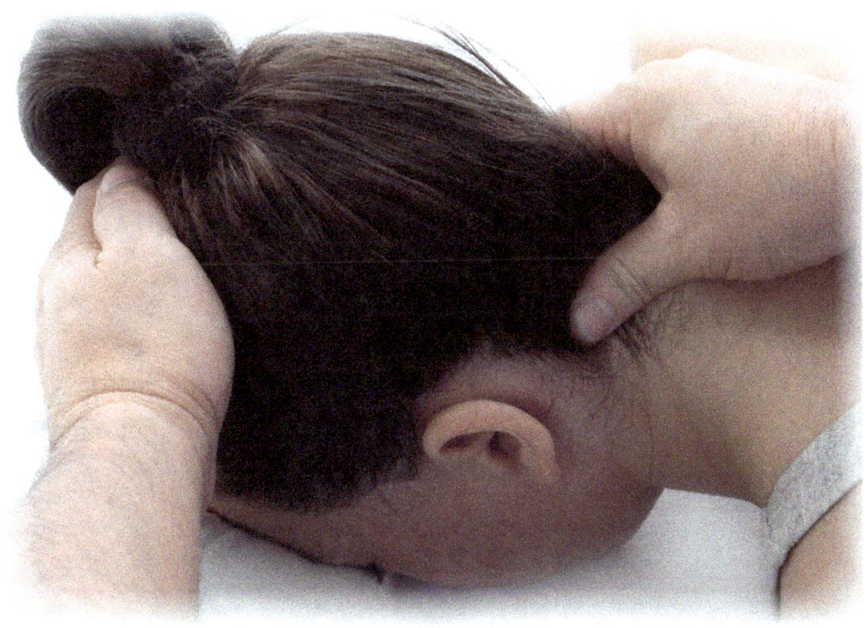

3.2. POSTERIOR CERVICAL REGION

PATIENT'S POSTURE: Prone, with the forehead resting on a pillow, shoulders in abduction and elbows bent.

THERAPIST'S POSITION: Basic, on the left side of the patient. Right knee at the level of the axillary region.

TYPE OF PRESSURE: Right thumb; the other fingers surround the neck. The other hand holds the top of the patient's head.

Nº. OF POINTS: A five-point line.

DIRECTION OF THE LINE: The first point below the occipital bone to C7-D1; the direction of the pressure is towards the trachea.

OBSERVATIONS:The thumb and little finger's work is very important. The pincer-style pressure avoids squashing the patient's face against the resting surface.

One of the complementary points to the Five Warning Points is located between the second and third cervical vertebrae, on the right side.

Three times for three seconds.

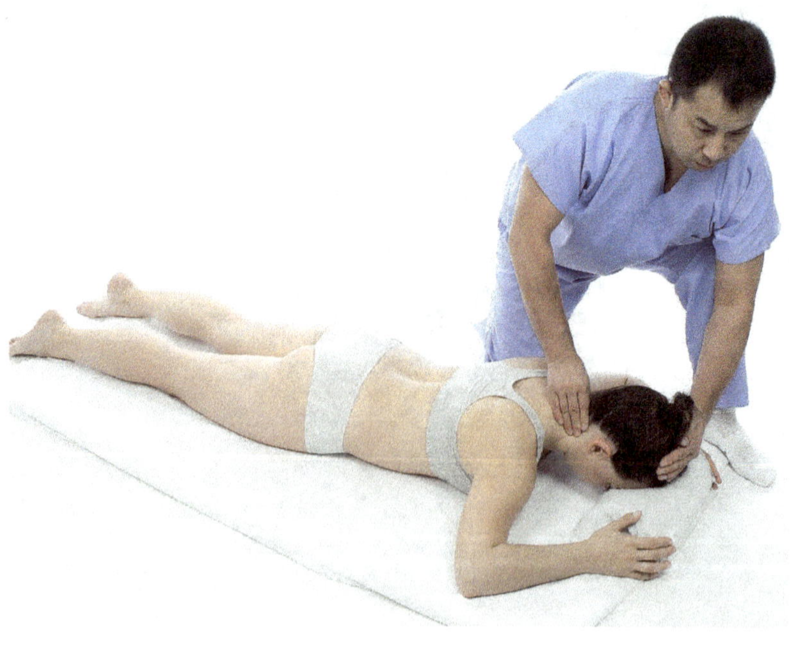

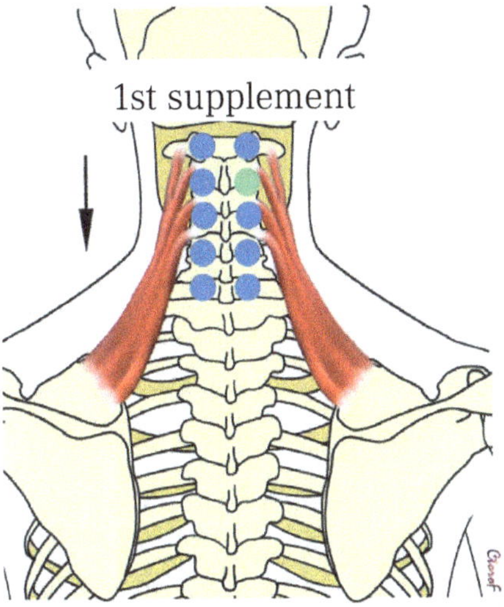

1st supplement

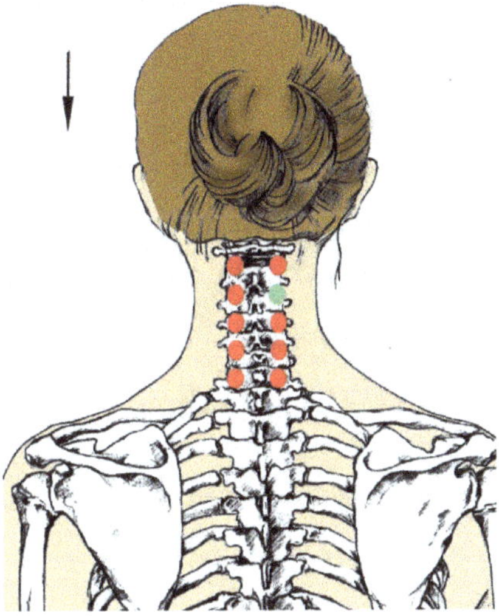

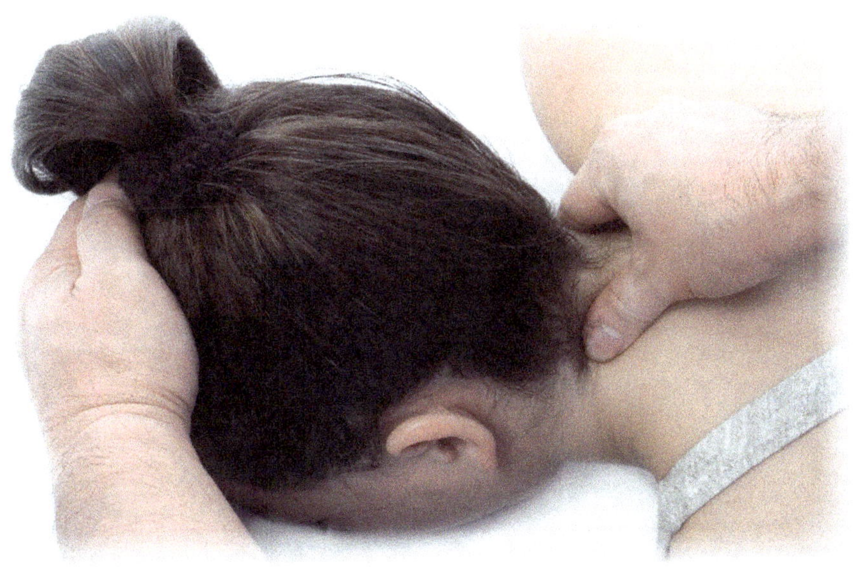

3.3. LATERAL CERVICAL REGION

PATIENT'S POSTURE: Prone, with the forehead resting on a pillow, shoulders in abduction and elbows bent.

THERAPIST'S POSITION: Basic, on the left side of the patient. Right knee at the level of the axillary region.

TYPE OF PRESSURE: Right thumb; the other fingers surround the neck. The other hand holds the top of the patient's head.

Nº. OF POINTS: A five-point line.

DIRECTION OF THE LINE: From under the mastoid tuberosity to the base of the neck; the direction is perpendicular to the neck.

OBSERVATIONS: The second point is suitable for treating insomnia.

Three times for three seconds.

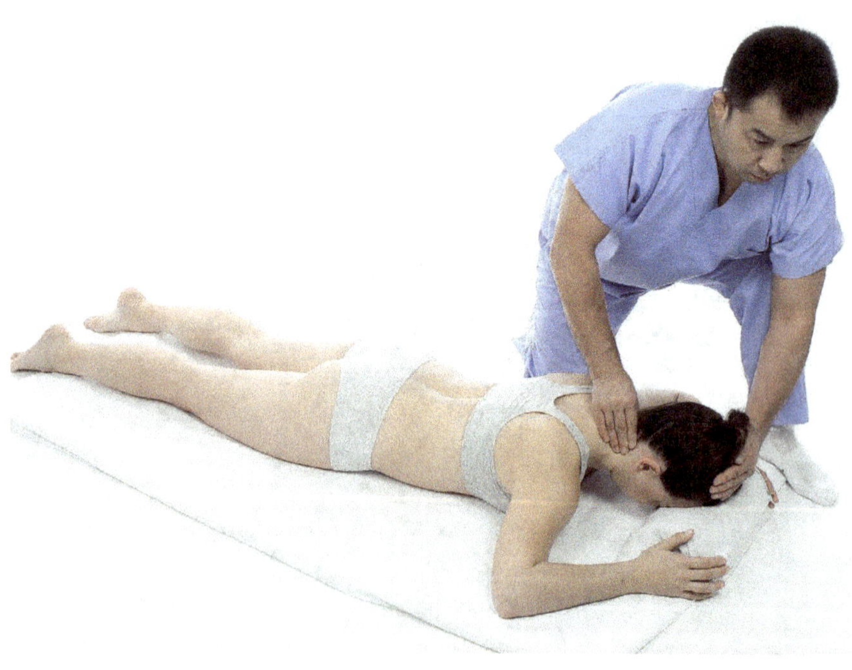

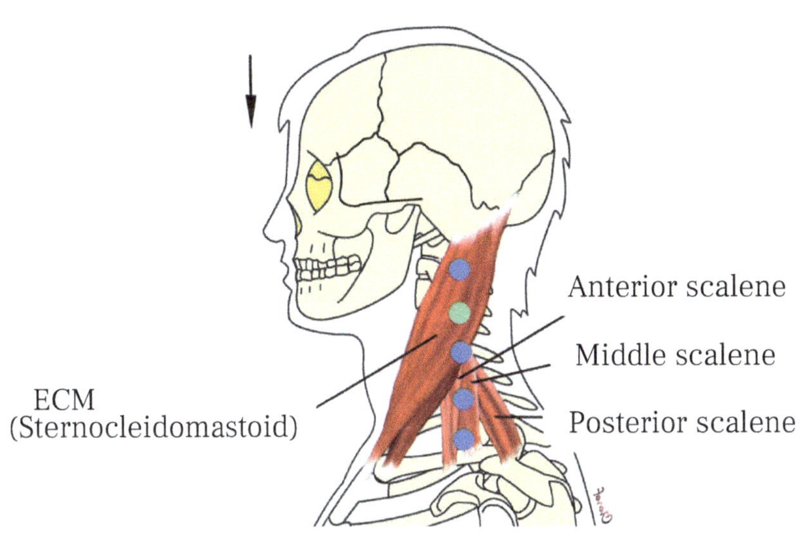

Anterior scalene
Middle scalene
Posterior scalene
ECM
(Sternocleidomastoid)

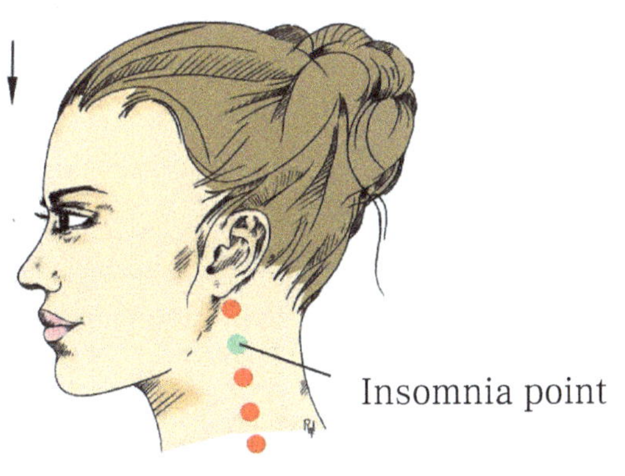

Insomnia point

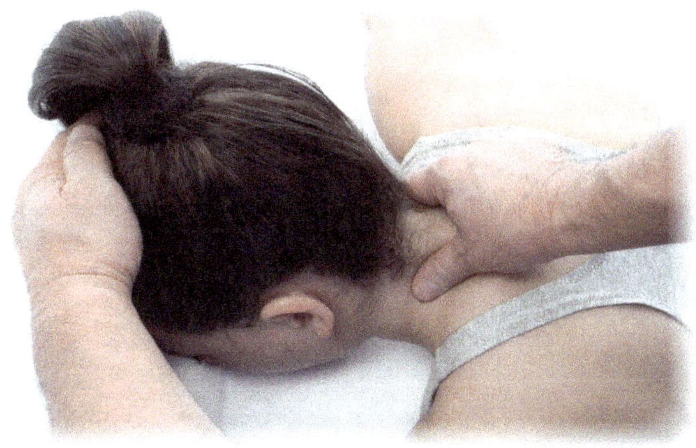

3.4. RACHIDIAN BULB REGION.

PATIENT'S POSTURE: Prone, with the forehead resting on a pillow, shoulders in abduction and elbows bent.

THERAPIST'S POSITION: Basic, on the left side of the patient. Right knee at the level of the axillary region.

TYPE OF PRESSURE: Work with the right thumb and the other fingers surround the neck. The other hand holds the top of the patient's head.

Nº. OF POINTS: One point.

DIRECTION OF THE LINE: Towards the space between the eyebrows with the hand holding the head.

OBSERVATIONS: This region is repeated for work the right side. It corresponds to key point *GV16 (Fuufu)*.

Three times for five seconds.

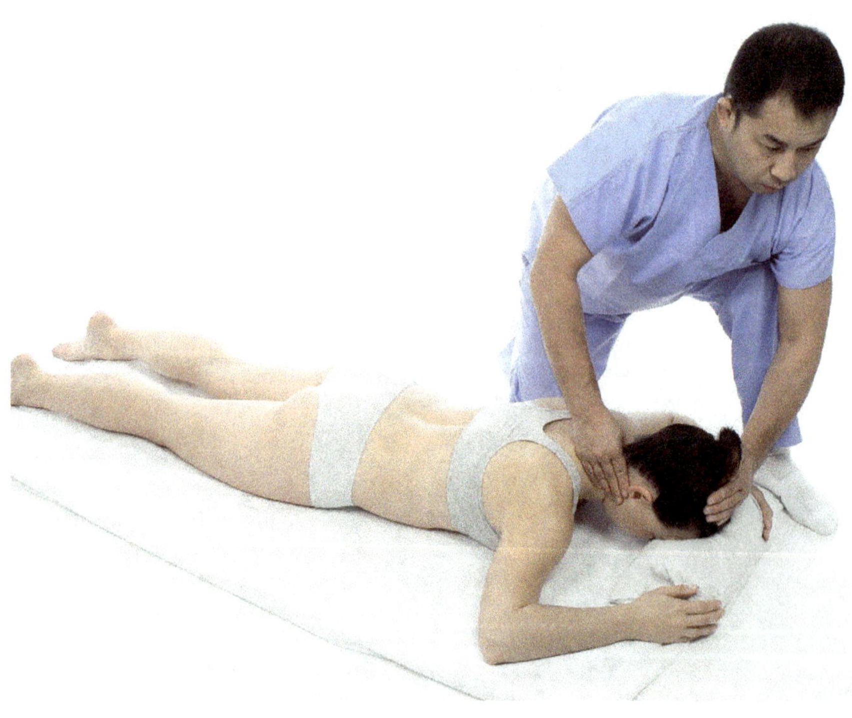

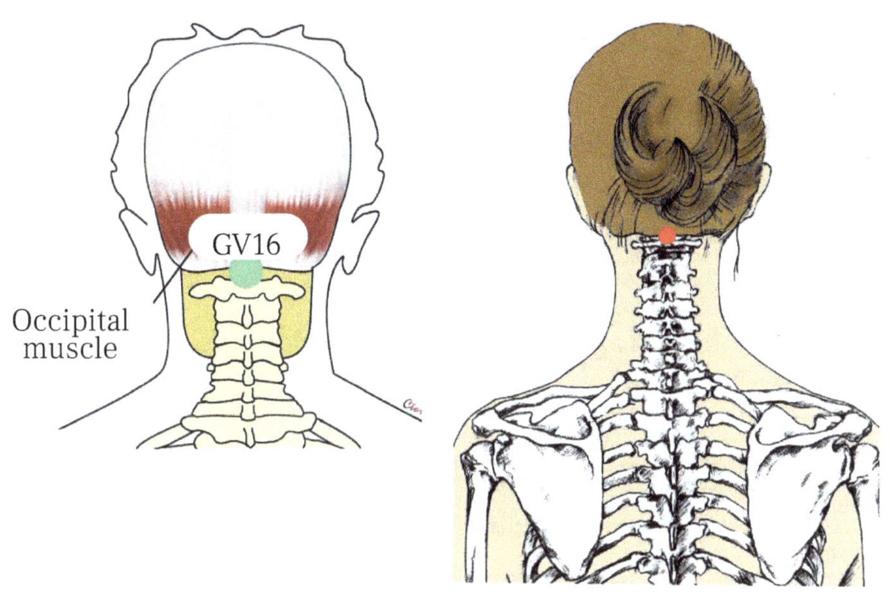

GV16
Occipital
muscle

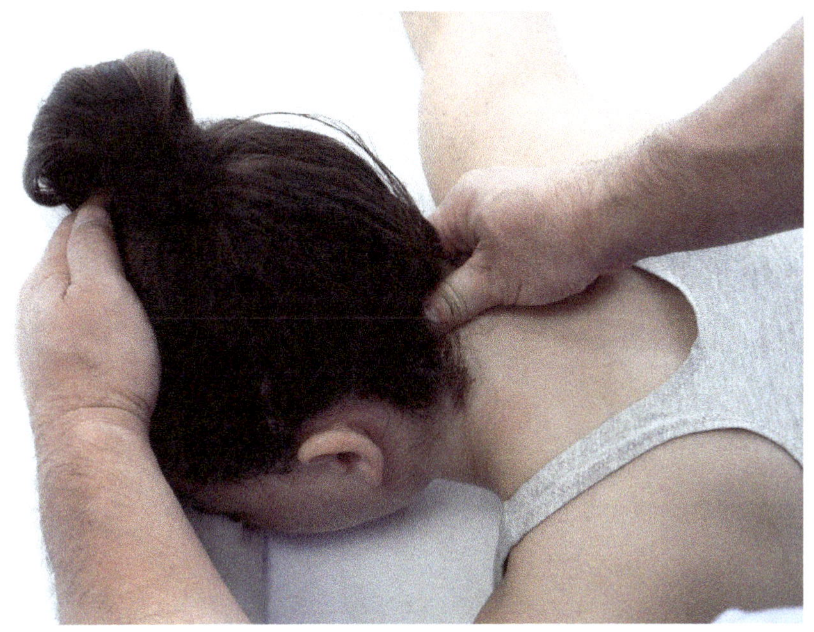

4. The Back (I)

Suprascapular region

4.1. Suprascapular point.

4.2. Suprascapular Region.

4.3. Base of the neck region.

Interscapular and scapula region

4.4. Interscapular region. 1st and 2nd lines.

4.5. Scapula region. Medial edge.

4.6. Scapula region. Central point.

4.7. Scapula region. Axillary fold.

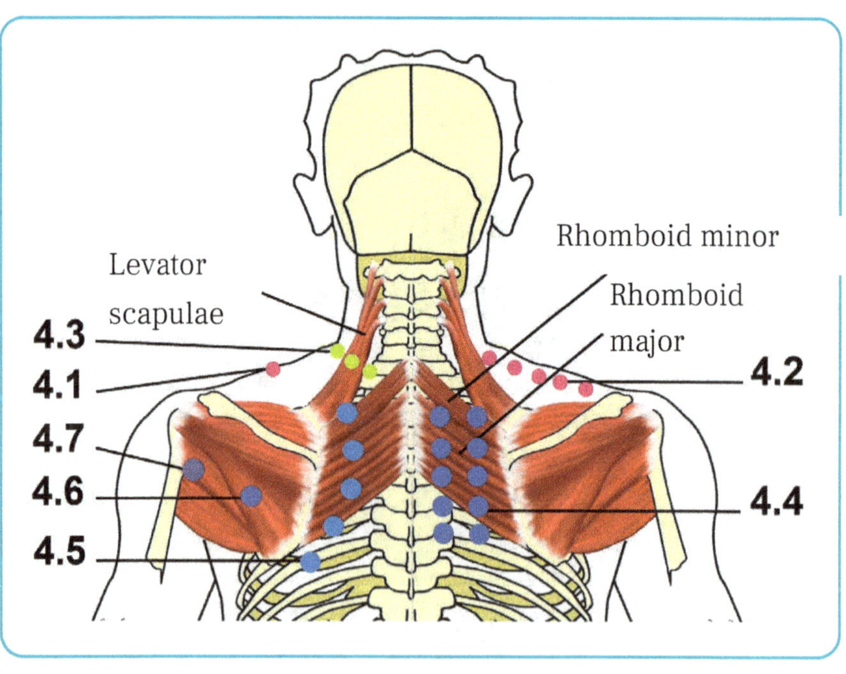

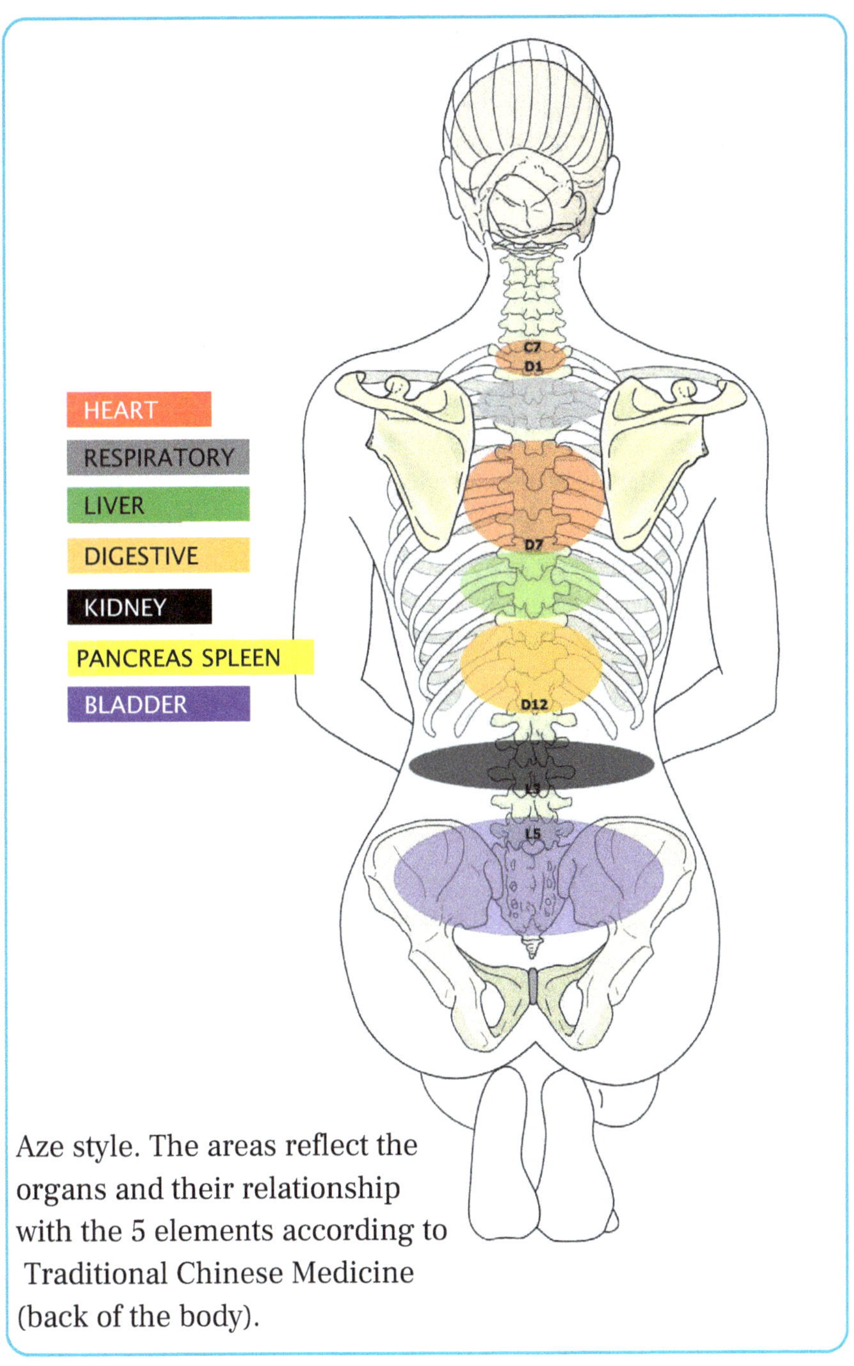

Aze style. The areas reflect the organs and their relationship with the 5 elements according to Traditional Chinese Medicine (back of the body).

4.1. SUPRASCAPULAR POINT

PATIENT'S POSTURE: Prone. Head turned towards the therapist, shoulders in abduction and elbows bent.

THERAPIST'S POSITION: Seiza facing the patient's head. Rotate on the arches and position yourself 45° relative to the centre line of the patient's body.

TYPE OF PRESSURE: Left thumb; middle finger on the spinal column. The other hand is supported on the floor to fix the posture.

Nº. OF POINTS: One point. Coincides with the second point of the suprascapular line: *GB21 (Kensei)*.

DIRECTION OF PRESSURE: Towards the centre of the body at the level of D7.

OBSERVATIONS: Tilt the body from the hara while maintaining the arm's position so that the pressure penetrates correctly. Slow and deep pressure. This point coincides with the second point of the Supraescapular Line (key point *GB21, Kensei*).

Three times for five seconds.

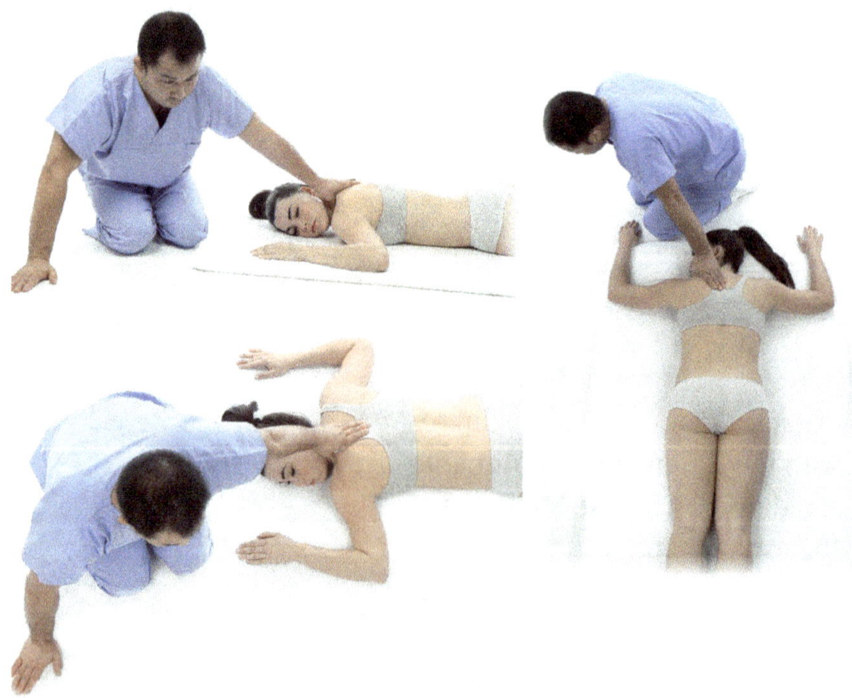

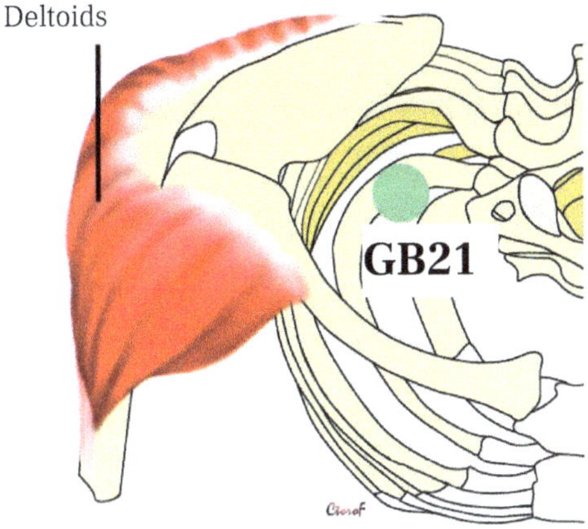

Deltoids
GB21

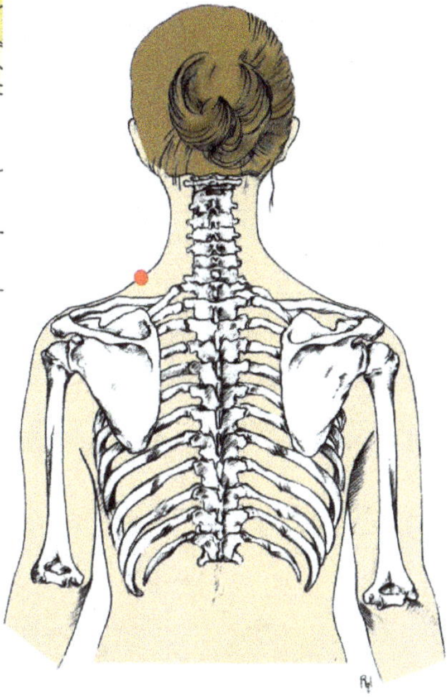

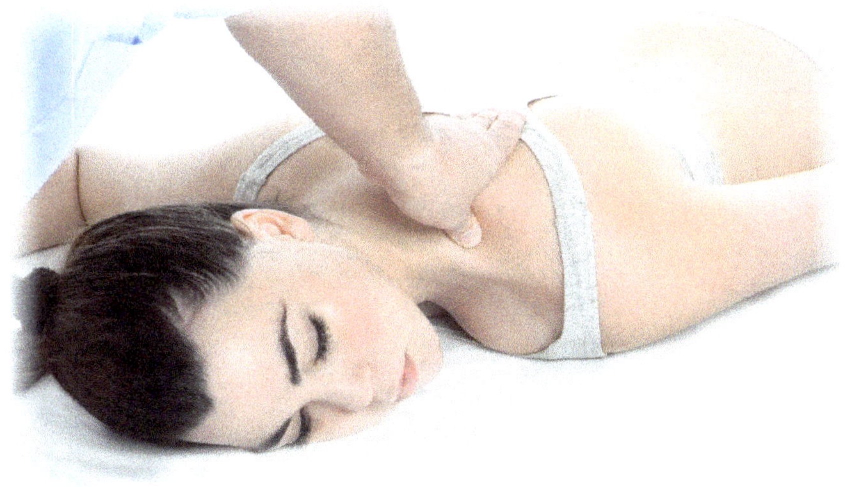

4.2. SUPRAESCAPULAR REGION

PATIENT'S POSTURE: Prone. Head turned towards the therapist, shoulders in abduction and elbows bent.

THERAPIST'S POSITION: Seiza, 45° above the patient's head.

TYPE OF PRESSURE: Left thumb. The other hand is supported on the floor.

Nº. OF POINTS: A five-point line.

DIRECTION OF THE LINE: Along the superior bundle of the trapezium muscle, from the base of the neck to the shoulder. Slow and deep pressure.

OBSERVATIONS: The second point in this region is the suprascapular point (see 4.1) and corresponds to key point *GB21 (Kensei)*.

Three times for three seconds.

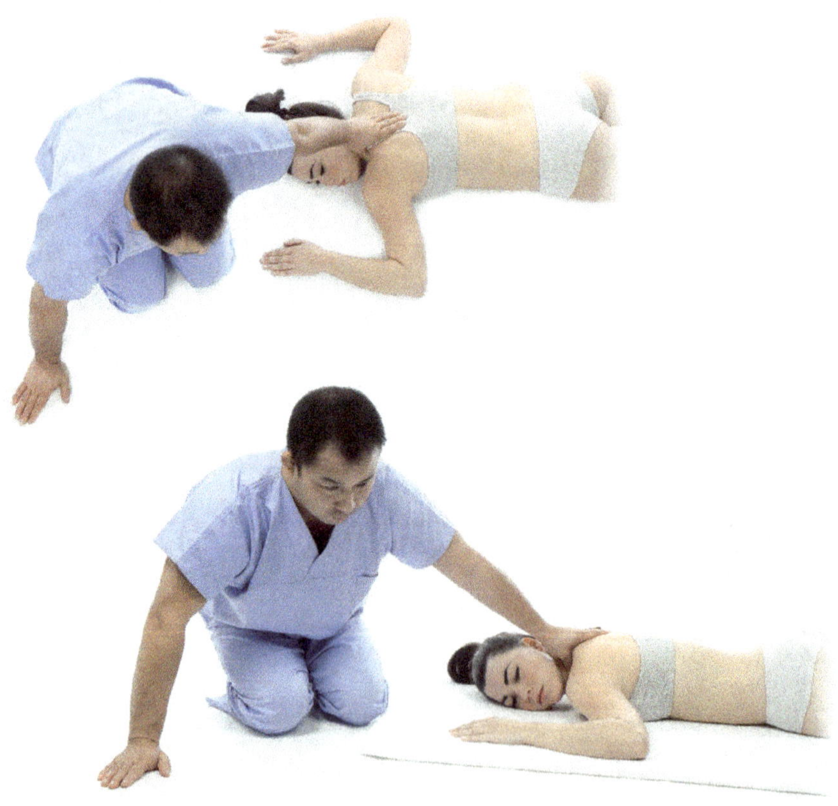

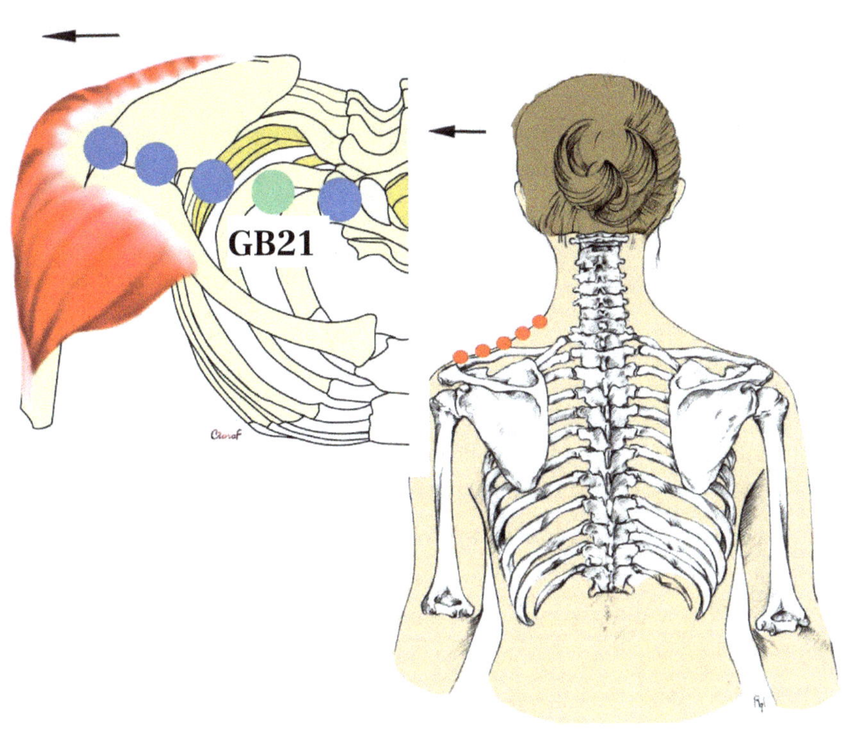

GB21

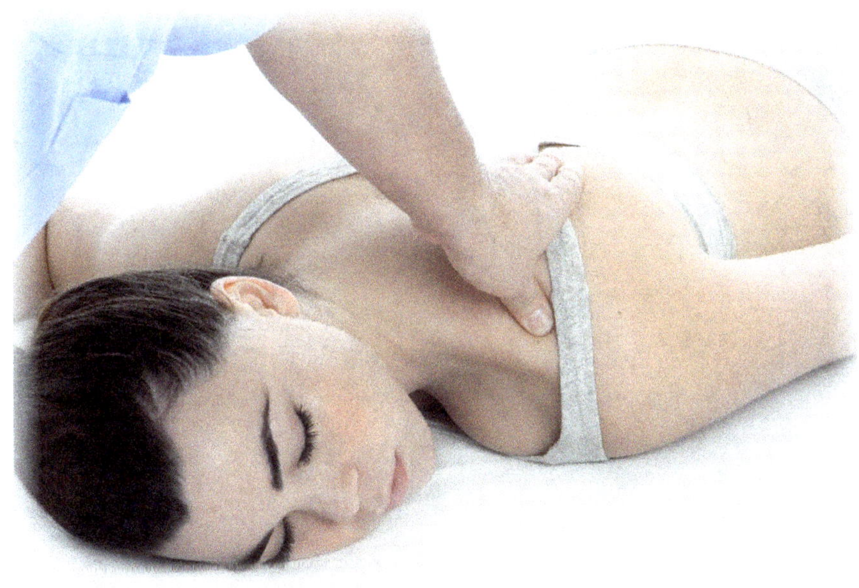

4.3. BASE OF THE NECK REGION

PATIENT'S POSTURE: Prone. Head turned towards the therapist, shoulders in abduction and elbows bent.

THERAPIST'S POSITION: Seiza, 45º above the patient's head.

TYPE OF PRESSURE: Left thumb. The other hand is supported on the floor.

Nº. OF POINTS: A five-point line.

DIRECTION OF THE LINE: Around the neck. The first point is located at the top of the middle third of the collarbone (esternocleidomastoid muscle insertion) and the last point on the levator scapulae muscle.

To treat the region we imagine a line between the described areas and we work on the scalene muscles.

The third point, in the centre of the line, is the last point of the Lateral Cervical Region and the first of the Suprascapular Region.

OBSERVATIONS: The position of the patient's arms tightens the area by pushing the contracture out to be better worked on.

Three times for three seconds.

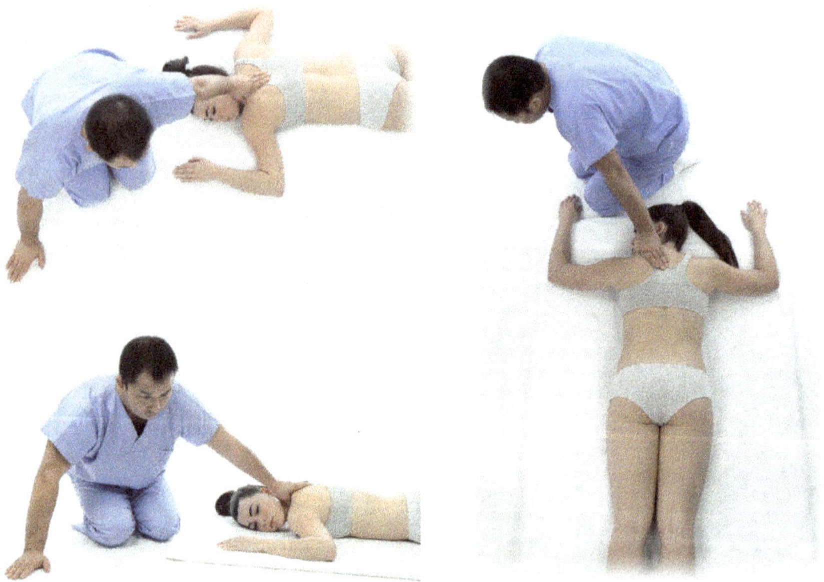

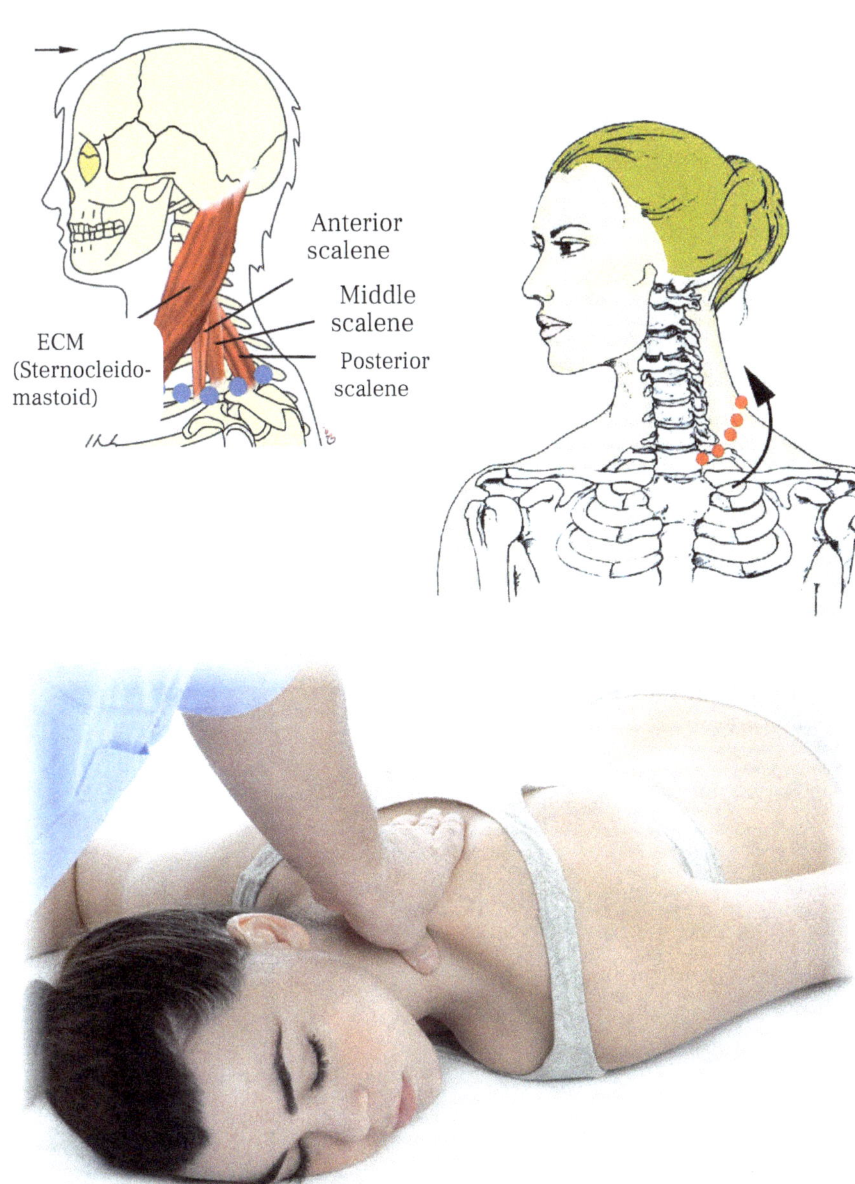

Anterior
scalene
Middle
scalene
Posterior
scalene
ECM
(Sternocleido-
mastoid)

4.4. INTERSCAPULAR REGION. 1st and 2nd LINES

PATIENT'S POSTURE: Prone. Head turned towards the therapist, shoulders in abduction and elbows bent.

THERAPIST'S POSITION: Basic, perpendicular to the working area. The right knee is on the ground, at the level of the patient's shoulder blade; left foot above the head.

TYPE OF PRESSURE: 1st and 2nd repetitions: Logo.

3rd Repetition: Thumb over thumb

(left one below).

Nº. OF POINTS: Two five-point lines.

DIRECTION OF THE LINE: The first line is located on the internal edge of the paravertebral muscles. The first point is located at D1 and the last point on the D7 line. The second line runs parallel to the previous line along the external edge of the paravertebral musculature. Repeat both lines alternatively.

OBSERVATIONS: When working thumb over thumb, the thumb of the hand holding the shoulder remains underneath. This is the best way to work on Western bodies that have more accentuated dorsal kyphosis.

Three times for three seconds.

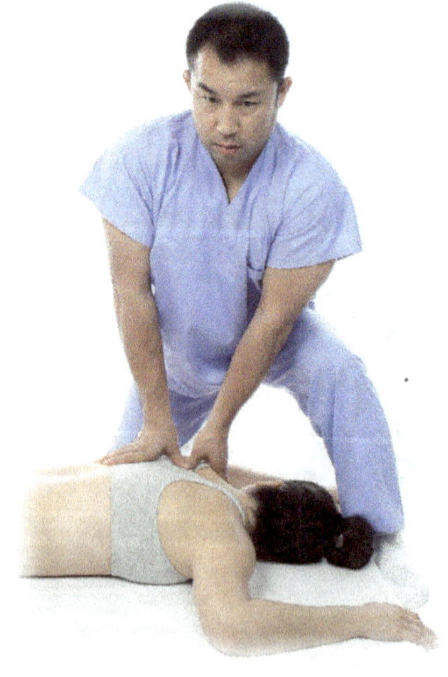

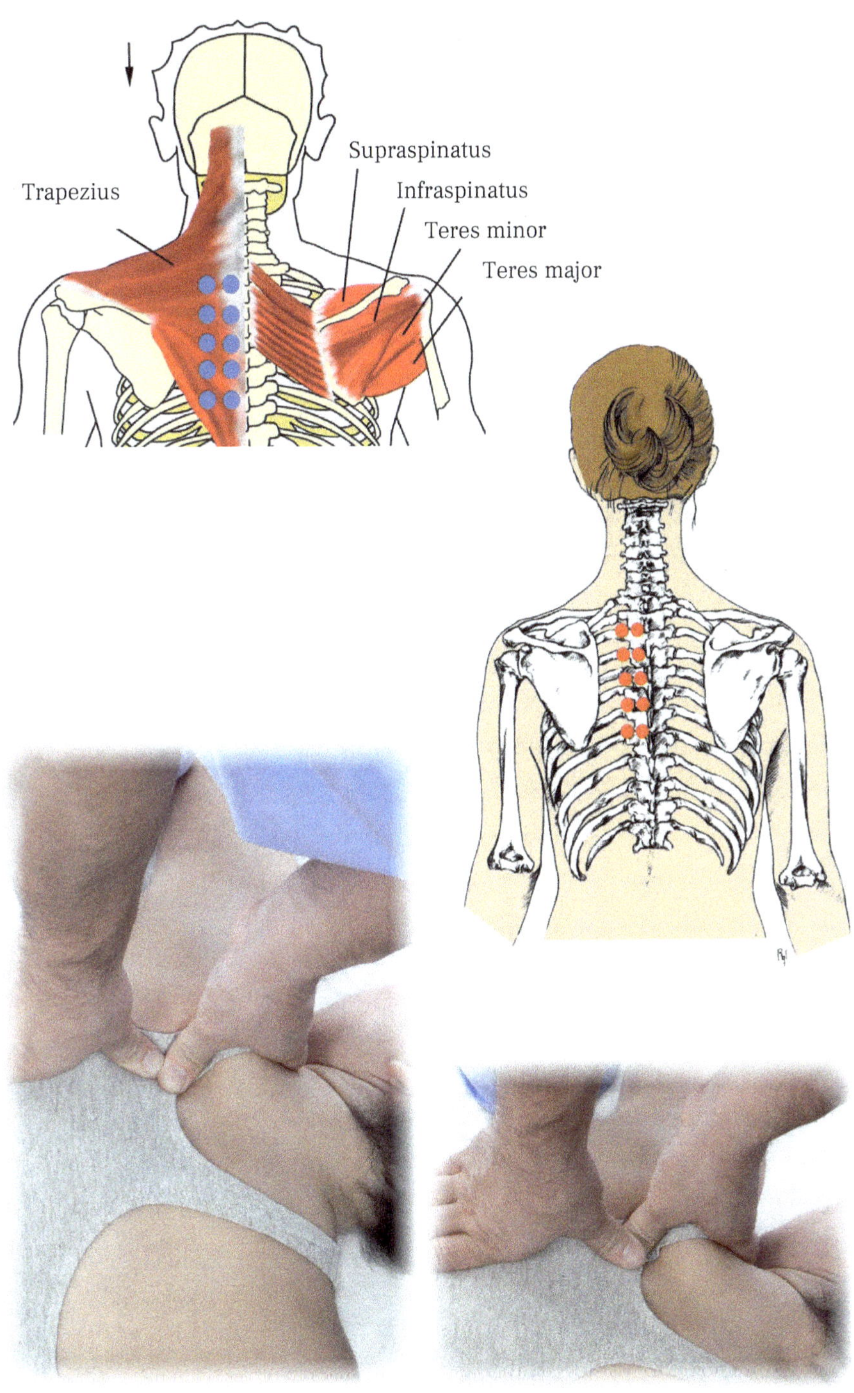

Trapezius
Supraspinatus
Infraspinatus
Teres minor
Teres major

4.5. SCAPULA REGION: MEDIAL EDGE

PATIENT'S POSTURE: Prone. Head turned towards the therapist, shoulders in abduction and elbows bent.

THERAPIST'S POSITION: Basic, right knee on the ground, at the level of the patient's shoulder blade; left foot above the head.

TYPE OF PRESSURE: 1st and 2nd repetitions: Logo.
3rd Repetition: Thumb over thumb (left one below).

If the scapula has low mobility and is stuck to the rib cage, the thumbs will be used in A.

Nº. OF POINTS: A five-point line.

DIRECTION OF THE LINE: Located around the vertebral edge, from the superior to inferior angle.

OBSERVATIONS: As in the previous case, the thumb of the hand holding the shoulder remains underneath. You have to look for the contracture in the third point area and work it for longer. This area roughly coincides with point *B43 (Koukou)*, which is one of the five warning points.

Three times for three seconds.

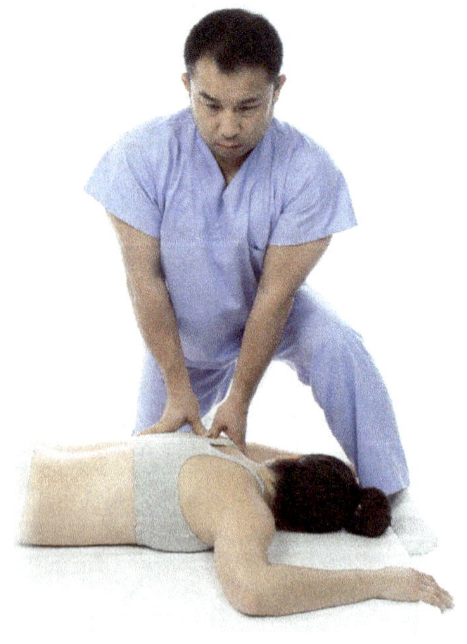

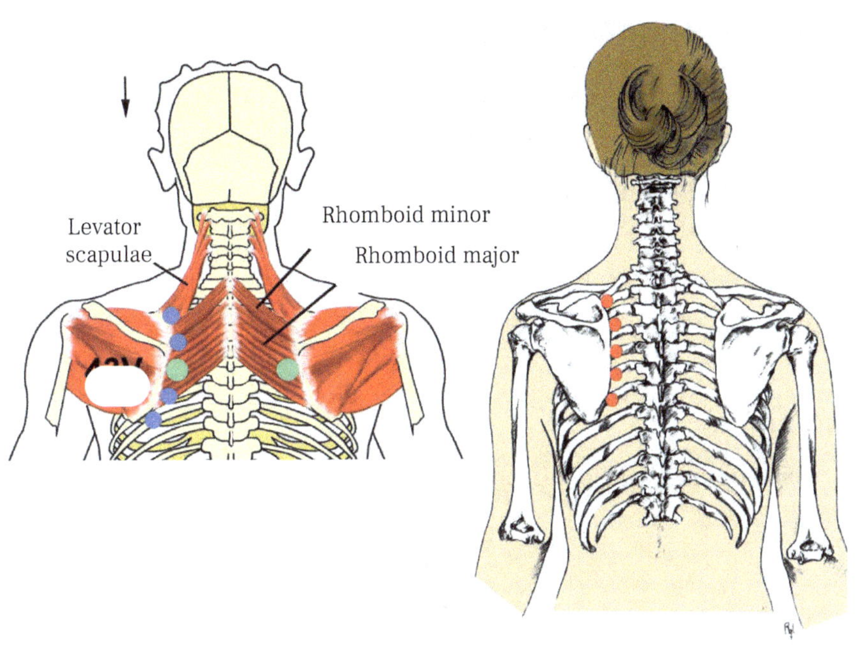

Levator
scapulae
Rhomboid minor
Rhomboid major

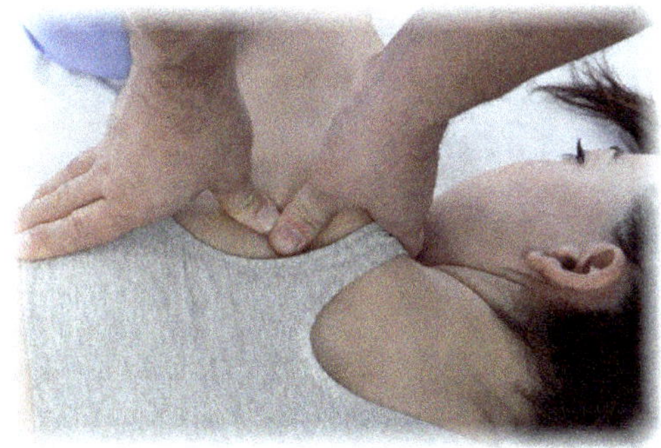

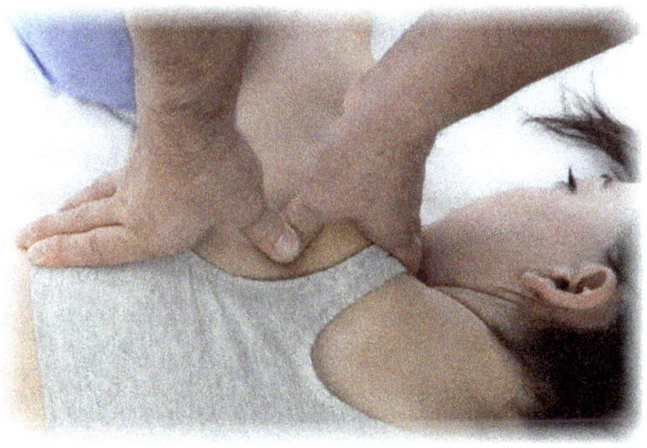

4.6. SCAPULA REGION: CENTRAL POINT

PATIENT'S POSTURE: Prone. Head turned towards the therapist, shoulders in abduction and elbows bent.

THERAPIST'S POSITION: Basic, right knee on the ground, at the level of the patient's shoulder blade; left foot above the head.

TYPE OF PRESSURE: Only one thumb. The other hand rests on the back.

Nº. OF POINTS: One point.

OBSERVATIONS:This point coincides to key point *SI11 (Tensou)*. Slow and deep pressure.

Three times for five seconds.

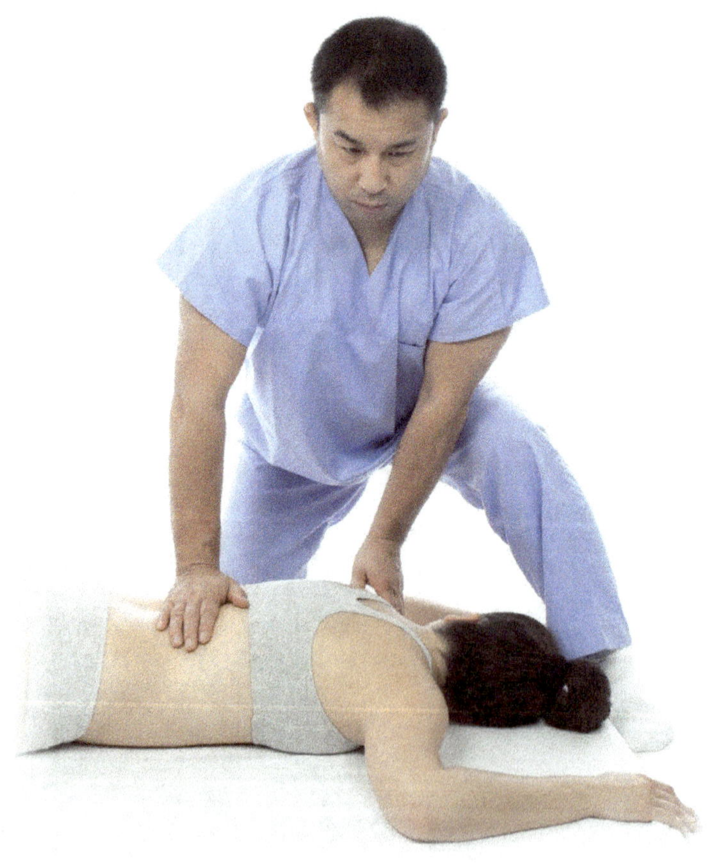

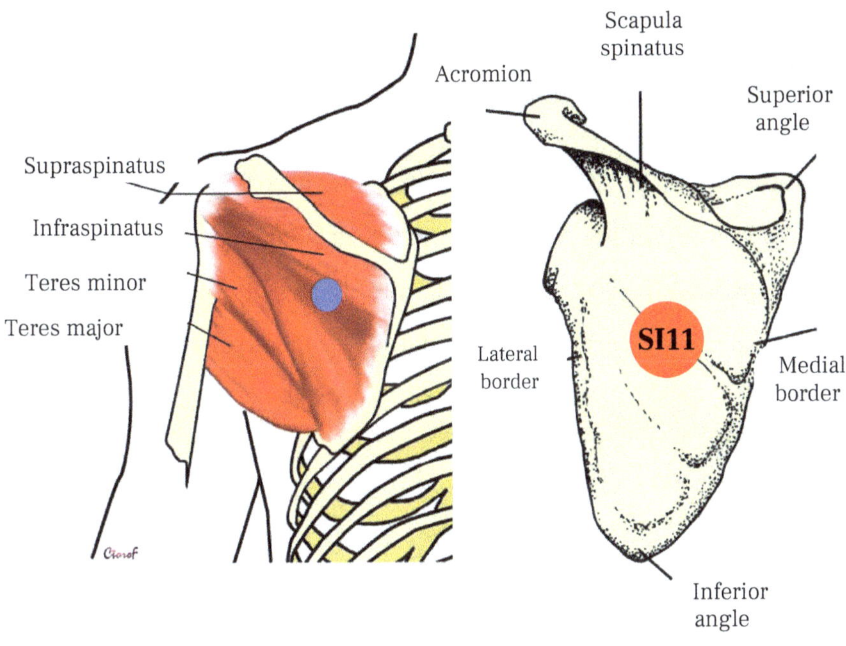

Supraspinatus
Infraspinatus
Teres minor
Teres major
Acromion
Scapula spinatus
Superior angle
Lateral border
SI11
Medial border
Inferior angle

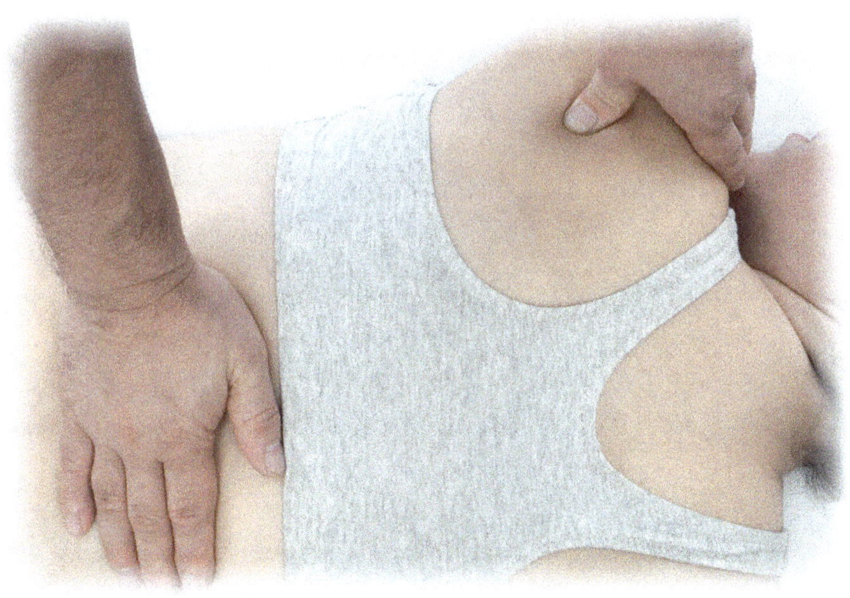

4.7. SCAPULA REGION: AXILLARY FOLD

PATIENT'S POSTURE: Prone. Head turned towards the therapist, shoulders in abduction and elbows bent.

THERAPIST'S POSITION: Basic, right knee on the ground, at the level of the patient's shoulder blade; left foot above the head.

TYPE OF PRESSURE: Only one thumb. The other hand rests on the back.

Nº. OF POINTS: One point. Dorsal side of the axillary fold.

OBSERVATIONS: This point coincides to key point *SI9 (Kentei)*. Slow and deep pressure.

Three times for three seconds.

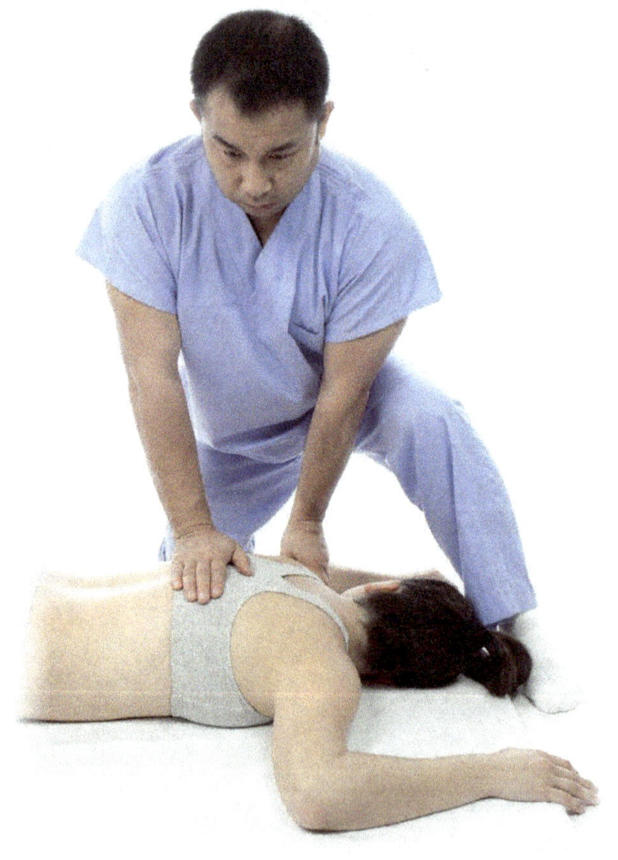

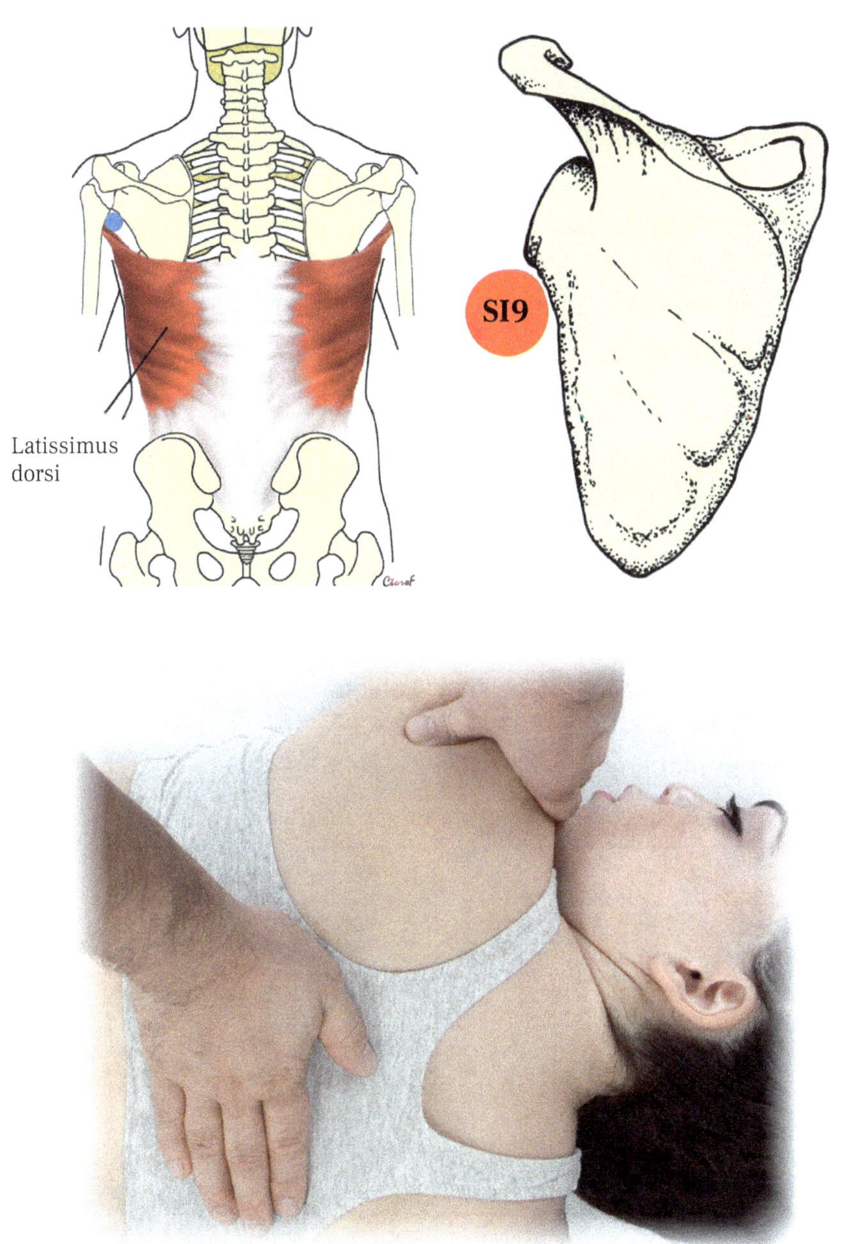

Repeat the Neck and Back work (I)
on the RIGHT SIDE.

5. The Back (II)

Infrascapular and lumbar region

5.1. Infrascapular and lumbar region. 1st and 2nd lines on both sides of the spinal column.

5.2. Infrascapular and lumbar region. 1st, 2rd and 3rd lines.

5.3. Lumbar region. B52 Line.

5.4. Iliac crest region.

Sacral and gluteus region

5.5. Sacral region.

5.6. Sacroiliac joint region (internal edge).

5.7. Sacroiliac joint region (external edge).

5.8. Gluteus maximus region.

5.9. Pyramidal point.

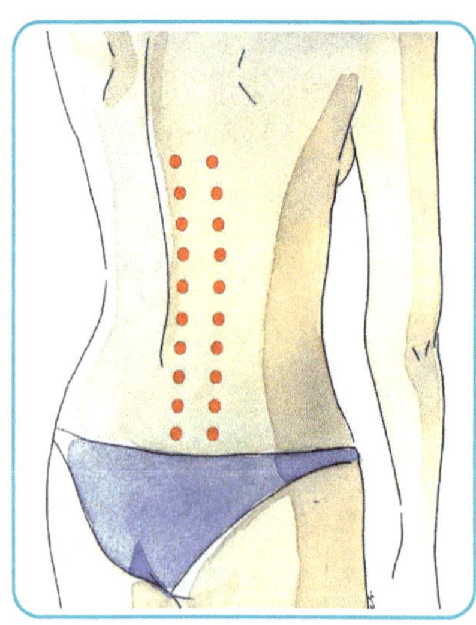
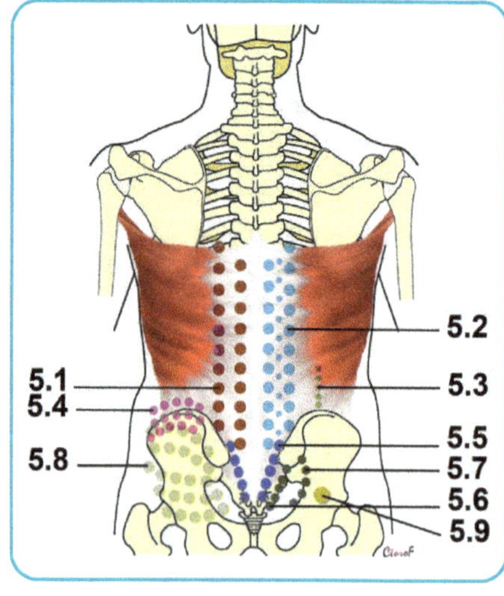

5.1. INFRACAPULAR AND LUMBAR REGION.
1st and 2nd LINES ON BOTH SIDES OF THE SPINAL COLUMN

PATIENT'S POSTURE: Prone. Head turned towards the therapist, shoulders in abduction and elbows bent.

THERAPIST'S POSITION: Basic. Left side of the patient, right knee at the level of the sacral region.

TYPE OF PRESSURE: Both thumbs at the same time.

Nº. OF POINTS: Two simultaneous lines of ten points on either side of the spinal column. The first line runs along the medial edge of the paravertebral musculature and the second line along the lateral edge.

DIRECTION OF THE LINE: From the inferior edge of the shoulder blade (D8-D9) until L5-S1. Pressure must be applied between the transverse process without touching the column. Repeat both lines alternatively.

OBSERVATIONS:Simultaneous work on both sides allows comparative diagnosis of the state of the back. The lumbar area is the centre of the body and a "thermometer" of its general state.

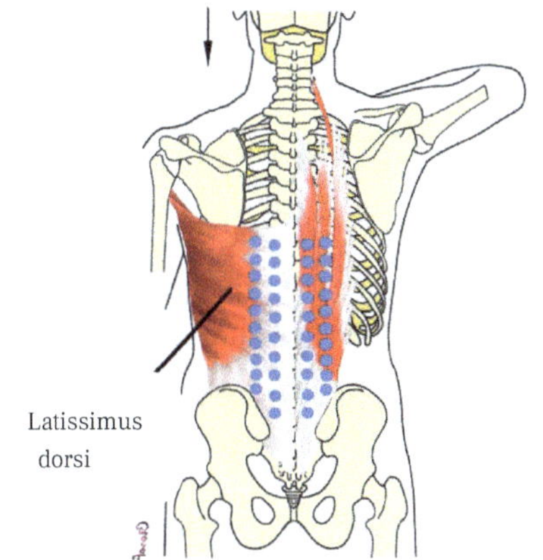

Three times for three seconds.

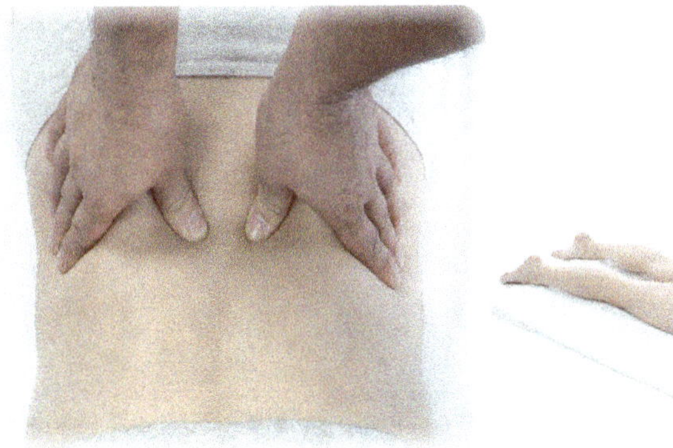

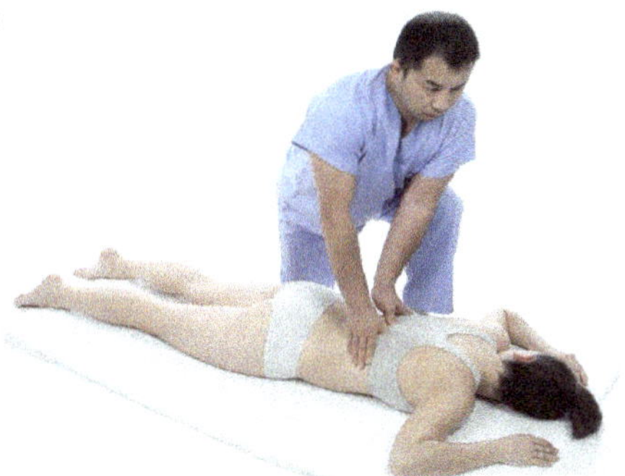

5.2. INFRACAPULAR AND LUMBAR REGION. 1st, 2nd and 3rd LINES

PATIENT'S POSTURE: Prone. Head turned towards the therapist, shoulders in abduction and elbows bent.

THERAPIST'S POSITION: Basic. Maintaining the previous position.

TYPE OF PRESSURE: 1st and 2nd repetitions: Logo.

3rd repetition: Thumb over thumb (right below).

Nº. OF POINTS: Three ten-point lines.
1st Line: 10 points (medial edge of paravertebral muscles).

2nd Line: 10 points (lateral edge of paravertebral muscles).

3rd Line: 10 points (in the centre of paravertebral muscles).

DIRECTION OF THE LINE: D8-D9 to L5–S1. First 1st and 2nd lines alternatively and then three repetitions of the 3rd Line.

OBSERVATIONS:When working the 3rd line, keep it perpendicular and work slowly. The fifth point *B21 (Iyu)* of the 3rd line is one of five warning points and serves to diagnose digestive problems.

The tenth point *B26 (Kangenyu)*, of the 3rd line is another warning point regarding the state of the lumbar area.

Three times for three seconds.
The tenth point 3 x 5 seconds at the end of the 1st line.

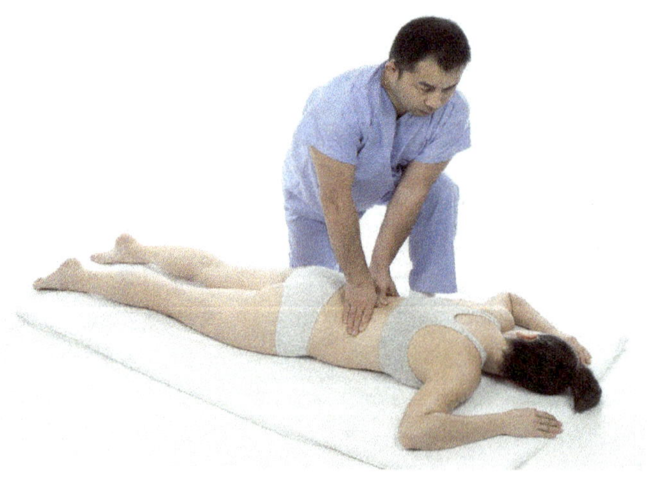

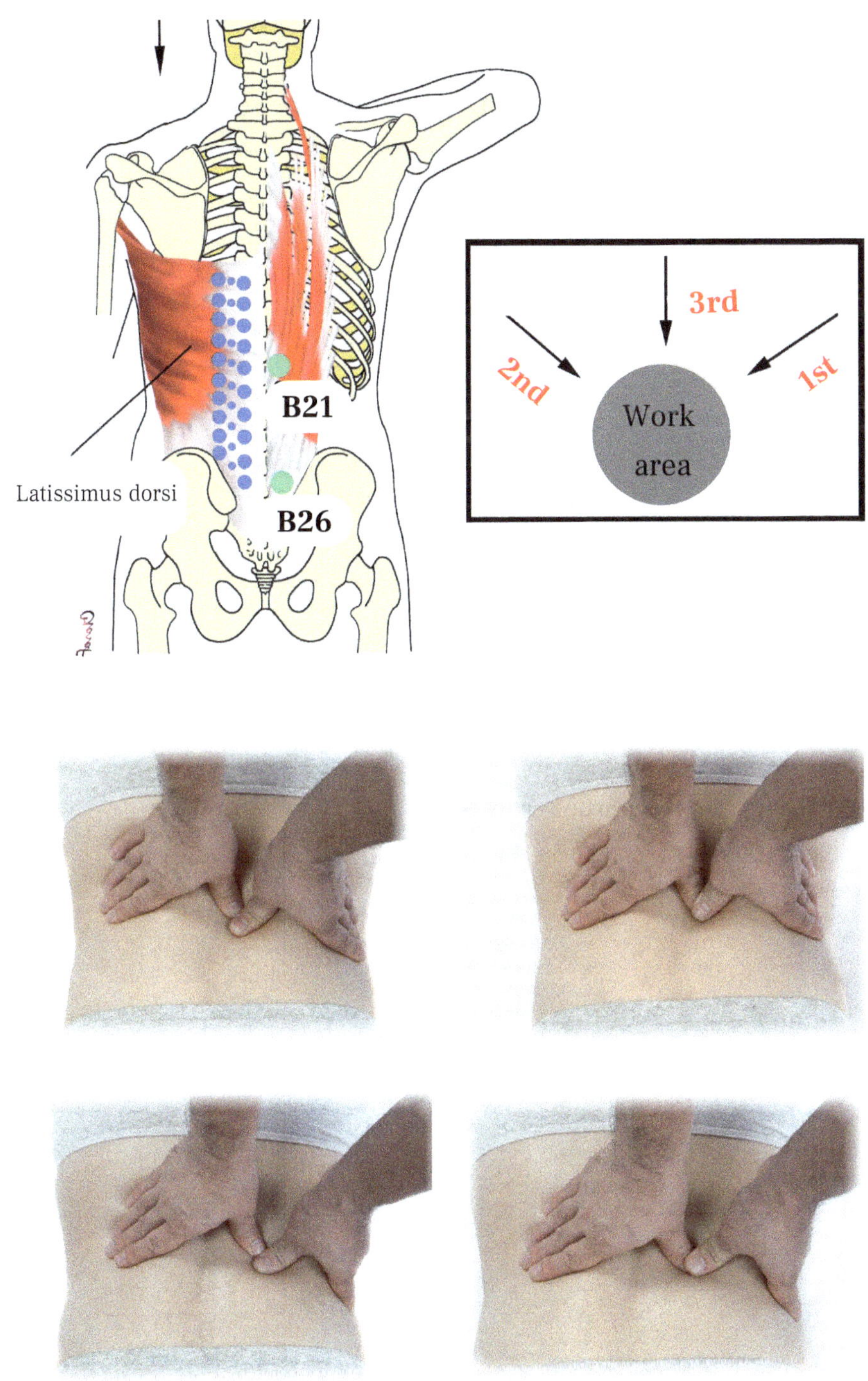

Latissimus dorsi
B21
B26
3rd
2nd
1st
Work
area

5.3. LUMBAR REGION. B52 LINE

PATIENT'S POSTURE: Prone. Head turned towards the therapist, shoulders in abduction and elbows bent.

THERAPIST'S POSITION: Seiza or kneeling, perpendicular to the patient's body.

TYPE OF PRESSURE: Thumb over thumb (right one below) with hands together and slightly overlapping. Slow pressure and towards the centre of the body.

Nº. OF POINTS: A five-point line.

DIRECTION OF THE LINE: It is located two fingers laterally from the second line of the Infraescapular and Lumbar Region. In a downward direction. Between the sixteenth rib and the iliac crest.

OBSERVATIONS: Forming a triangle to locate the warning points *B52 (Shishitsu, third point)*, which relates to the state of the lumbar zone, the *ovarian* point (fifth point), related to the genital tract and a third warning point, *B26 (Kangenyu,* tenth of the lumbar area) and which in turn signals in the centre of the body.

In the centre of the triangle we have formed, we can imagine a more important central point.

Three times for three seconds.

Third point: Three times for five seconds.

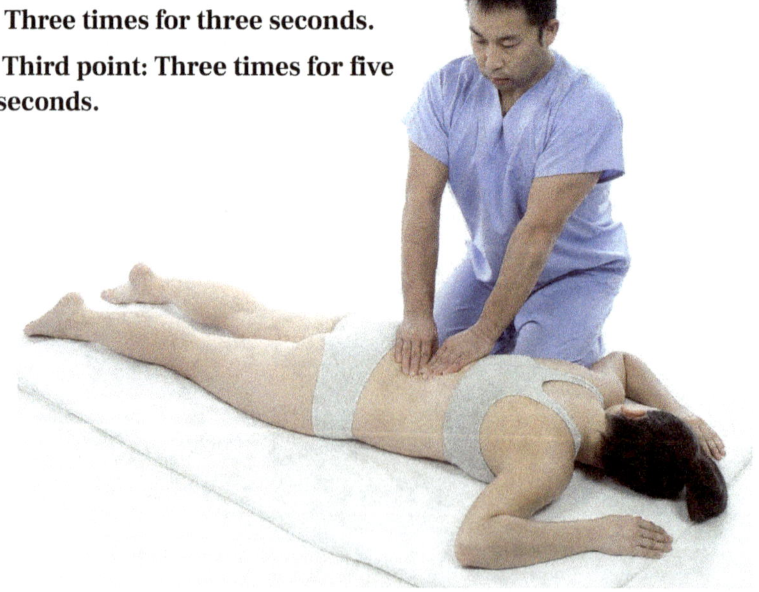

Quadratus lumborum

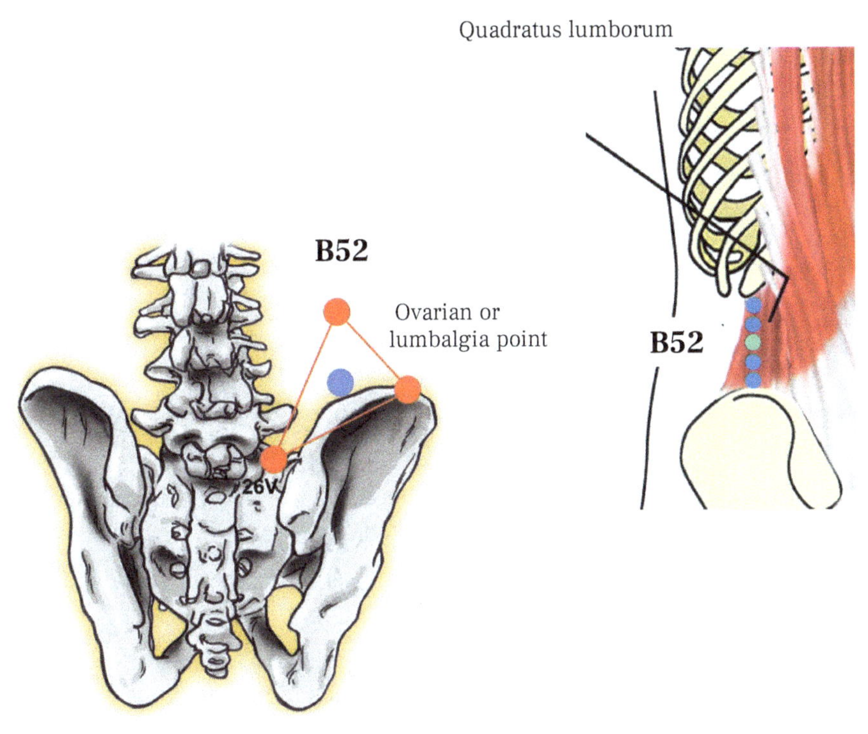

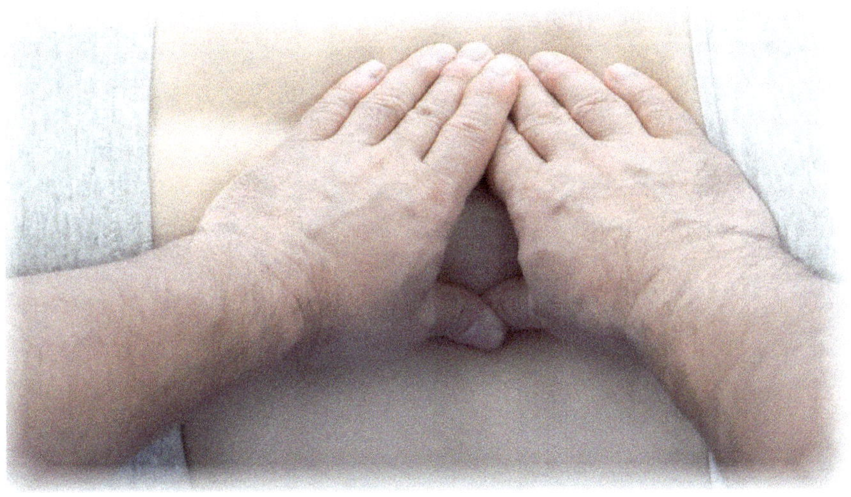

5.4. ILIAC CREST REGION

PATIENT'S POSTURE: Prone. Head turned towards the therapist, shoulders in abduction and elbows bent.

THERAPIST'S POSITION: Basic. Left side of the patient, the right knee at the level of the major trochanter.

TYPE OF PRESSURE: Thumb over thumb (aspa).
        1st and 2nd repetitions: Logo.
        3rd repetition: Thumb over thumb (right below).

Nº. OF POINTS: Three five-point lines:
1st line: Following the edge of the iliac crest.

2nd line: One finger above the previous one, over the quadratus lumborum muscle.

3rd line: Along the bony edge of the iliac crest, in the quadratus lumborum's insertion area and the gluteus medius and maximus.

DIRECTION OF THE LINE: From the sacrum laterally. Repeat alternately in this order: 1st line, 2nd line, and 3rd line.

OBSERVATIONS: The warning point for lumbalgia or the ovaries can be found at the 3rd point of any of the three lines mentioned above. It is used for lumbar and hormonal problems.

On the third line, along the bony edge of the iliac crest, contractures can be found easily if the person has lumbar problems.

Three times for three seconds.

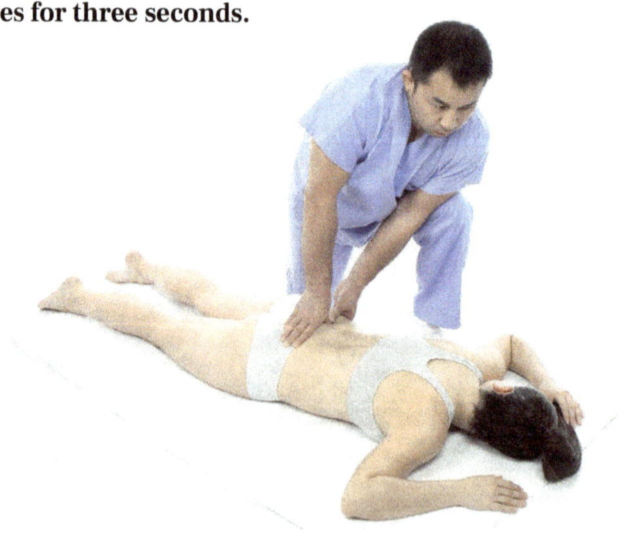

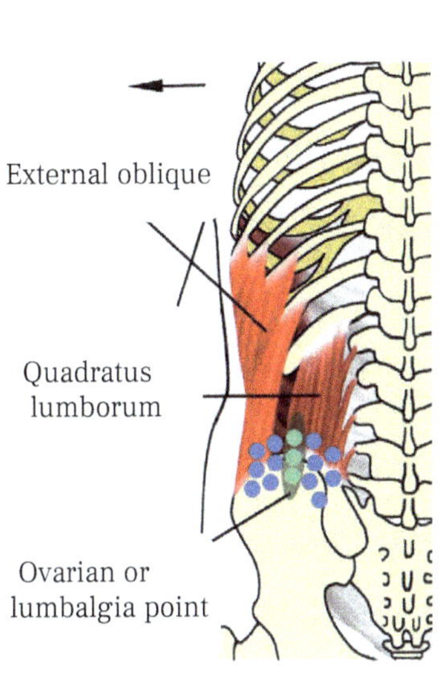

External oblique
Quadratus
lumborum
Ovarian or
lumbalgia point

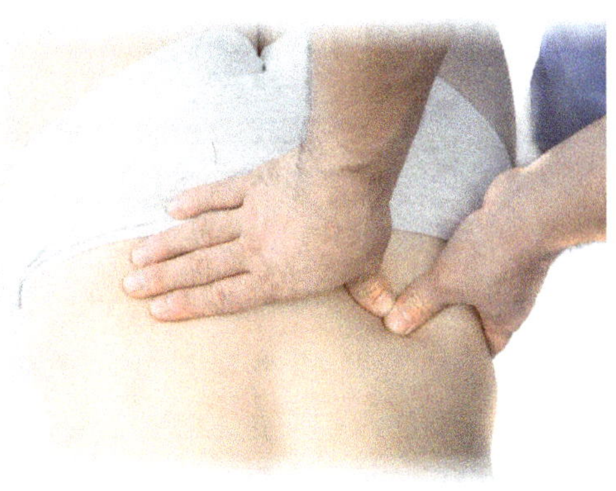

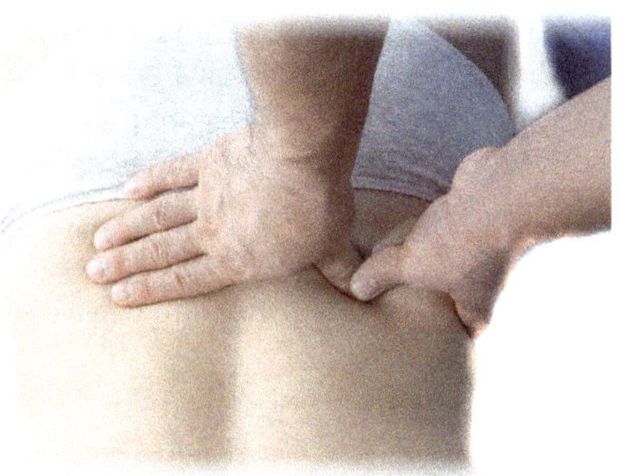

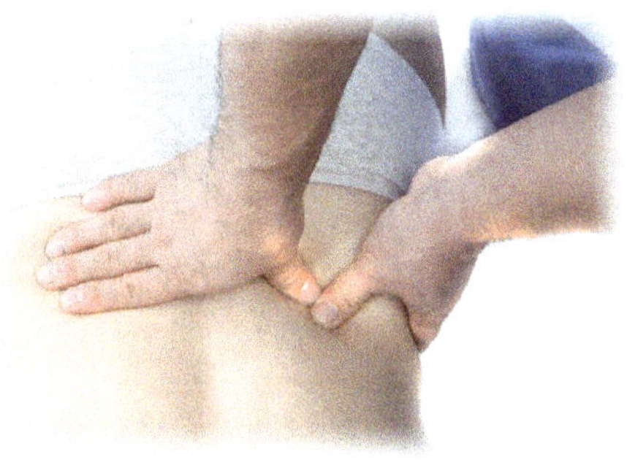

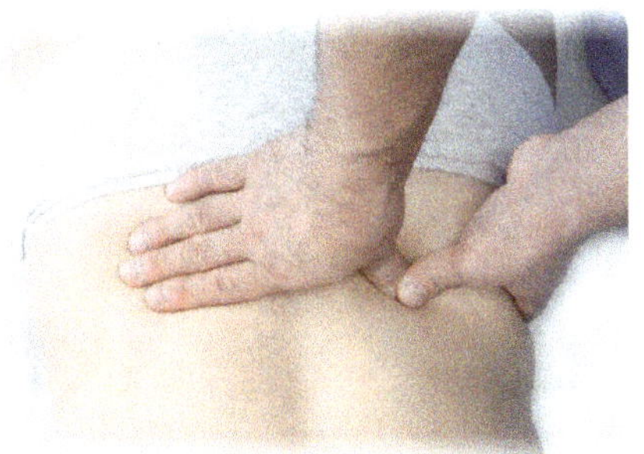

5.5. SACRAL REGION

PATIENT'S POSTURE: Prone. Head turned towards the therapist, shoulders in abduction and elbows bent.

THERAPIST'S POSITION: Basic, maintaining the previous position.

TYPE OF PRESSURE: Both thumbs, with a slightly bent right arm.

Nº. OF POINTS: Two five-point lines.

DIRECTION OF THE LINE: Descending lines (V-shaped), the two lines at once, from the first sacral notch to the fourth.

OBSERVATIONS: Points four and five are very close together, around the fourth sacral foramen. We can find contractures at this level if the patient has sciatica or herniated discs in L5-S1. Western people suffer more in this area due to a more accentuated hyperlordosis which causes the area to touch the surface when in repose, becoming red as circulation is limited.The second point of this region, on the second sacral foramen, corresponds to key point *B32 (Jiryou)*.

The triangle formed by the 2nd and 3rd lumbar which coincides with point *GV4 (Meimon)*, is essential for treating lumbalgia and genital tract disorders.

Three times for three seconds.

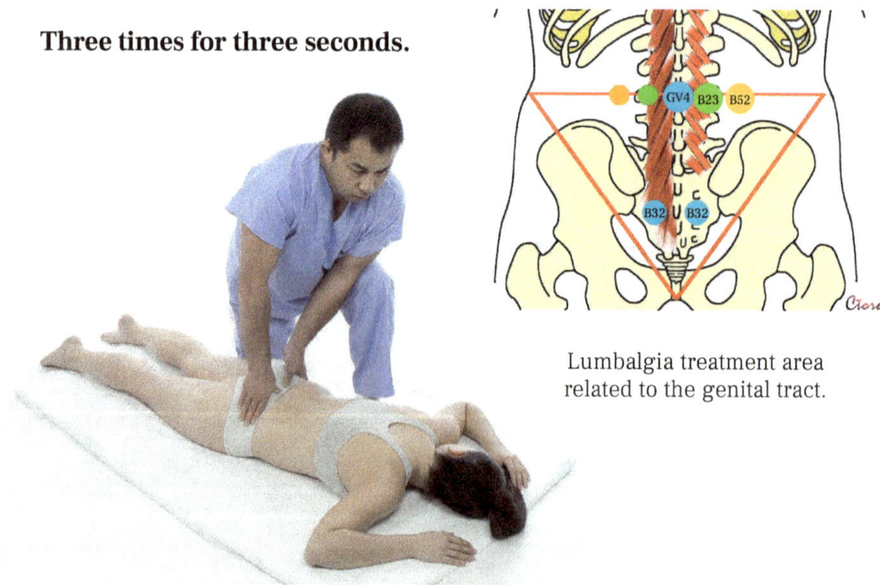

Lumbalgia treatment area
related to the genital tract.

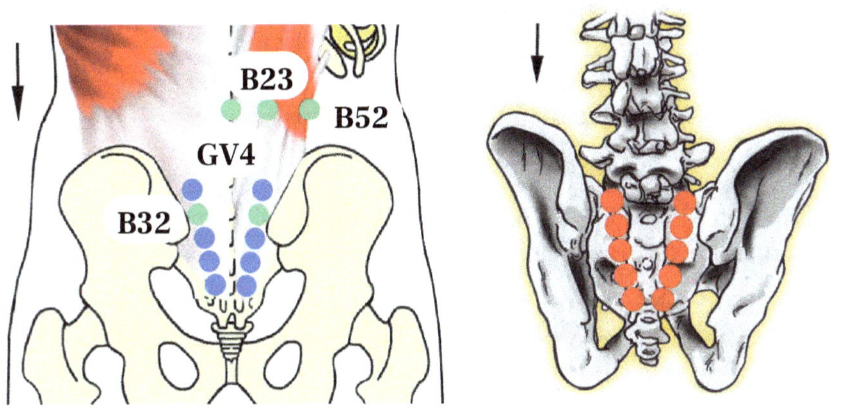

B23
B52
GV4
B32

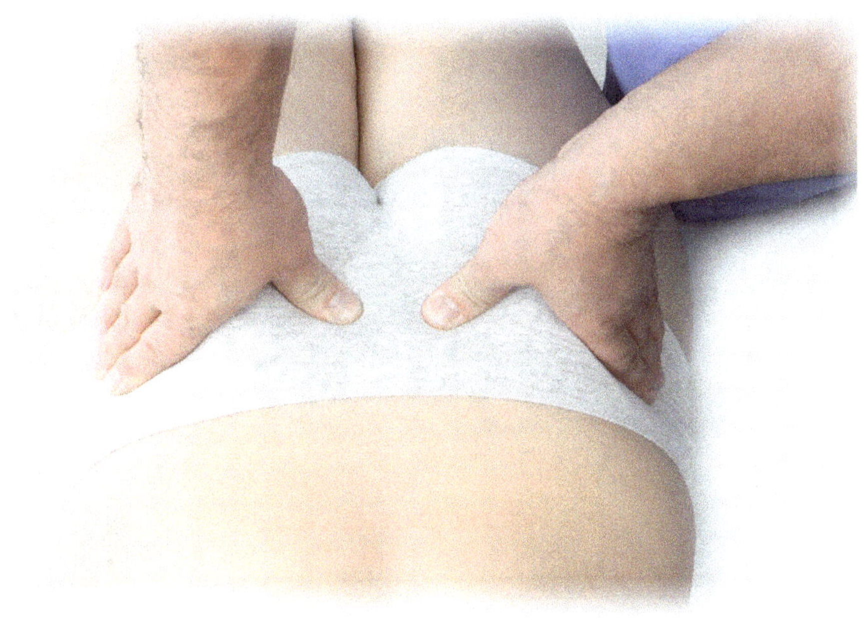

5.6. SACROILIAC JOINT REGION (INTERNAL EDGE)

PATIENT'S POSTURE: Prone. Head turned towards the therapist, shoulders in abduction and elbows bent.

THERAPIST'S POSITION: Basic, maintaining the previous position.

TYPE OF PRESSURE: Thumb over thumb (aspa).

Nº. OF POINTS: A five-point line.

DIRECTION OF THE LINE: Along the internal edge of the sacroiliac joint. From the PSIS (posterior superior iliac spine) to the coccyx.

OBSERVATIONS:The work of the sacroíliac joint is very important because of its relationship to the lower back and the leg muscles and nerves.

This region works on the insertion of the gluteus maximus and posterior sacroíliac ligaments; in addition to the inferior portion of the thorolumbar aponeurosis.

Three times for three seconds.

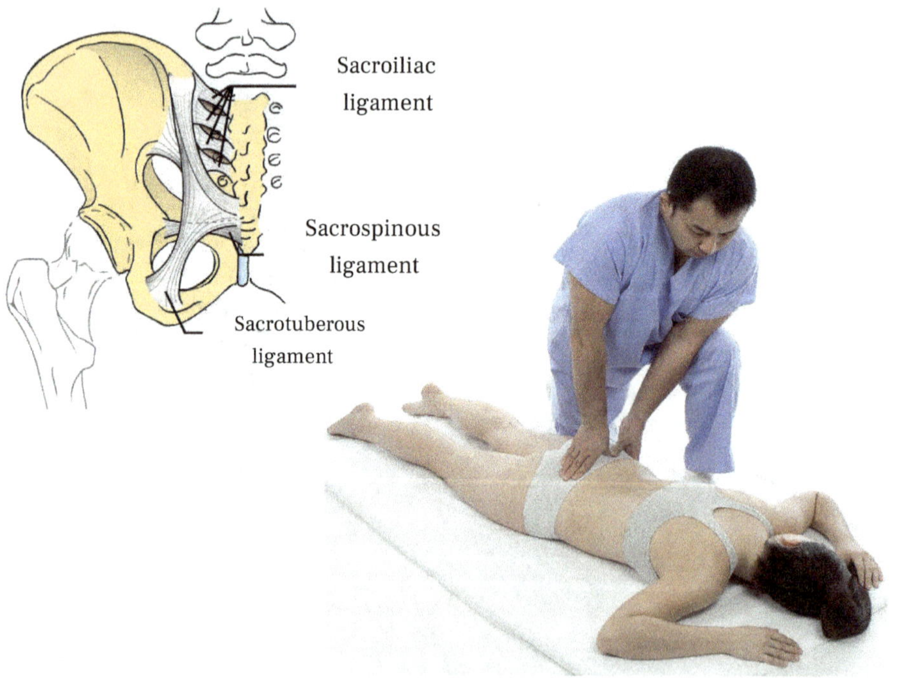

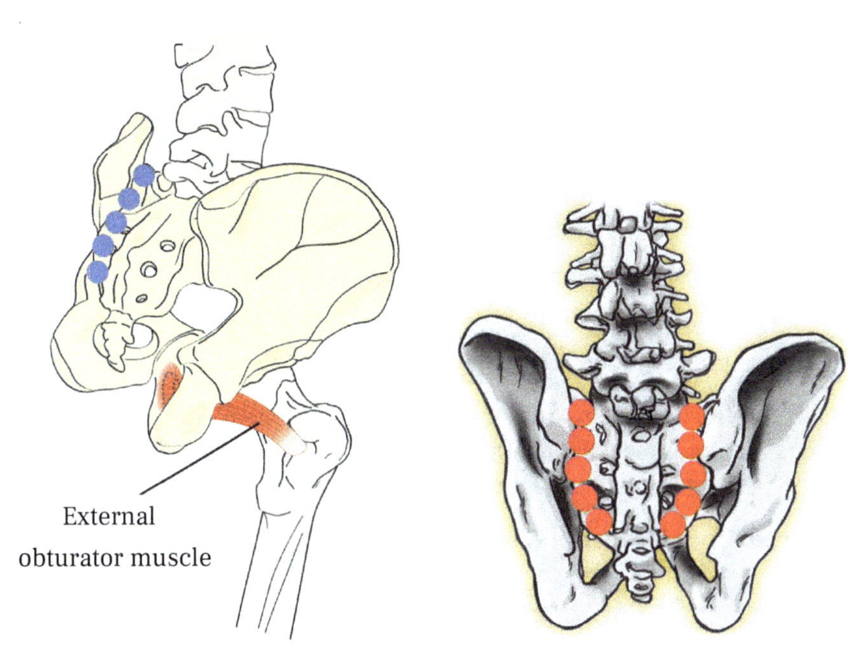

External
obturator muscle

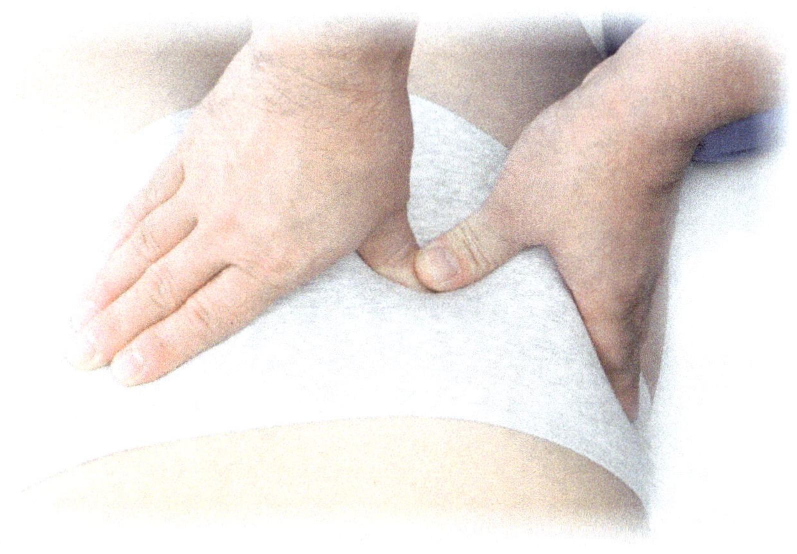

5.7. SACROILIAC JOINT REGION (EXTERNAL EDGE)

PATIENT'S POSTURE: Prone. Head turned towards the therapist, shoulders in abduction and elbows bent.

THERAPIST'S POSITION: Seiza, perpendicular to the patient's body.

TYPE OF PRESSURE: Thumb over thumb (right below).

Nº. OF POINTS: A five-point line.

DIRECTION OF THE LINE: Along the external edge of the sacroiliac joint. From the PSIS (posterior superior iliac spine) to the coccyx.

OBSERVATIONS: This region works on the pyramidal insertions, the gluteus maximus, as well as the sacrotuberous ligament and the inferior portion of thorolumbar aponeurosis.

Three times for three seconds.

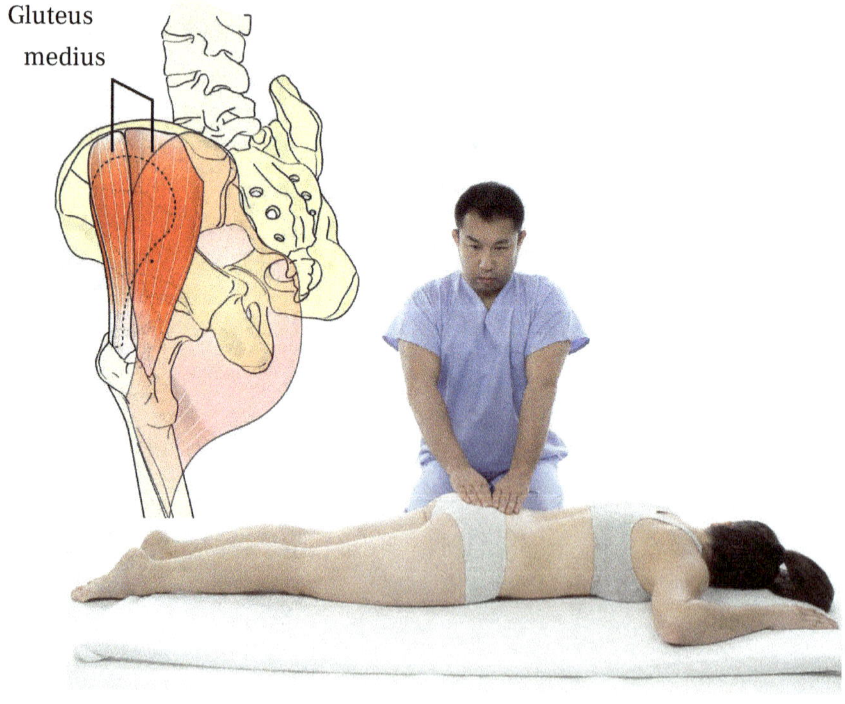

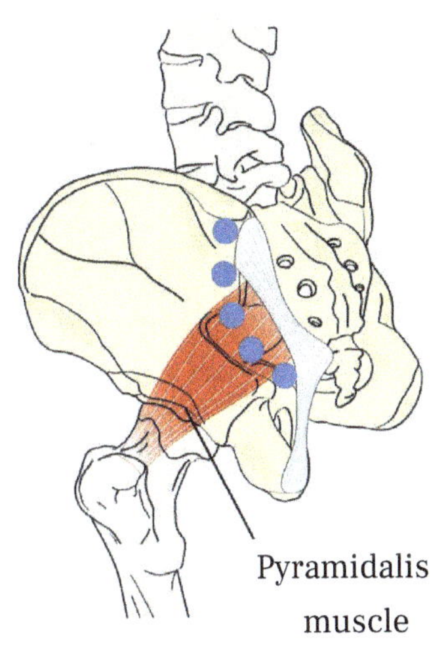

Pyramidalis
muscle

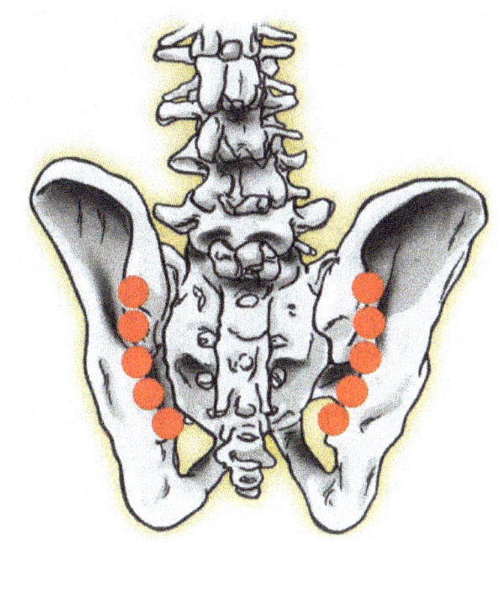

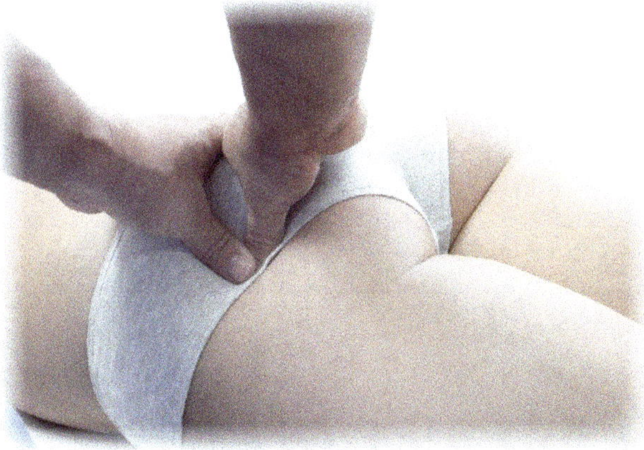

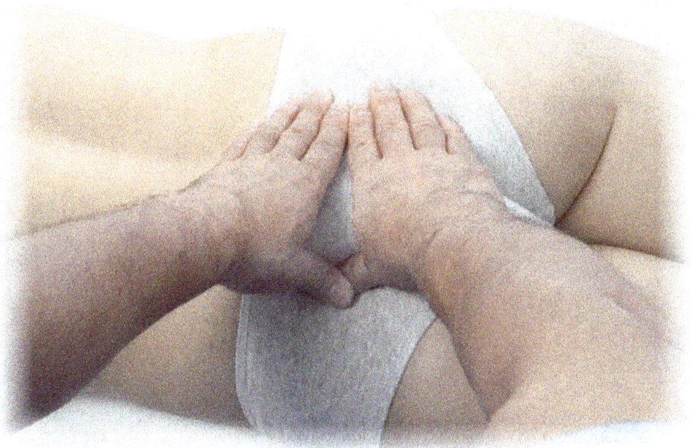

5.8. GLUTEUS MAXIMUS REGION

PATIENT'S POSTURE: Prone. Head turned towards the therapist, shoulders in abduction and elbows bent.

THERAPIST'S POSITION: Seiza, perpendicular to the patient's body.

TYPE OF PRESSURE: Thumb over thumb (right below). Fan-shaped, taking the tip of both middle fingers as an axis of the movement.

Nº. OF POINTS: Five five-point lines.

DIRECTION OF THE LINE: From the iliac crest at the end of the sacrum, and from the sacroiliac joint to the greater trochanter.

OBSERVATIONS: The first line coincides with the previous region.

Three times for three seconds.

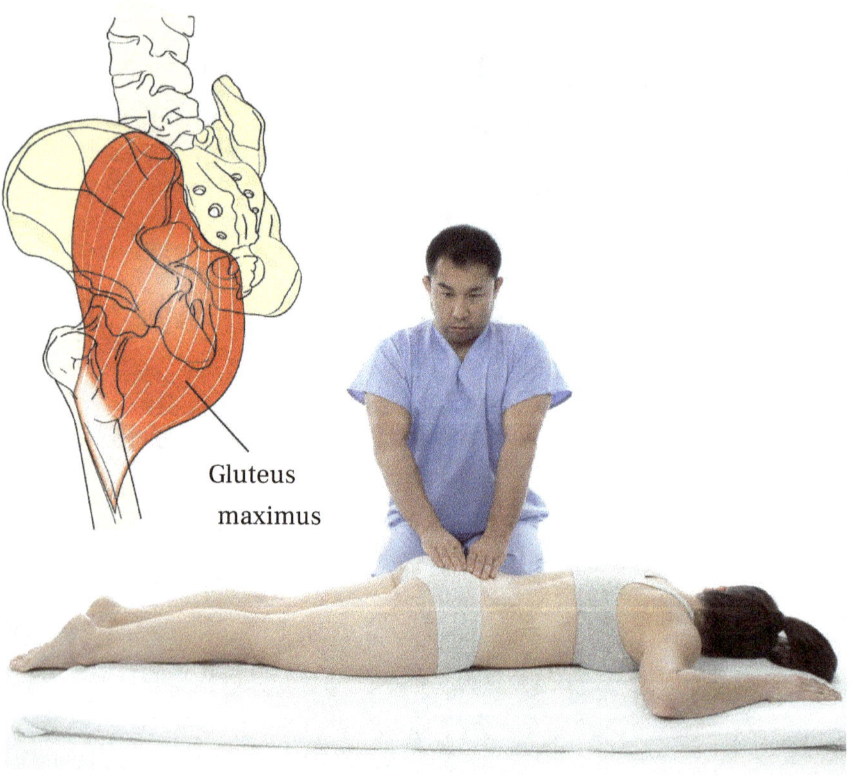

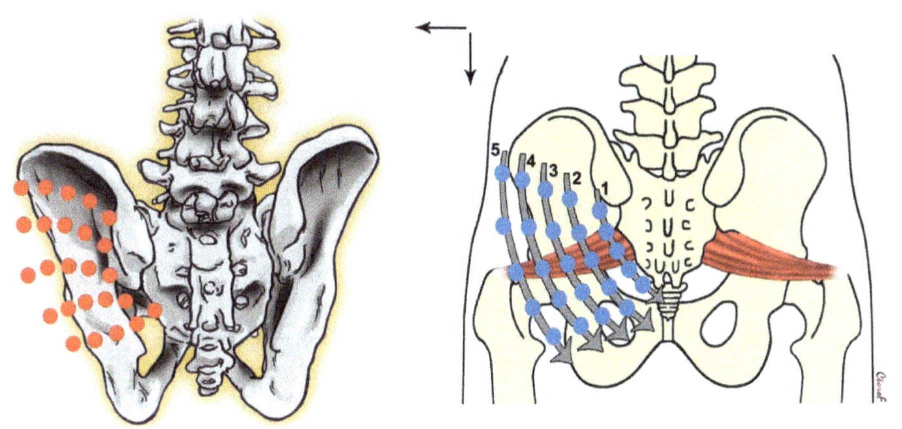

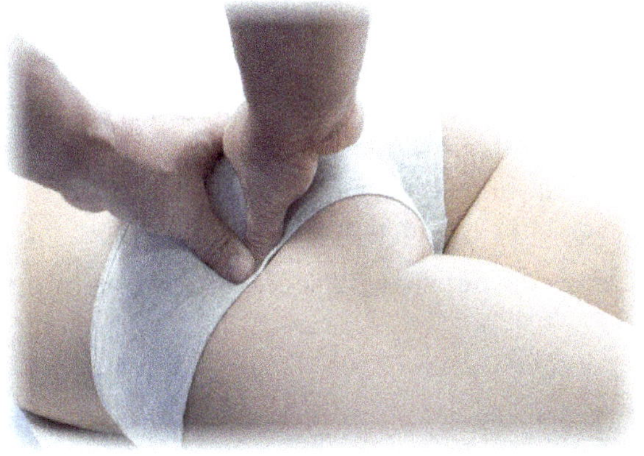

5
4
3
2
1

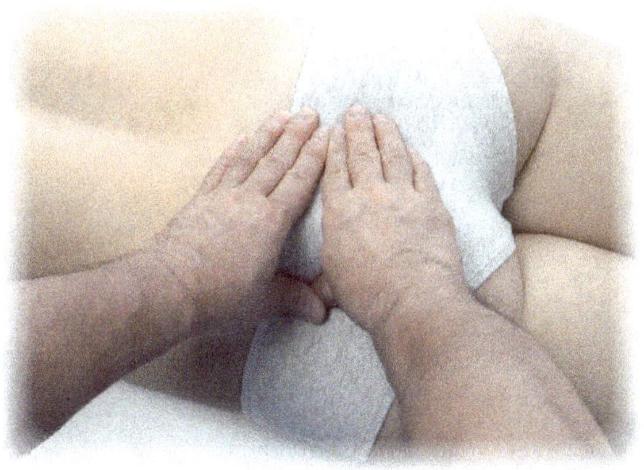

5.9. PIRAMIDAL POINT

PATIENT'S POSTURE: Prone. Head turned towards the therapist, shoulders in abduction and elbows bent.

THERAPIST'S POSITION: Kneeling or seiza, perpendicular to the patient's body.

TYPE OF PRESSURE: Thumb over thumb (right below). Hands supported on the sacrum to focus the pressure which should be light and maintained for between 30 seconds and one minute. If the area is very sensitive, apply pressure with thumbs in V.

Nº. OF POINTS: One point.

DIRECTION OF THE LINE: This point is located approximately halfway between the pyramidal or pyriform muscle (the origin is on the sacrum's anterior surface and the insertion in the greater trochanter).

OBSERVATIONS: Located below the pyramidal muscle, we can look for point *GB30 (Kanchou)* that is located between the greater trochanter of the femur and the sacral hiatus in the third closest to the greater trochanter. This point is used for numerous ailments: diarrhea, indigestion, constipation, lumbalgia, erectile dysfunction and infertility.

Apply pressure for between 30 seconds and one minute.

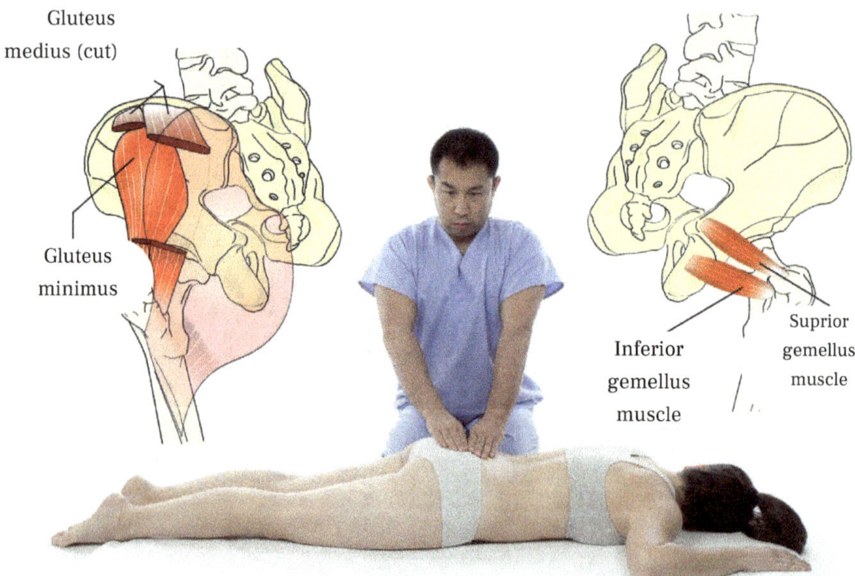

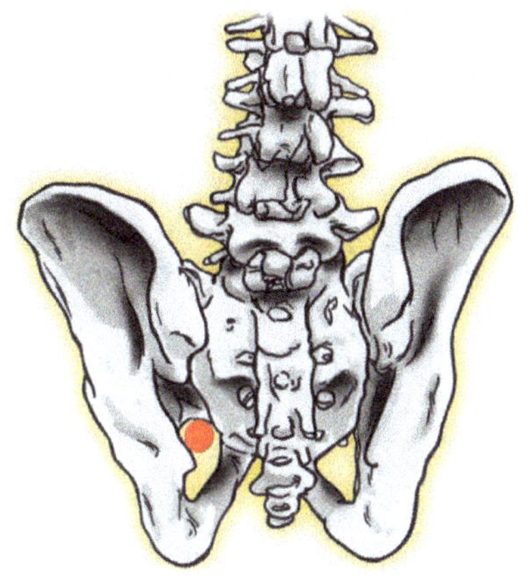

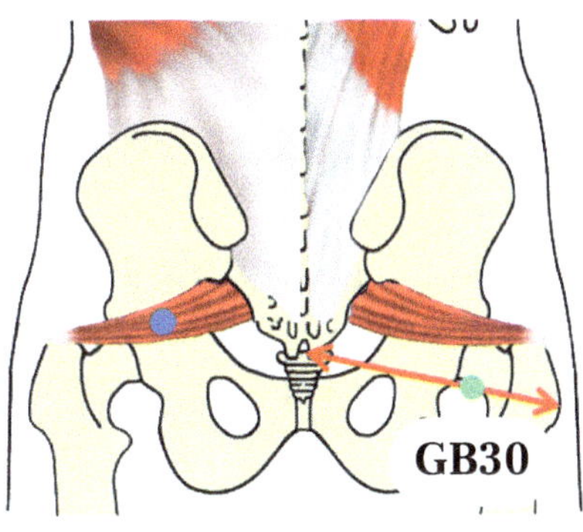

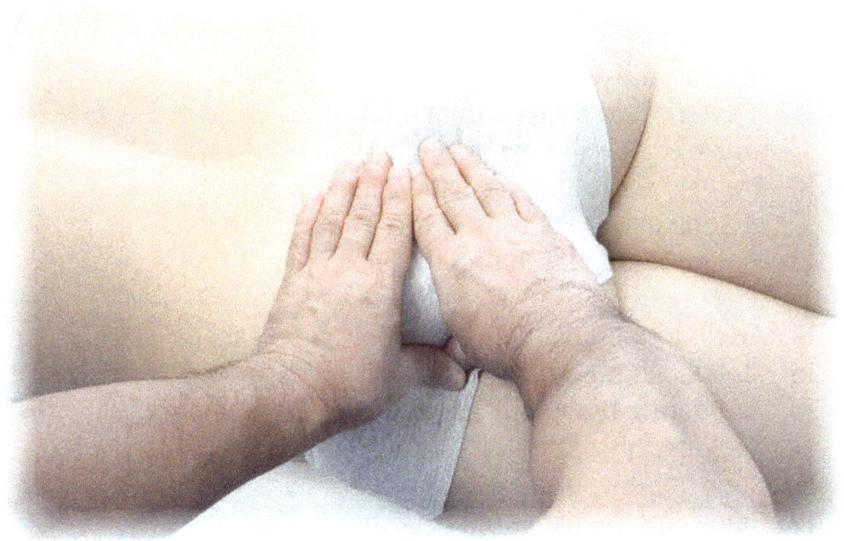

Repeat the Back (II)
routine on the RIGHT SIDE.

6. Lower limbs

Leg

6.1. Posterior femoral region. Central, internal and external line.
6.2. Popliteal fossa region.
6.3. Posterior sural region.
6.4. Lateral and medial sural region
6.5. B60-K3 region. Both sides.
6.6. Lateral and medial calcaneal region. Both sides.
6.7. Calcaneal tubercule region.

Plantar aspect and stretches

6.8. Plantar region. Centre line.
6.9. Plantar region. External arch line.
6.10. Plantar region. Internal arch line.
6.11. Plantar region. Line of the inferior area of the first metatarsal.
6.12. Plantar region. Line of the metatarsophalangeal joint spaces.
6.13. Extending and rotating the toes (circumduction).
6.14. Ankle rotation.
6.15. Metatarsal region.
6.16. Elongating the Achilles tendon.
6.17. Rocking the ankle.
6.18. Relaxing the sural triceps.
6.19. Releasing the leg joints.

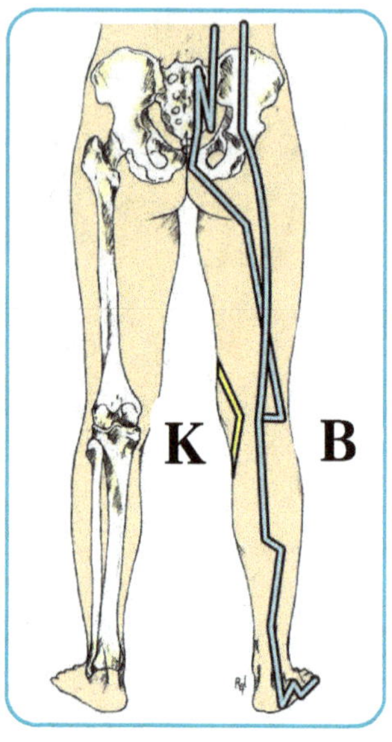

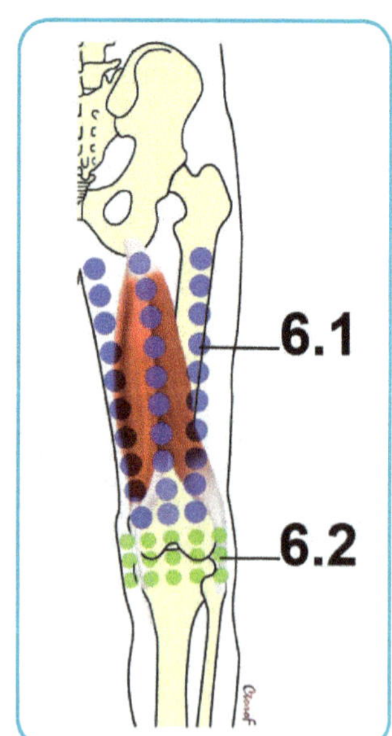

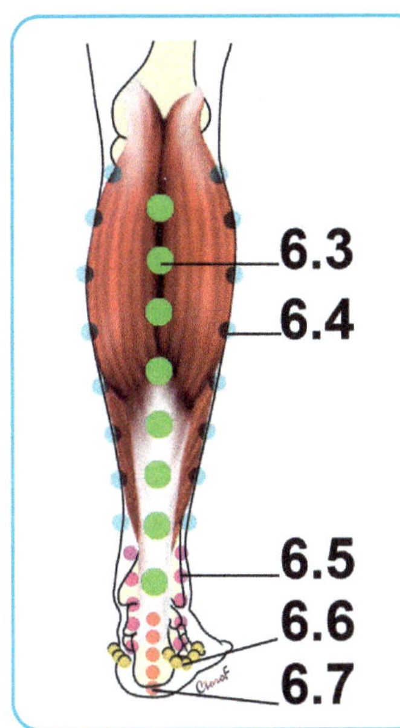

6.3
6.4
6.5
6.6
6.7

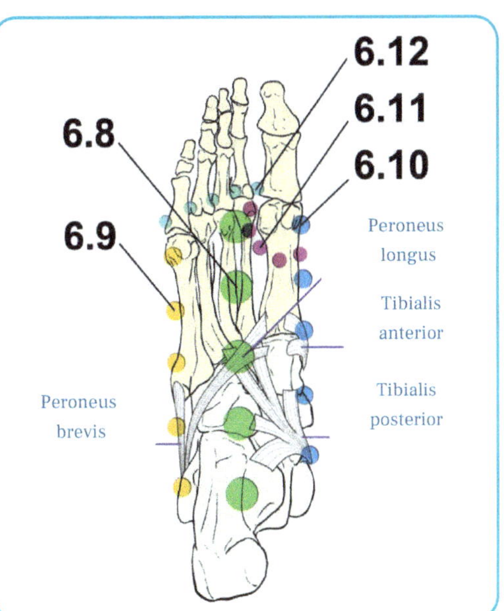

6.12
6.11
6.10
6.8
6.9
Peroneus
longus
Tibialis
anterior
Tibialis
posterior
Peroneus
brevis

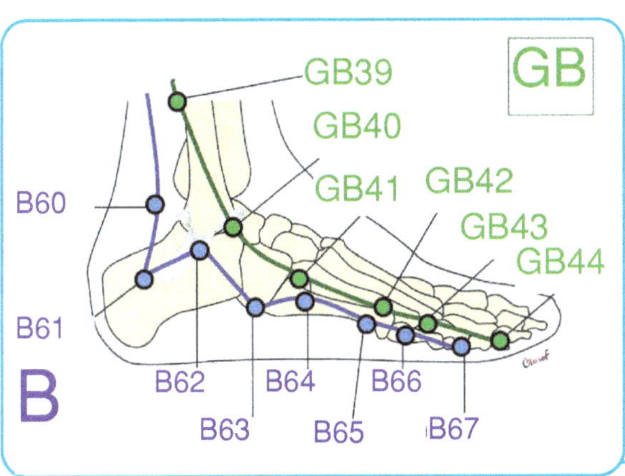

GB
GB39
GB40
GB41
GB42
GB43
GB44
B60
B61
B62
B63
B64
B65
B66
B67
B

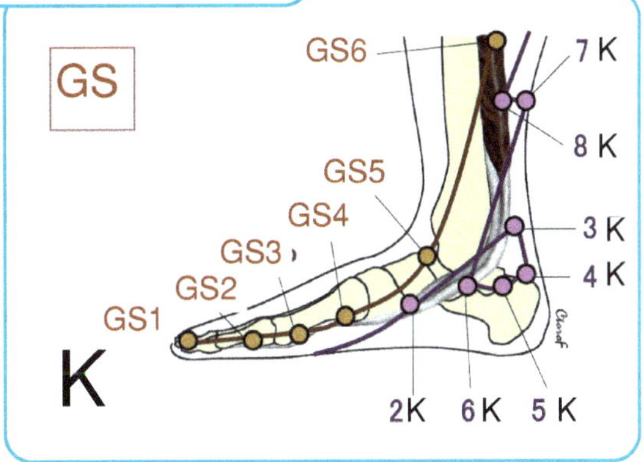

GS
GS6
GS5
GS4
GS3
GS2
GS1
7 K
8 K
3 K
4 K
2 K 6 K 5 K
K

6.1. POSTERIOR FEMORAL REGION.
CENTRAL, INTERNAL AND EXTERNAL LINES

PATIENT'S POSTURE: Prone. Head turned towards the therapist, shoulders in abduction and elbows bent.

THERAPIST'S POSITION: Basic.

TYPE OF PRESSURE: 1st and 2nd repetitions: Logo.
                           3rd repetition: Thumb over thumb (not aspa).

Nº. OF POINTS: Three ten-points lines.
Central line: From the ischial tuberosity to the centre of the popliteal fossa.

Medial line: Two fingers medially from the previous line towards the extreme medial of the popliteal fossa.

Lateral line: From the lesser trochanter to the extreme lateral of the popliteal fossa.

DIRECTION OF THE LINE: From the gluteal fold to the popliteal fossa. Repeat alternately in this order: central line, medial line, lateral line.

OBSERVATIONS:The first point of the first line corresponds to **key point** *B36 (Shoufu)*; useful when the sciatic nerve is affected. The fifth point of the same line corresponds to key point *B37 (Inmon)*; this area is reflective of the suprascapular region.

Maintain proper perpendicular pressure when working the second and third lines.

Three times for three seconds.
First point of 1st Line,
3 x 5 seconds the first time.

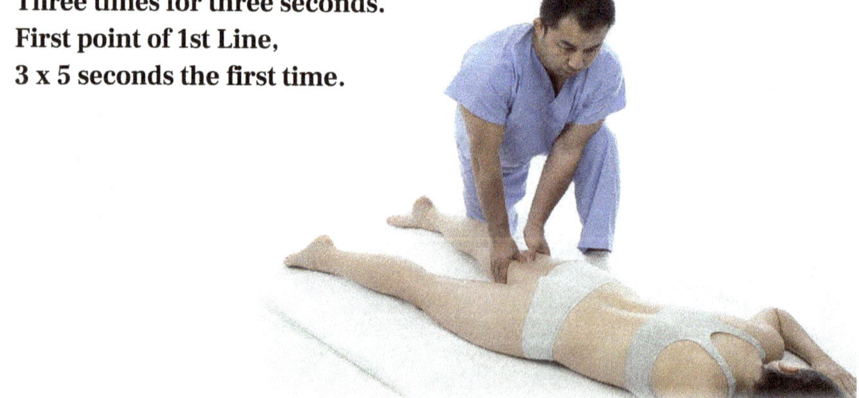

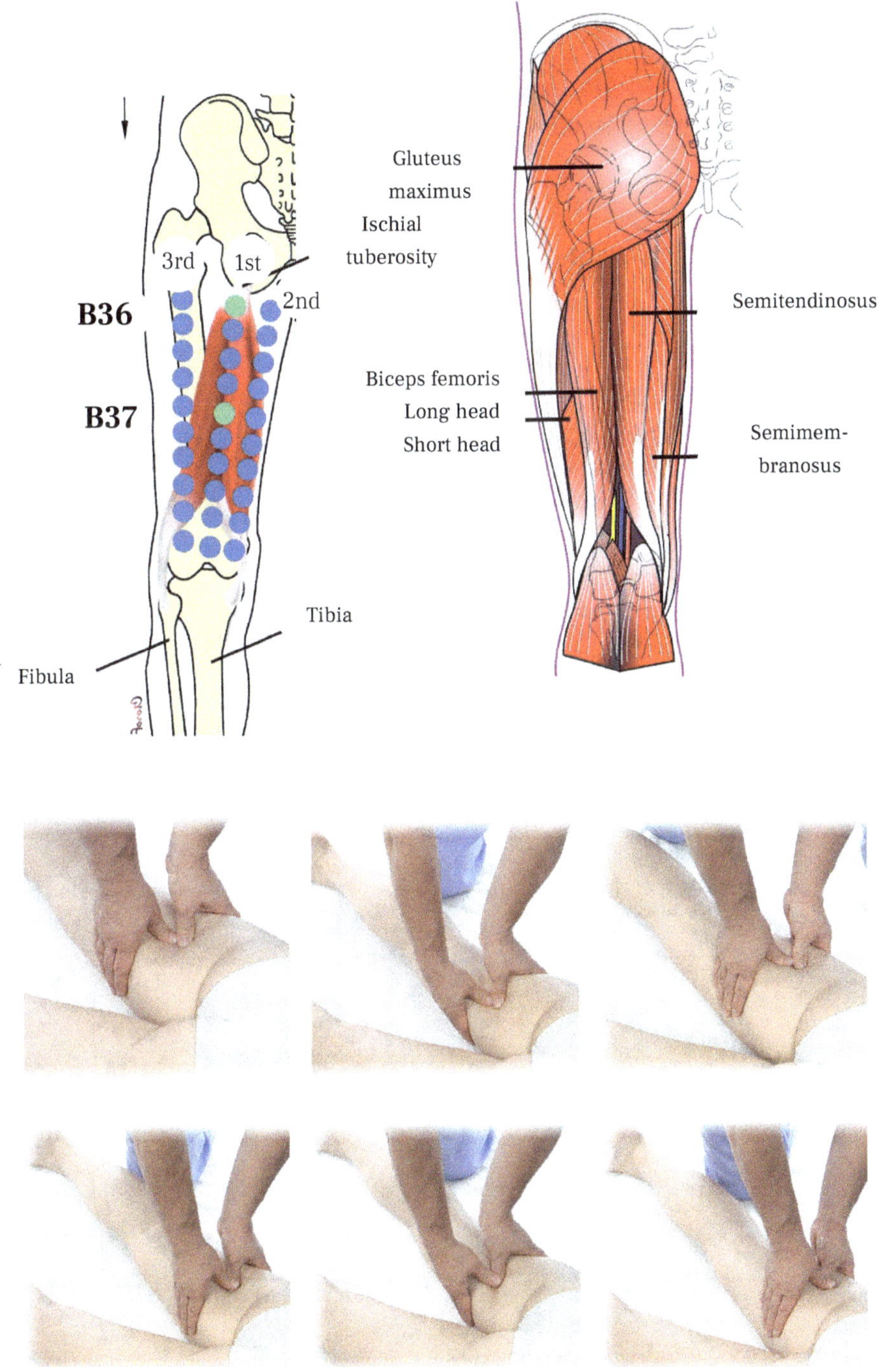

3rd
1st
2nd
B36
B37
Fibula
Tibia
Gluteus
maximus
Ischial
tuberosity
Biceps femoris
Long head
Short head
Semitendinosus
Semimem-
branosus

6.2. POPLITEAL FOSSA REGION

PATIENT'S POSTURE: Prone. Head turned towards the therapist, shoulders in abduction and elbows bent.

THERAPIST'S POSITION: Basic, on the left side of the patient. Right knee at ankle level.

TYPE OF PRESSURE: Thumbs in A shape.

N°. OF POINTS: Three five-point lines.

1st line: On the crease of the knee.

2nd line: One finger above the first line. 3rd line: One finger below the first line.

DIRECTION OF THE LINE: From lateral to medial, between the tendons of the hamstring muscles. Repeat alternately in this order: 1st line, 2nd line, and 3rd line.

OBSERVATIONS:Several important key points are located in this region. On the first line are located the *B39 (Iyou, first point), the B40 (Ichuu, third point)* and the *K10 (Inkoku, fifth point)*. On the third line, just below the *K10 (fifth point)*, there is one of the supplementary points of the Five Warning Points.

Three times for three seconds.

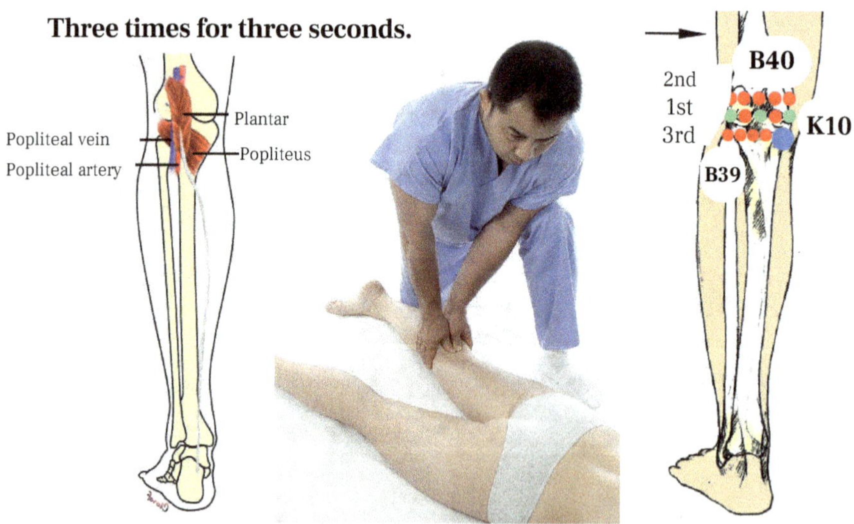

6.3. POSTERIOR SURAL REGION

PATIENT'S POSTURE: Prone. Head turned towards the therapist, shoulders in abduction and elbows bent.

THERAPIST'S POSITION: Basic, on the patient left side. Right knee at the level of the patient's toe.

TYPE OF PRESSURE: Thumbs in A shape. The rest of the hand surrounds the leg.

Nº. OF POINTS: An eight-point line.

DIRECTION OF THE LINE: It starts below the popliteal fossa and ends on the Achilles tendon (above the calcaneal bone).

OBSERVATIONS:If the patient's foot is not facing inwards, the position must be corrected, so as to maintain perpendicular pressure.

This region is reflective of the heart muscle and therefore the state of cardiac function. Key points *B56 (Syoukin, second point)* and *B57 (Syouzan, fourth point)* are located in this region.

Three times for three seconds.

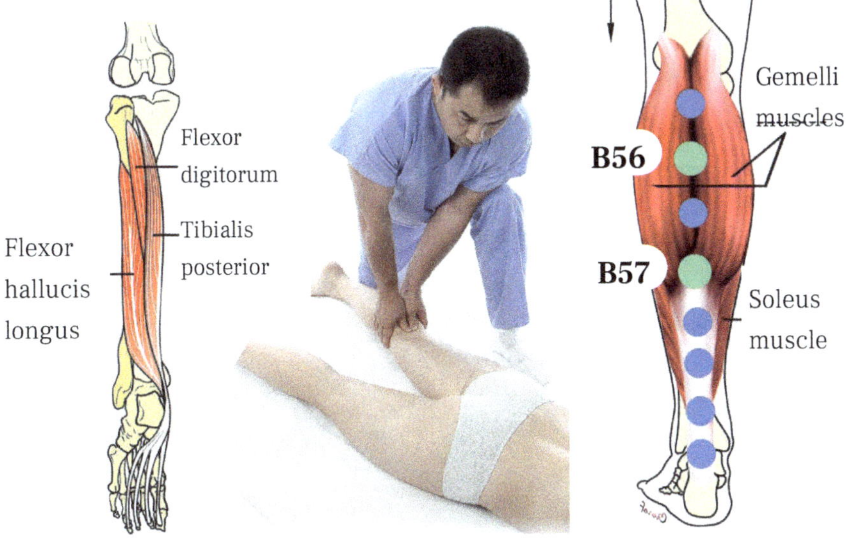

6.4. LATERAL AND MEDIAL SURAL REGION

PATIENT'S POSTURE: Prone. Head turned towards the therapist, shoulders in abduction and elbows bent.

THERAPIST'S POSITION: Seiza facing the area.

TYPE OF PRESSURE: In pincer, with V-shaped thumbs.

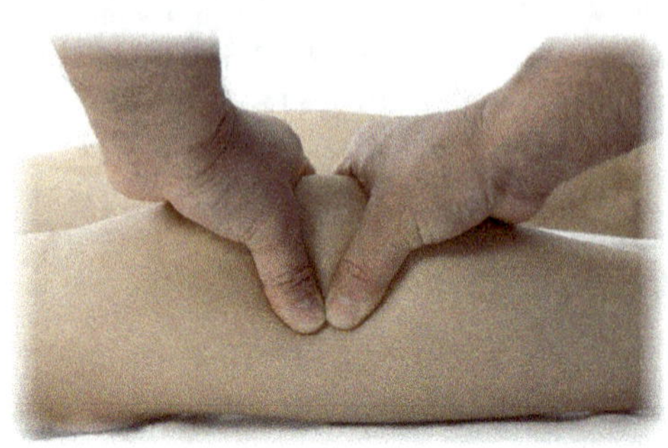

Nº. OF POINTS: Two eight-point lines.

DIRECTION OF THE LINE: Below the knee and towards the calcaneal bone. The lateral line runs along the belly of the muscle following the posterior edge of the fibula. The medial line runs along the belly of the muscle following the medial edge of the tibia. The first four pressures are applied on the muscle belly and the remaining four on the tendon area.

OBSERVATIONS: As in the previous case, this area is reflective of the state of the heart muscle.

Three times for three seconds.

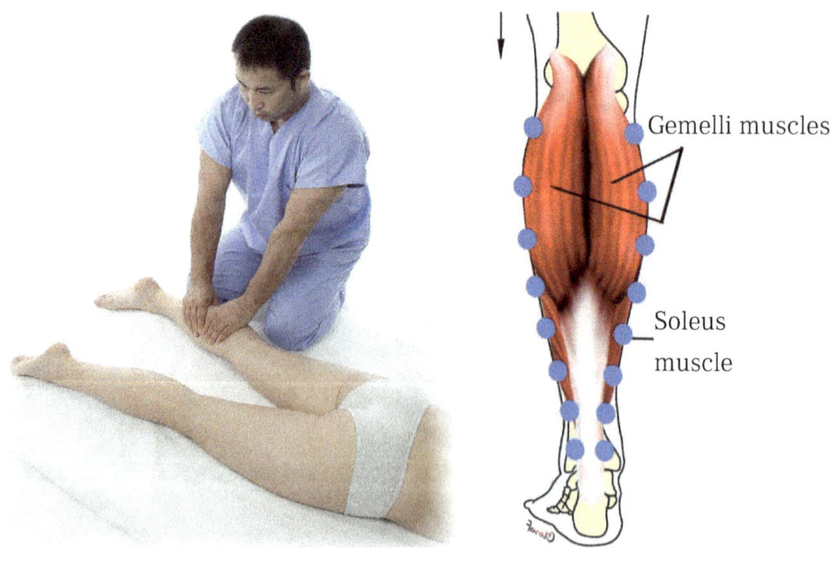

6.5. B60-K3 REGION. BOTH SIDES

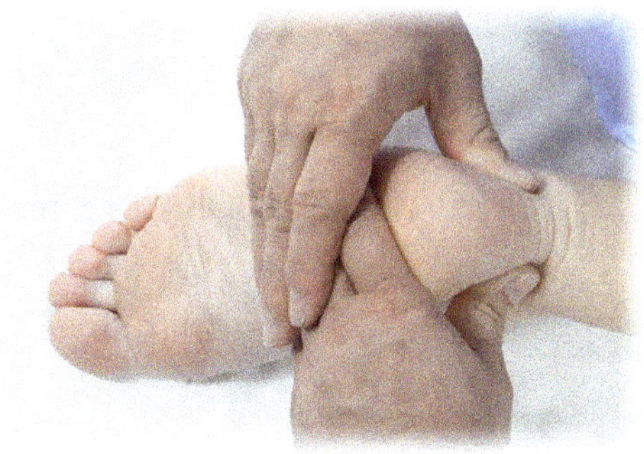

PATIENT'S POSTURE: Prone. Head turned towards the therapist, shoulders in abduction and elbows bent.

THERAPIST'S POSITION: Seiza, facing the patient's heels. Straight back with slightly bent arms. Hands are around the sole of the foot.

TYPE OF PRESSURE: Both thumbs. Pressure is applied to both sides at the same time, countering the direction of both thumbs.

Nº. OF POINTS: Two five-point lines.

DIRECTION OF THE LINE: Towards the sole of the foot, along the internal edge of the calcaneal tendon. The third point on each side coincides with *K3 (Taikei, internal)* and *B60 (Konron, external)*. The first and last points respectively are three fingers above and below the previous ones.

Three times for three seconds.

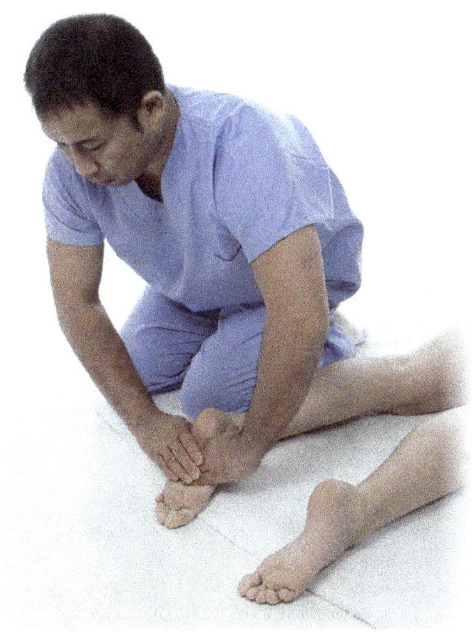

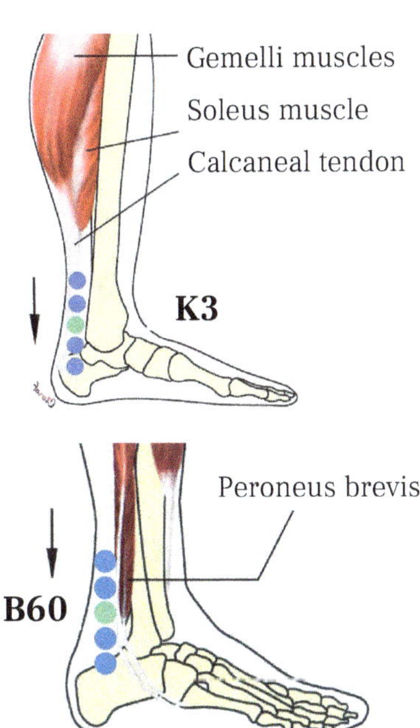

6.6. LATERAL AND MEDIAL CALCANEAL REGION. BOTH SIDES

PATIENT'S POSTURE: Prone. Head turned towards the therapist, shoulders in abduction and elbows bent.

THERAPIST'S POSITION: Seiza, maintaining the previous position.

TYPE OF PRESSURE: Both thumbs. Pressure is applied to both sides at the same time, countering the direction of both thumbs.

Nº. OF POINTS: Two five-point lines.

DIRECTION OF THE LINE: From the calcaneal tendon to the arch, bordering both maleolos. The first point on each side matches the *K3* (*Taikei*, internal) and *B60* (*Konron*, external).

OBSERVATIONS: Several key points are located in this region. On the side are *B60 (Konron, first point)*, *B62 (Shinmyaku, third point)* and *GB40 (Kyuukyo, fourth point)*. To locate the medial part's key points see 1.10. MEDIAL CALCANEAL REGION in supine decubitus.

Three times for three seconds.

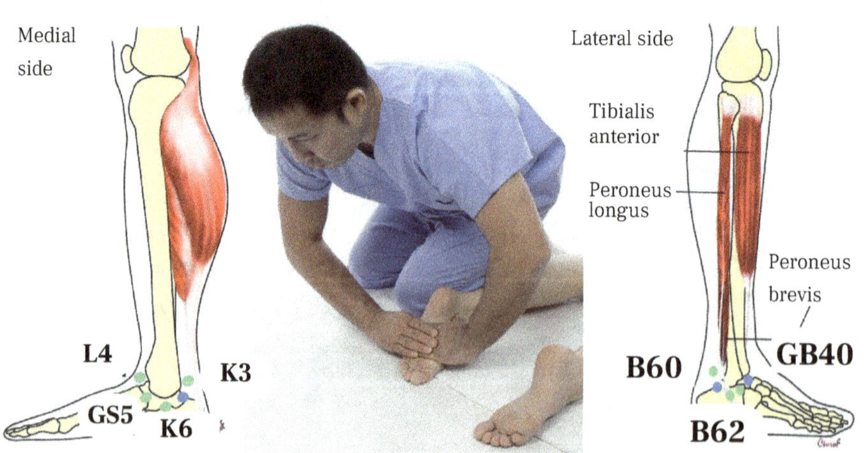

6.7. CALCANEAL TUBERCLE REGION

PATIENT'S POSTURE: Prone. Head turned towards the therapist, shoulders in abduction and elbows bent.

THERAPIST'S POSITION: Seiza, holding the leg with both hands below the ankle.

TYPE OF PRESSURE: Thumbs in an A shape; pressure will be accompanied by a dorsiflexion of the foot.

Nº. OF POINTS: One five-point line.

DIRECTION OF THE LINE: From the heel to the maleolos.

Three times for three seconds.

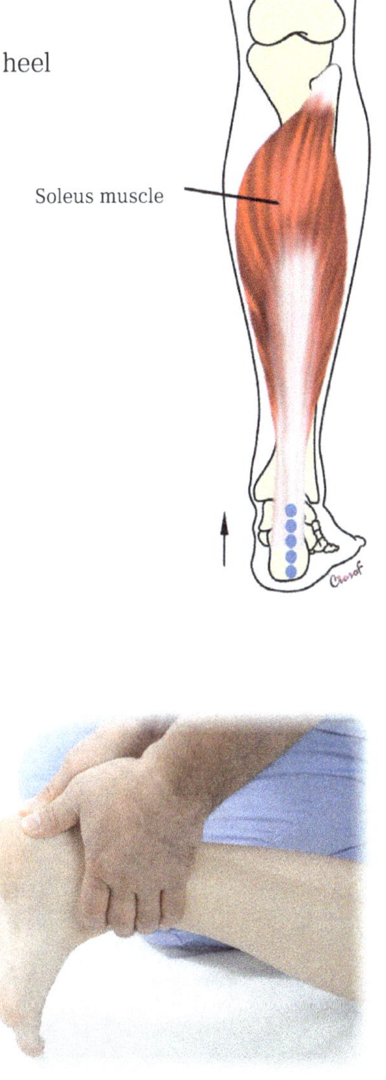

119

6.8. PLANTAR REGION. CENTRAL LINE

PATIENT'S POSTURE: Prone. Head turned towards the therapist, shoulders in abduction and elbows bent.

THERAPIST'S POSITION: Seiza, perpendicular to the area, placing the patient's left foot on the therapist's right thigh.

TYPE OF PRESSURE: Holding the ankle with the left hand and applying pressure with the right thumb.

Nº. OF POINTS: One five-point line.

DIRECTION OF THE LINE: From the heel to the toes.

OBSERVATIONS:On the central plantar line we can focus on point *K1* (*Yuusen,* fourth point), used to treat urine retention, headaches and vertigo.

Three times for three

seconds.

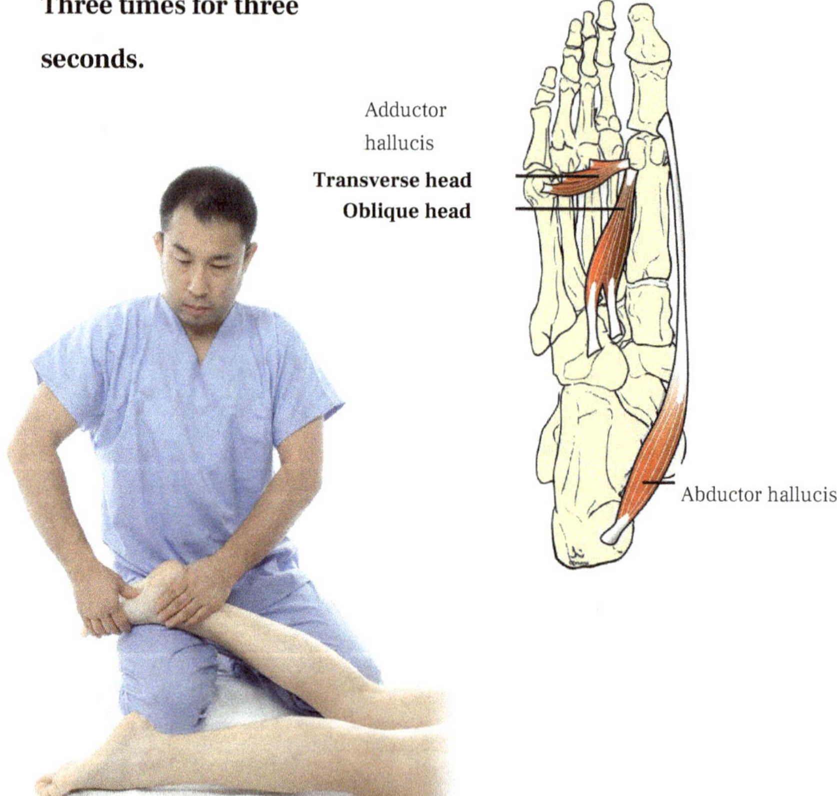

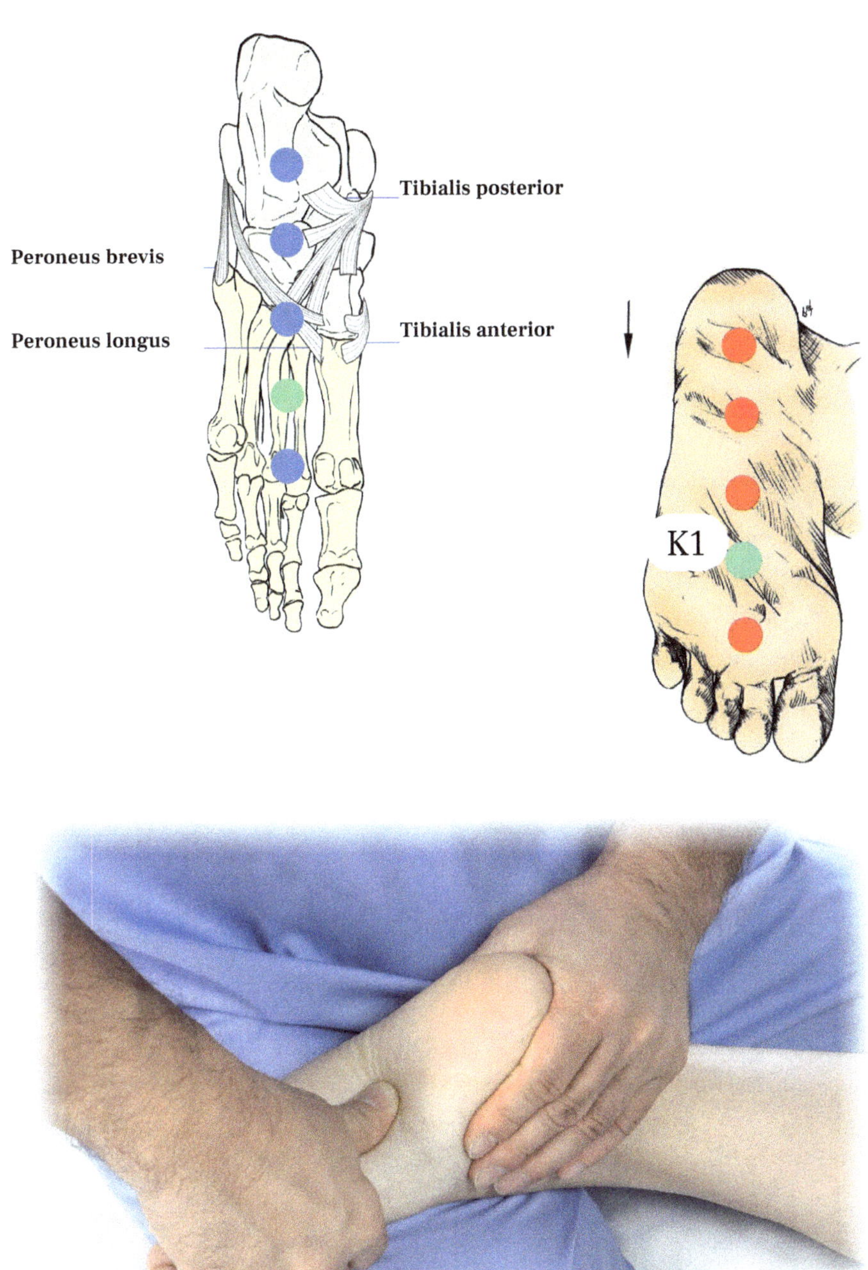

Tibialis posterior
Peroneus brevis
Peroneus longus
Tibialis anterior
K1

6.9. PLANTAR REGION. EXTERNAL ARCH LINE

PATIENT'S POSTURE: Prone. Head turned towards the therapist, shoulders in abduction and elbows bent.

THERAPIST'S POSITION: Seiza, perpendicular to the area, placing the patient's left foot on the therapist's right thigh.

TYPE OF PRESSURE: Holding the ankle with the left hand and applying pressure with the right thumb.

Nº. OF POINTS: One five-point line.

DIRECTION OF THE LINE: From the heel to the toes, along the lateral edge of the sole of the foot.

OBSERVATIONS: On the lateral plantar edge are two key points *B63 (Kinmon,* third point) and *B66 (Ashitsuukoku,* fifth point).

Point *B63* is used for treating lumbalgia, while point *B66* helps in psychic and psychosomatic disorders.

Three times for three seconds.

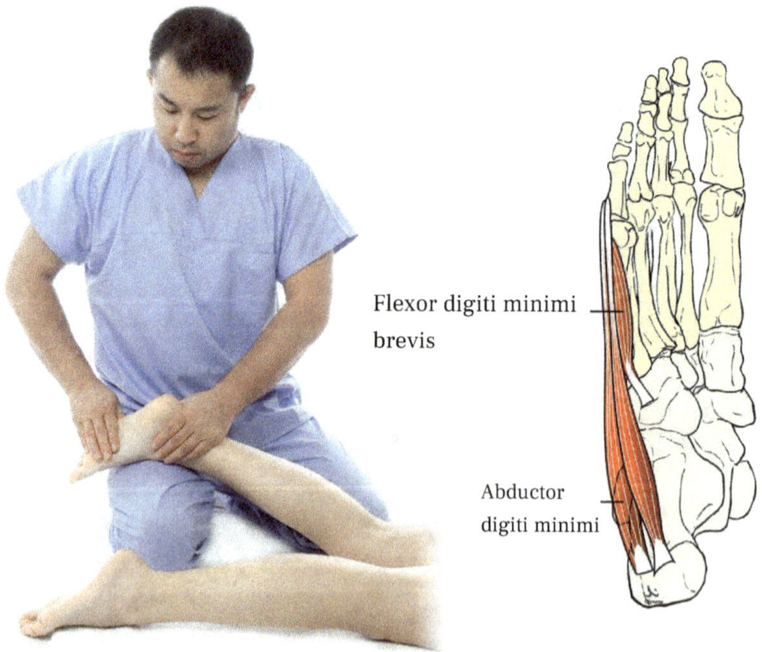

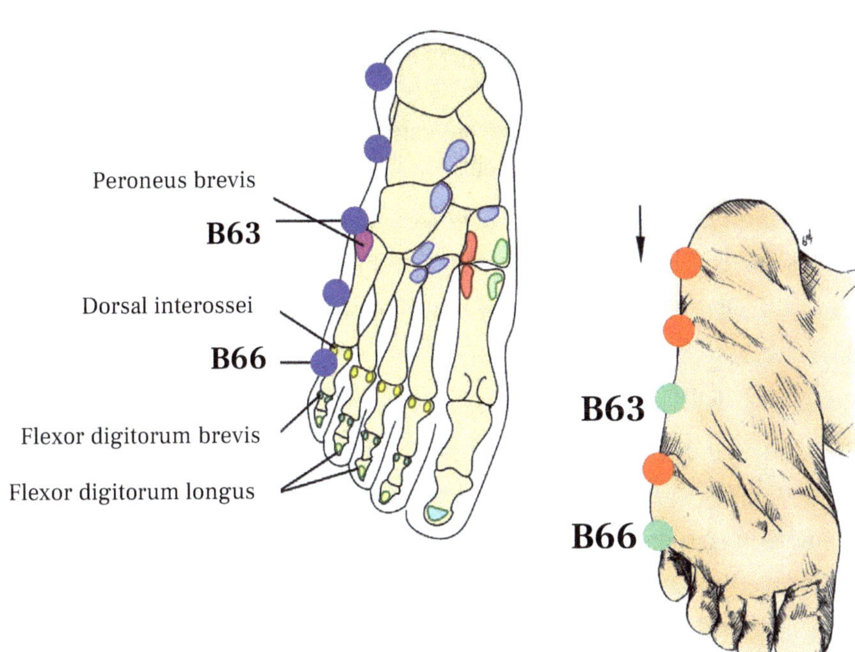

Peroneus brevis
B63
Dorsal interossei
B66
Flexor digitorum brevis
Flexor digitorum longus
B63
B66

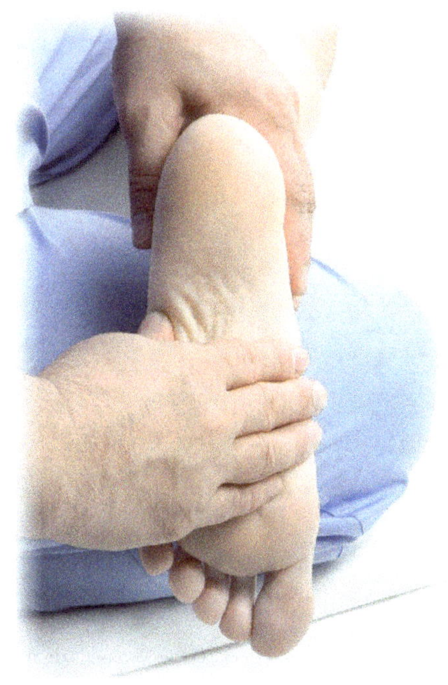

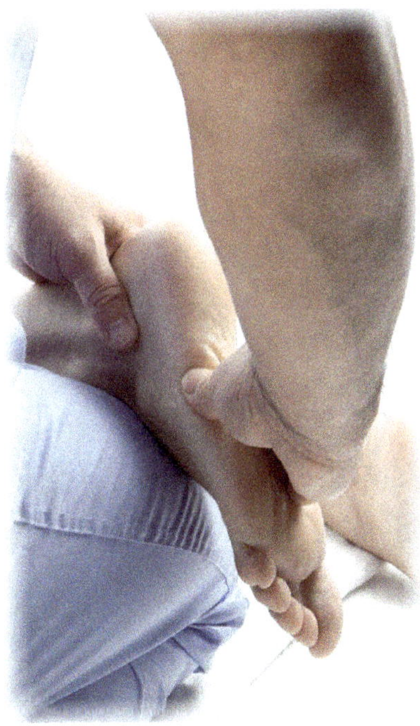

6.10. PLANTAR REGION. INTERNAL ARCH LINE

PATIENT'S POSTURE: Prone. Head turned towards the therapist, shoulders in abduction and elbows bent.

THERAPIST'S POSITION: Seiza, perpendicular to the area, placing the patient's left foot on the therapist's right thigh.

TYPE OF PRESSURE: Holding the ankle with the left hand and applying pressure with the right thumb.

Nº. OF POINTS: One five-point line.

DIRECTION OF THE LINE: From the heel to the toes, along the medial edge of the sole of the foot.

OBSERVATIONS: The third *point K2 (Nenkoku)*, is for treating gynaecological disorders.

The fourth and fifth point, *GB4 (Kouson)* and *GB2 (Daito)*, improve digestive disorders, strengthen the spleen and harmonize the stomach.

Three times for three seconds.

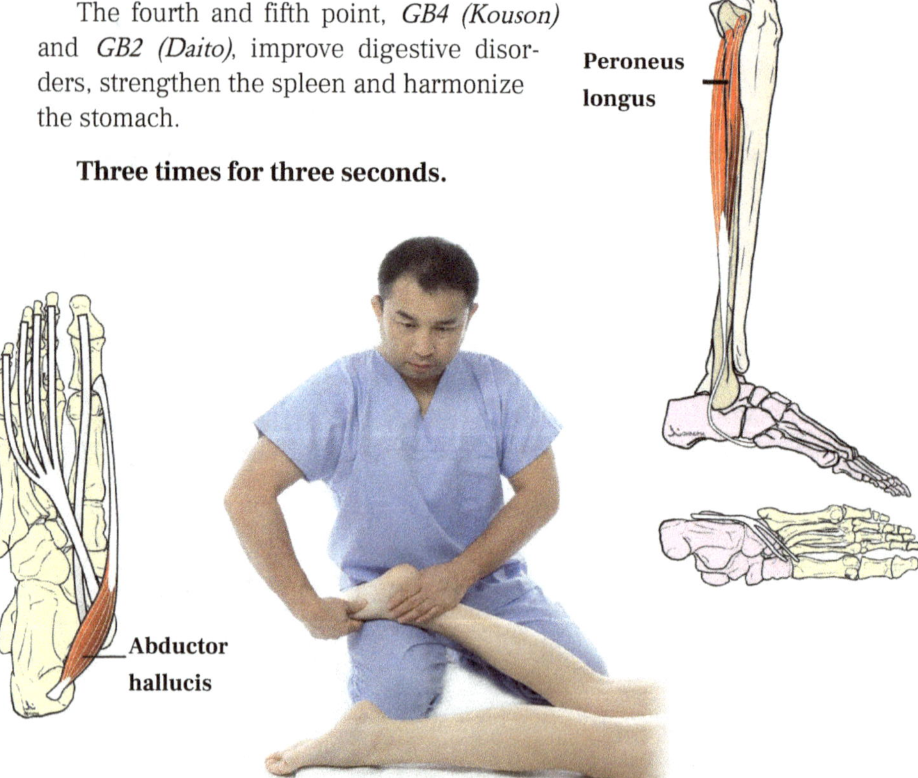

Reflective areas of the spinal column

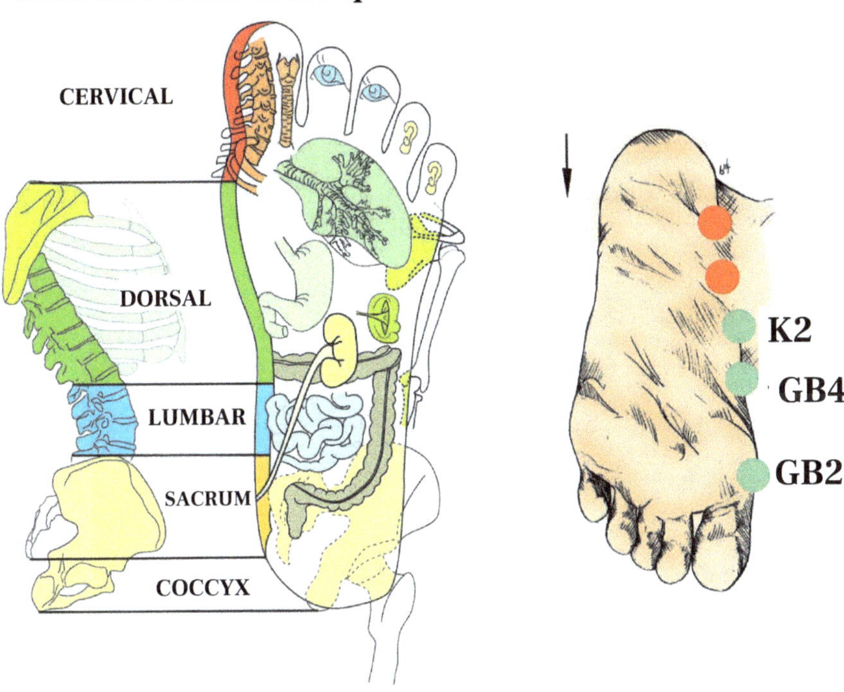

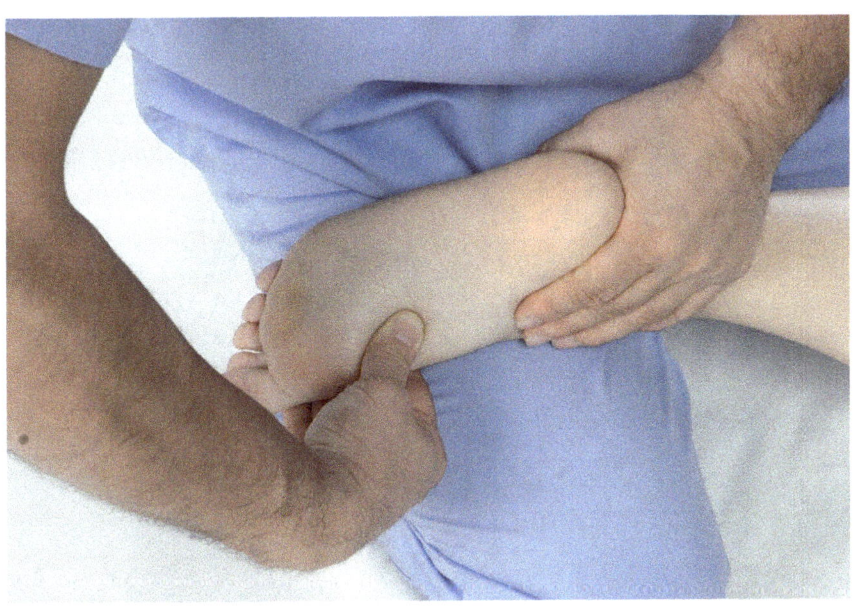

6.11. PLANTAR REGION. LINE OF THE INFERIOR FIRST METATARSAL

PATIENT'S POSTURE: Prone. Head turned towards the therapist, shoulders in abduction and elbows bent.

THERAPIST'S POSITION: Seiza, perpendicular to the area, placing the patient's left foot on the therapist's right thigh.

TYPE OF PRESSURE: Holding the ankle with the left hand and applying pressure with the right thumb.

Nº. OF POINTS: One five-point line.

DIRECTION OF THE LINE: From the internal plantar arch to the interdigital space of the first and second toe; around the metatarsophalangeal joint of the first toe.

OBSERVATIONS: The first point corresponds to key point *GB3 (Taihaku)*, indicated to combat gastroenteritis and general digestive disorders.

Three times for three seconds.

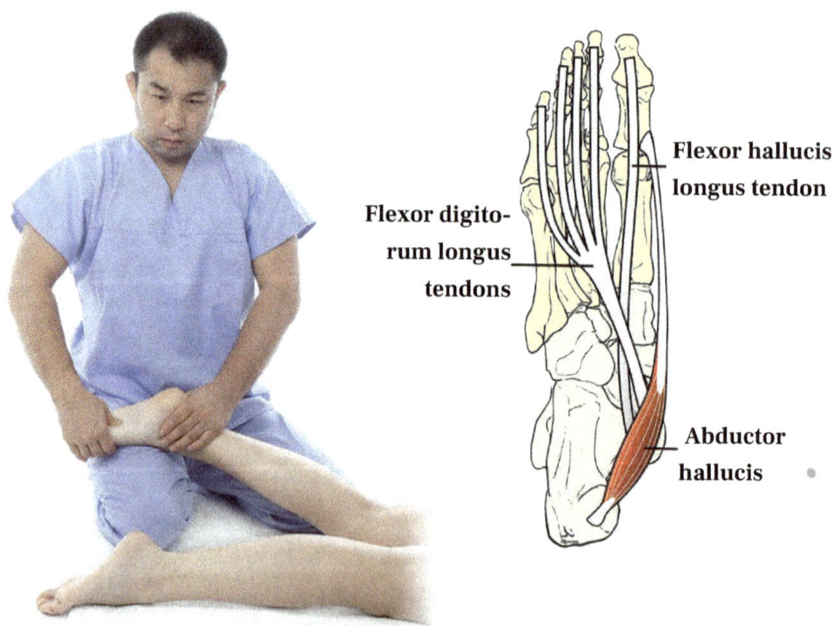

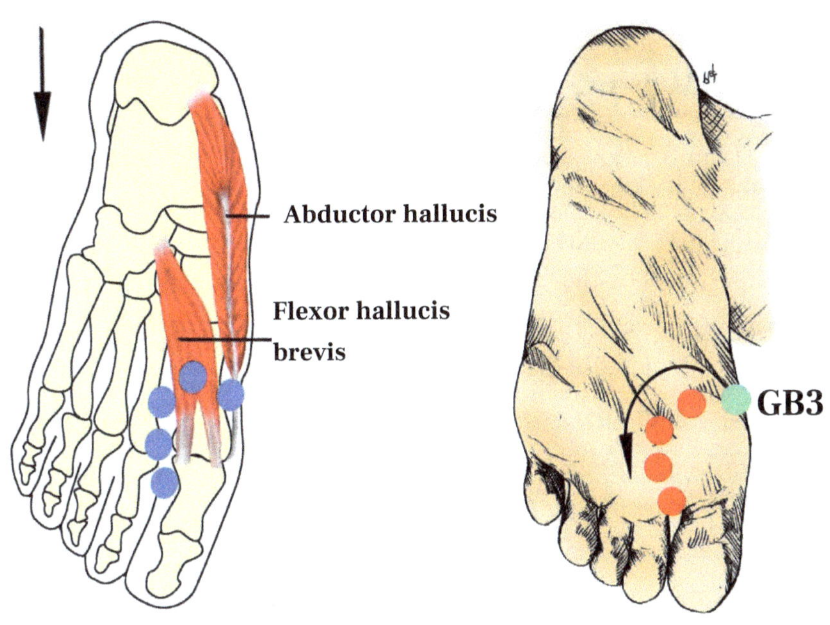

Abductor hallucis
Flexor hallucis
brevis
GB3

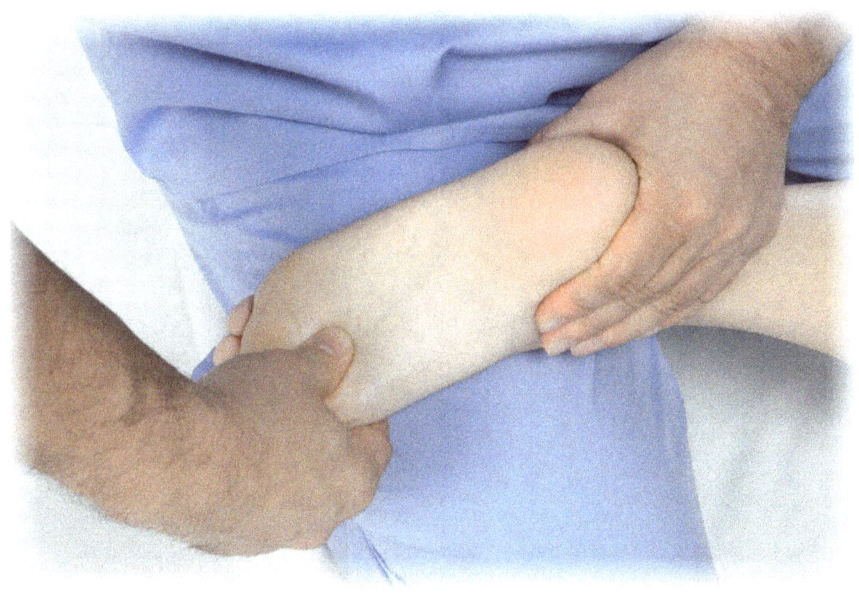

6.12. PLANTAR REGION. LINE OF METATARSOPHALAN-

GEAL JOINT SPACES

PATIENT'S POSTURE: Prone. Head turned towards the therapist, shoulders in abduction and elbows bent.

THERAPIST'S POSITION: Seiza, perpendicular to the area, placing the patient's left foot on the therapist's right thigh.

TYPE OF PRESSURE: Holding the ankle with the left hand and applying pressure with the right thumb.

Nº. OF POINTS: One five-point line.

DIRECTION OF THE LINE: From the big toe to the little one, in the interdigital spaces, except for the last point that is located on the external edge of the foot.

OBSERVATIONS: The fifth point corresponds to key point *B66 (Ashitsuukoku)* and is used to treat headaches, cephalea, neck stiffness, vertigo and epistaxis (nasal hemorrhaging).

Three times for three seconds.

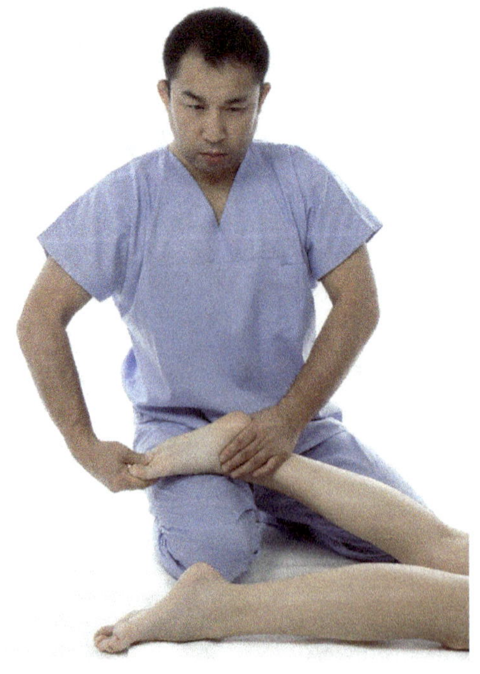

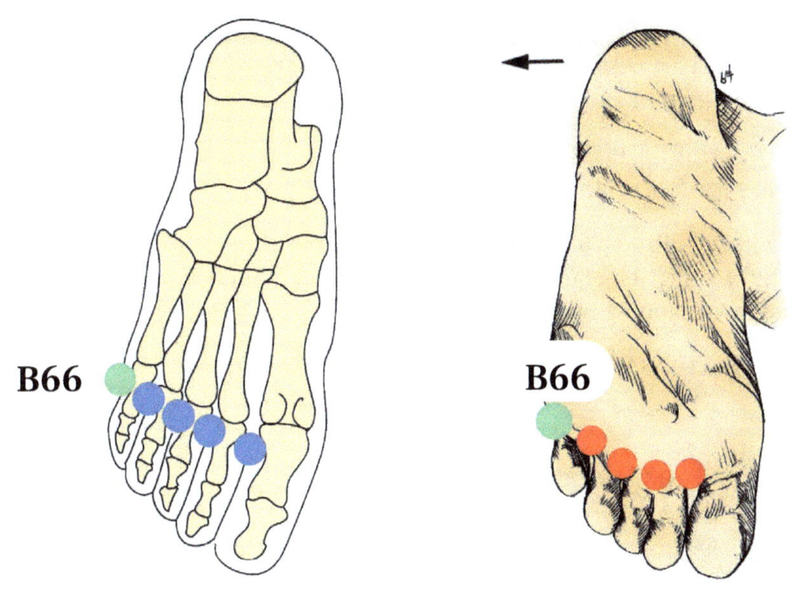

B66
B66

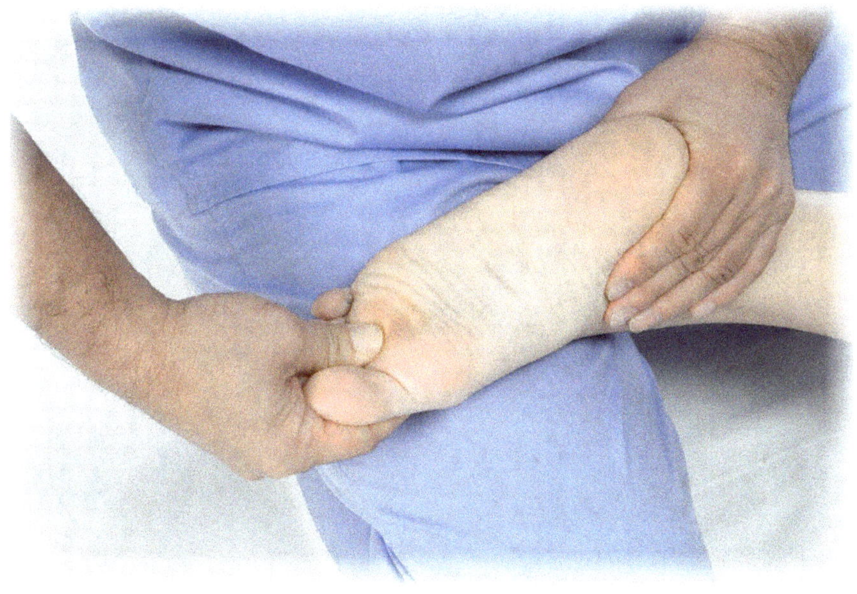

6.13. STRETCHING AND ROTATING THE TOES (Circumduction)

PATIENT'S POSTURE: Prone. Head turned towards the therapist, shoulders in abduction and elbows bent.

THERAPIST'S POSITION: Seiza, perpendicular to the area, placing the patient's left foot on the therapist's right thigh.

TYPE OF PRESSURE: Hold the base of the metatarsals with the left hand. The right hand hooks the proximal phalanx next to the metarsophalangeal joint. Stretch and widely rotate (circumduction) each toe.

Nº. OF POINTS: Ten rotations per toe and direction.

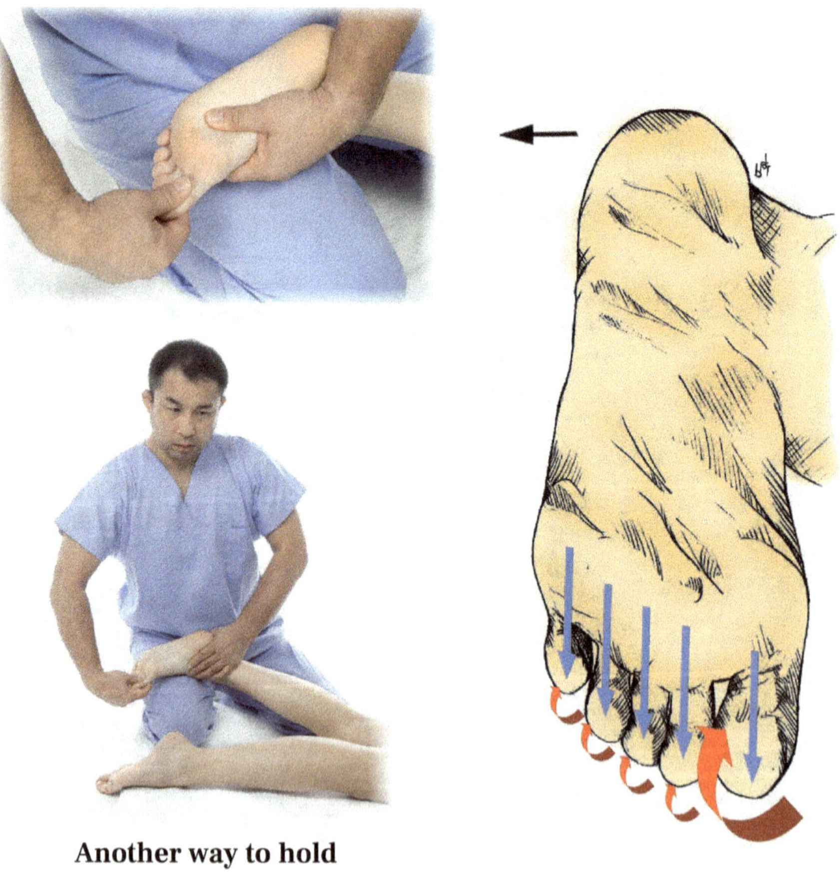

Another way to hold

6.14. ANKLE ROTATION

PATIENT'S POSTURE: Prone. Head turned towards the therapist, shoulders in abduction and elbows and knees bent.

THERAPIST'S POSITION: Seiza, facing the treatment area.

TYPE OF PRESSURE: Hold the ankle with your left hand. With the right perform wide circles while holding the metatarsophalangeal joints.

OBSERVATIONS: Each circle must be performed to the full range of ankle mobility. This movement works on key points *B62 (Shinmyaku) and GB40 (Kyuukyo)*; the latter is very important for treating a sprained ankle.

Ten times to each side.
Ten times more to the side of greater resistance.

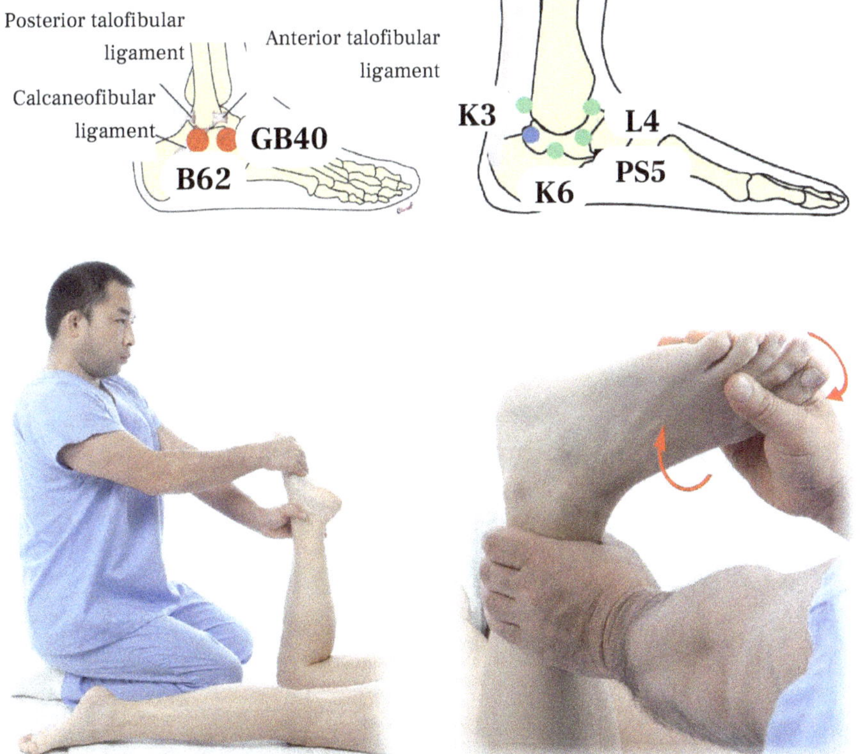

6.15. METATARSAL REGION

PATIENT'S POSTURE: Prone. Head turned towards the therapist, shoulders in abduction and elbows and knees bent.

THERAPIST'S POSITION: Seiza, facing the treatment area.

TYPE OF PRESSURE: Movement of flexi-extension of the metatarsus. Each hand holds adjacent metatarsus and performs the movement in the opposite direction: one hand flexes a metatarsus and, the other, extends the adjacent one.

Nº. OF POINTS: Four areas.

DIRECTION OF THE LINE: From the big toe to the little toe.

OBSERVATIONS: Locally, this exercise helps improve the mobility of the foot joints. Generally helping to improve blood circulation throughout the body. We can highlight two key points between the metatarsus of the foot: point *GB41 (Ashirinkyuu)*, which calms headache and lumbalgia pains, and point *L3 (Taishou)*, for menstrual and urinary disorders.

Ten repetitions per area.

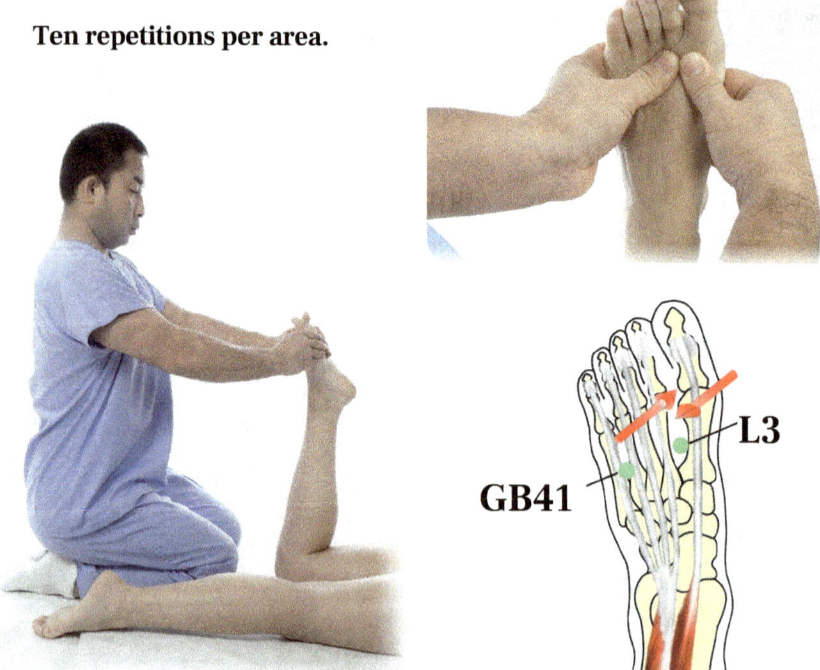

6.16. ELONGATING THE ACHILLES TENDON

PATIENT'S POSTURE: Prone. Head turned towards the therapist, shoulders in abduction and elbows and knees bent.

THERAPIST'S POSITION: Seiza, facing the treatment area.

TYPE OF PRESSURE: Hold the ankle with the left hand and stretch with the opposite arm by levering with the forearm.

Nº. OF POINTS: Two stretches. The first time it is done with the patient's knee bent 90º. The second time, it flexes approximately 120º so that the stretch on the calcaneal tendon is intensified.

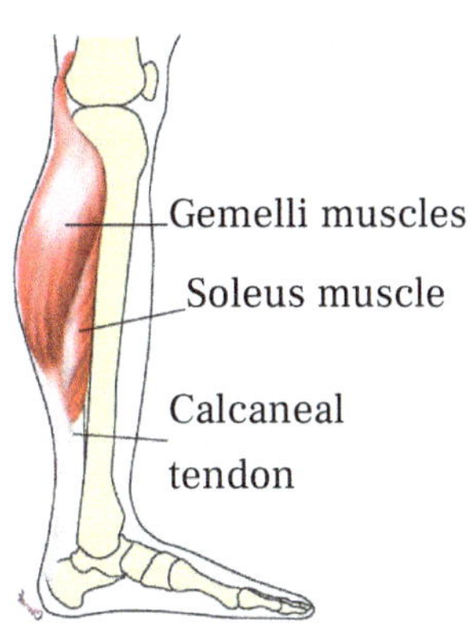

OBSERVATIONS: This work also performs the stretching of the soleus muscle, the innermost of the triceps sural group. The calf muscles are not stretched. This is only possible with the knee in extension; this exercise is carried out in supine decubitus. Work slowly, stretching to the patient's limit.

Once for each stretch for five seconds.

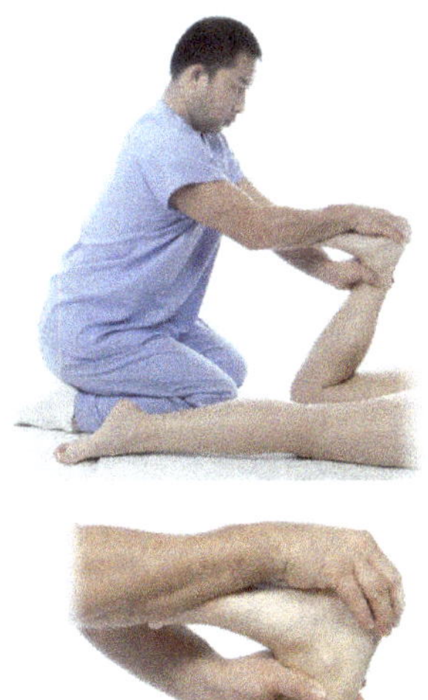
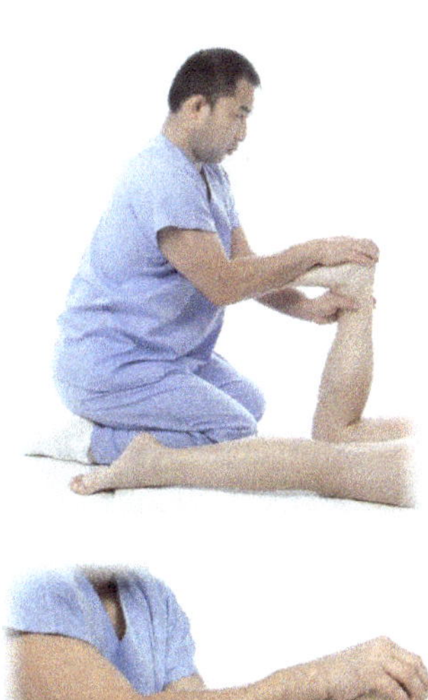
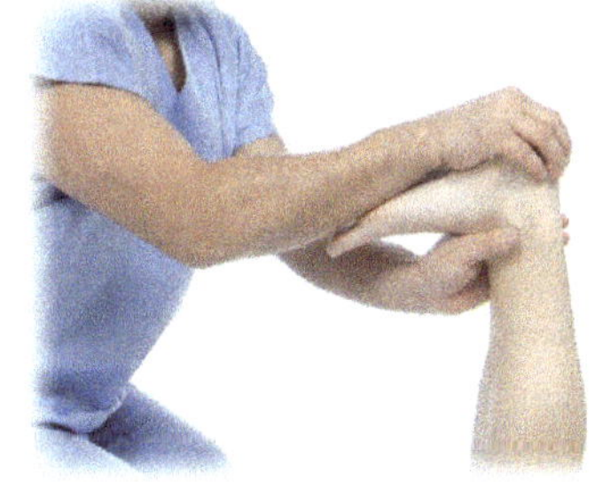

6.17. ROCKING THE ANKLE

PATIENT'S POSTURE: Prone. Head turned towards the therapist, shoulders in abduction and elbows and knees bent.

THERAPIST'S POSITION: Seiza, maintaining the previous position.

TYPE OF PRESSURE: Thumbs in A, on the centre of the ankle. Rock the foot, alternately flexing the plantar and dorsal.

OBSERVATIONS: The point where the thumbs are placed corresponds to key point *S41 (Kaikei)*.

Once for ten seconds.

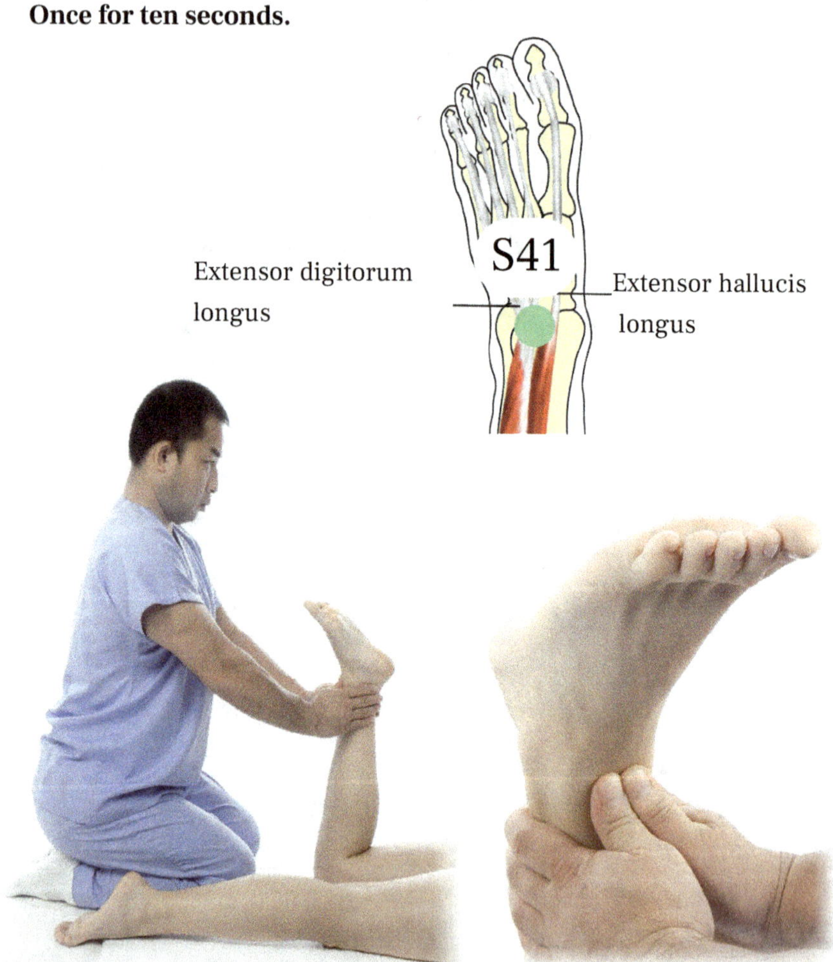

6.18. RELAXING THE SURAL TRICEPS

PATIENT'S POSTURE: Prone. Head turned towards the therapist, shoulders in abduction and elbows and knees bent.

THERAPIST'S POSITION: Seiza, maintaining the previous position.

TYPE OF PRESSURE: Hold the foot by the toes with the left hand (on the left side) and shake the leg moving the sural triceps.

Two or three times for ten seconds.

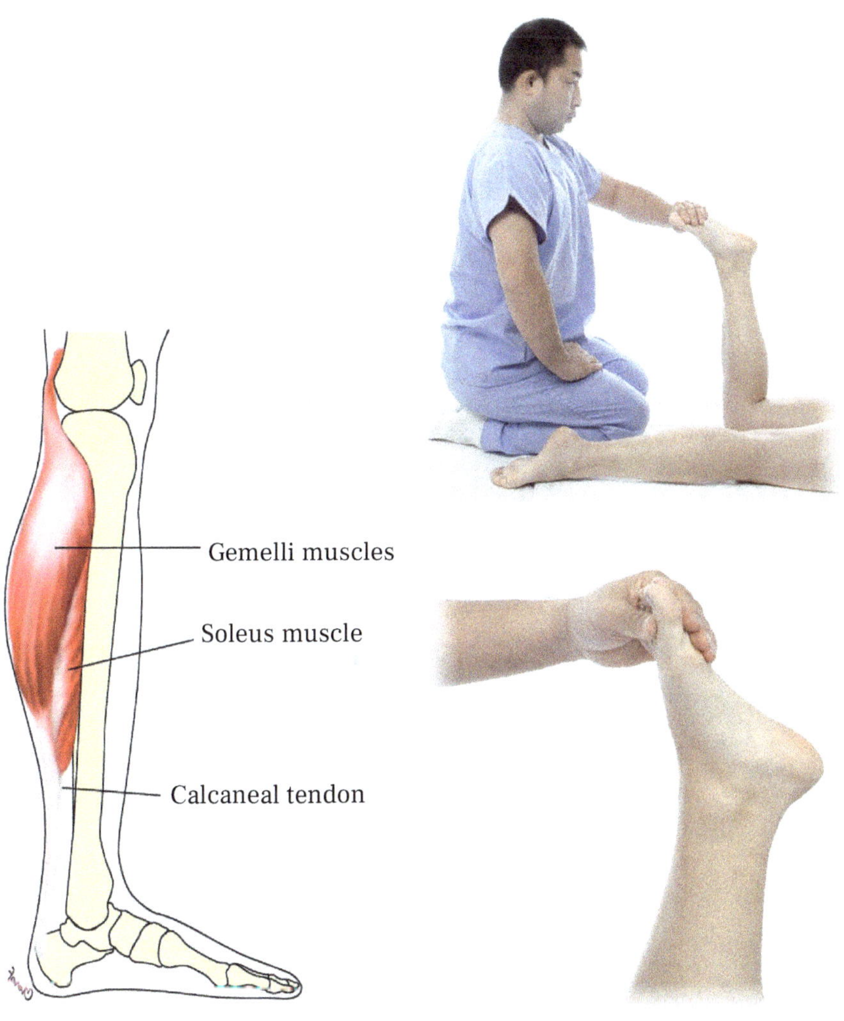

6.19. RELEASING THE LEG JOINTS

PATIENT'S POSTURE: Prone. Head turned towards the therapist, shoulders in abduction and elbows bent.

THERAPIST'S POSITION: Seiza, maintaining the previous position.

TYPE OF HANDLING: Embrace the patient's ankle by placing the left hand on the calcaneus and the right hand on the arch (on the left side). Extension is performed with the movement of the therapist's body by leaning slightly back.

OBSERVATIONS:The goal of this exercise is to release the leg joints, especially the hip joint; traction should reach the hip and gluteal muscles.

Three times for five seconds.

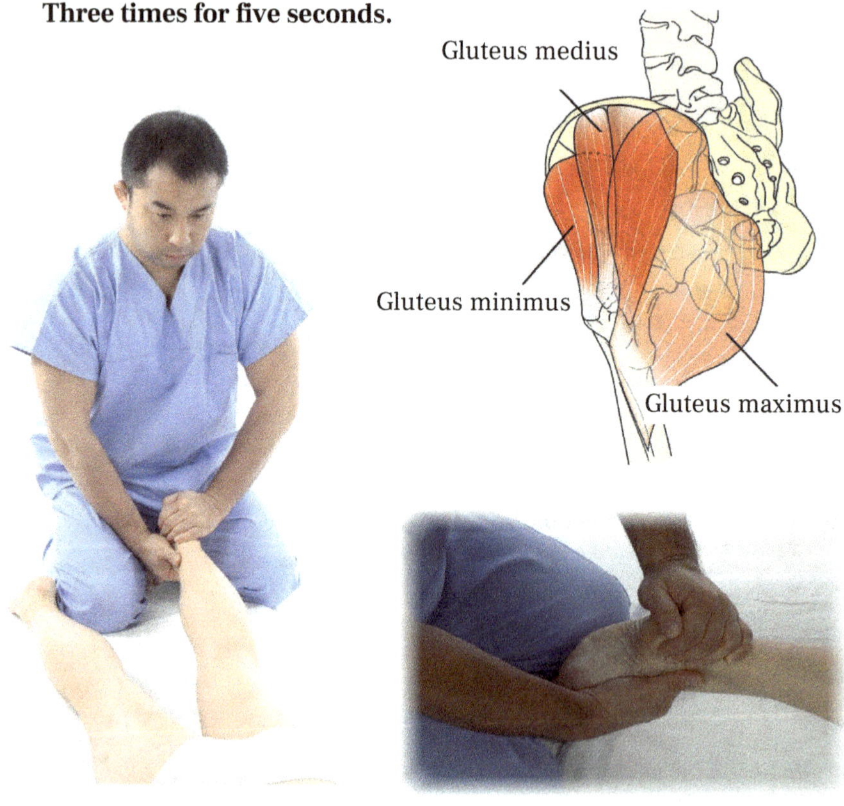

Repeat the same routine on the RIGHT LEG.

7. Back adjustments

7.1. Scapulas.

7.2. Gluteus.

7.3. Spinous process.

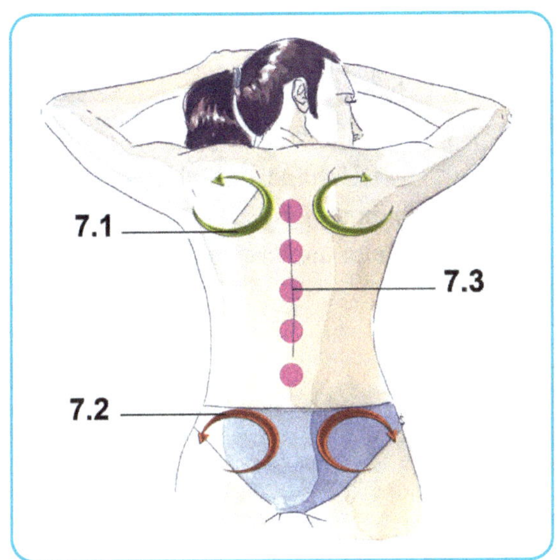

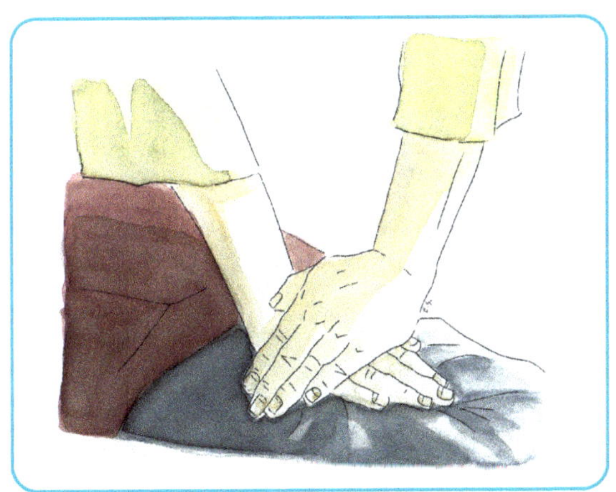

7.1. SCAPULAS

PATIENT'S POSTURE: Prone. Head turned towards the therapist, shoulders in abduction and elbows bent.

THERAPIST'S POSITION: Basic, on the right side of the patient. Left knee at the level of the patient's hip.

TYPE OF PRESSURE: Palms of the hands on each of the scapulas, pressing down firmly.

Nº. OF POINTS: Two areas, on the scapulas.

OBSERVATIONS: Work deeply, with the body weight.

Five outward turns. First left hand and then right hand.
Five outward turns with both hands at once.
Five inward turns with both hands at once.

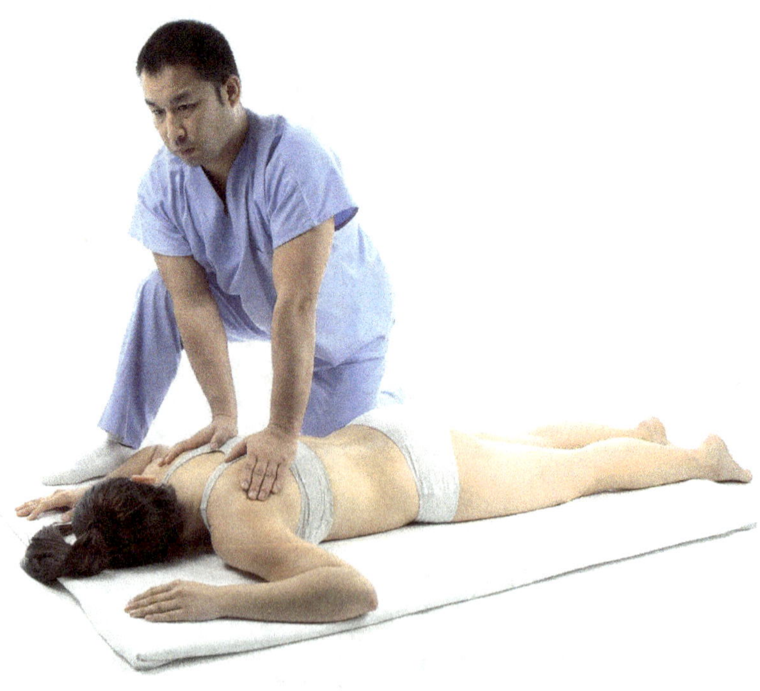

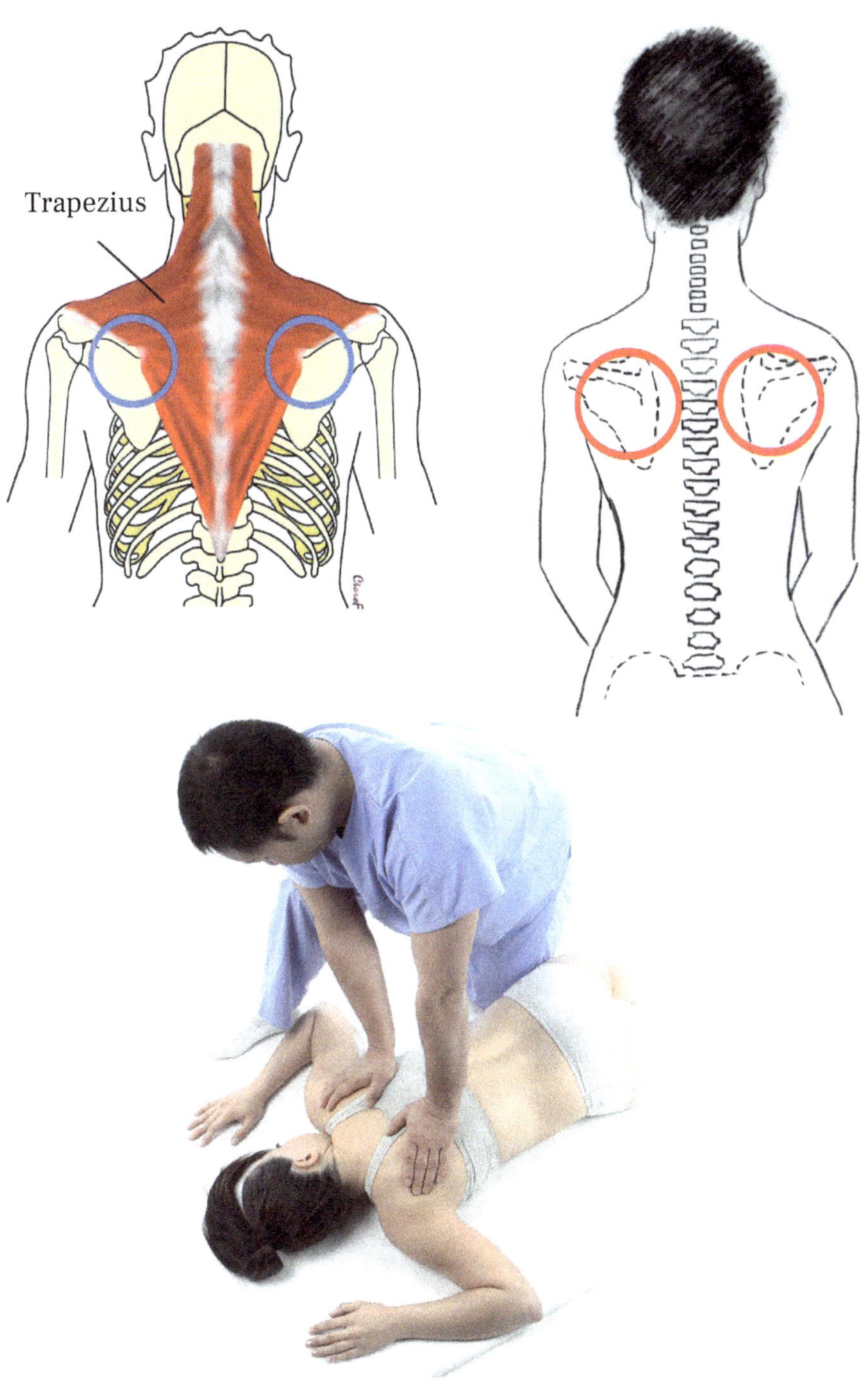

Trapezius

7.2. GLUTEUS

PATIENT'S POSTURE: Prone. Head turned towards the therapist, shoulders in abduction and elbows bent.

THERAPIST'S POSITION: Basic, on the right side of the patient. Left knee at the level of the patient's greater trochanter.

TYPE OF PRESSURE: Palms of hands on hips, pressing firmly on the gluteus.

Nº. OF POINTS: Two areas, on both gluteus maximus.

OBSERVATIONS: Work deeply, with the body weight.

Five outward turns. First left hand and then right hand.
Five outward turns with both hands at once.
Five inward turns with both hands at once.

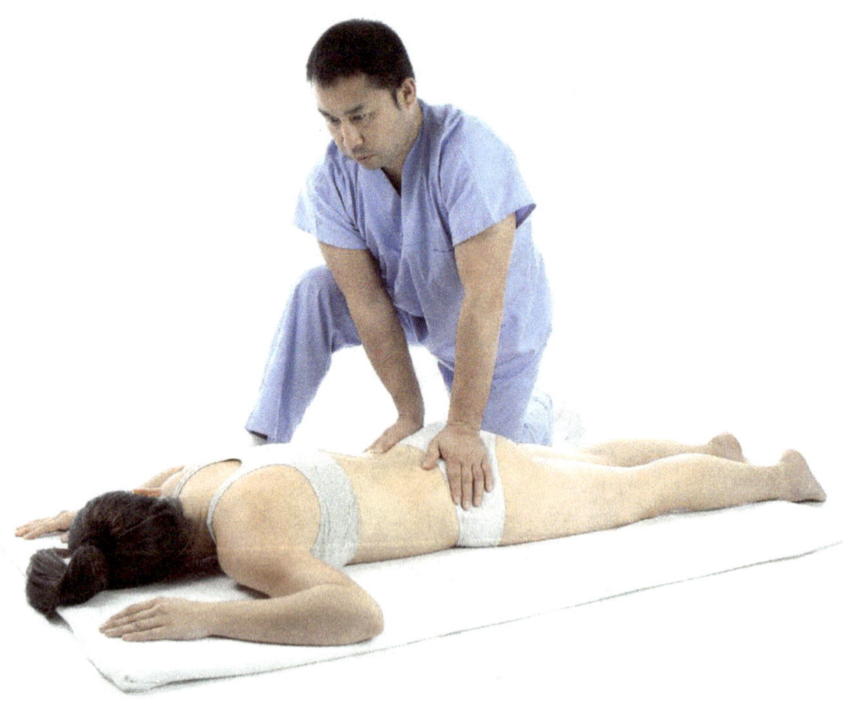

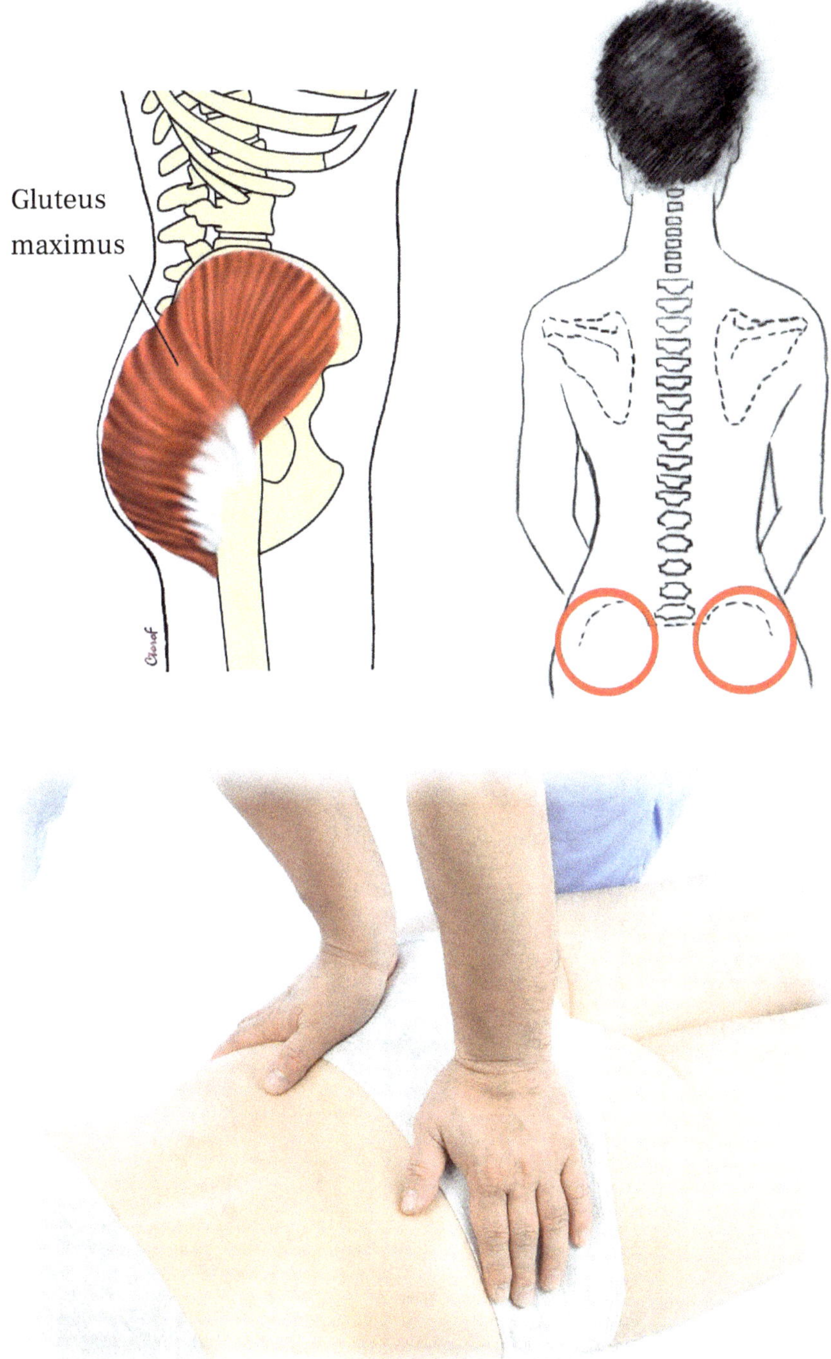
Gluteus
maximus

7.3. SPINOUS PROCESS

PATIENT'S POSTURE: Prone. Head turned towards the therapist, shoulders in abduction and elbows bent.

THERAPIST'S POSITION: Basic, on the right side of the patient. Left knee at the level of the patient's hip.

TYPE OF PRESSURE: Crossed palms. Left over the spinal column between the shoulder blades, resting the middle finger on the spinous process of the seventh cervical vertebra; the right is crossed over the left.

Nº. OF POINTS: Five pressures and two frictions.

DIRECTION OF THE LINE: From the interscapular area to the sacral region.

OBSERVATIONS:The last pressure is applied on the sacrum. The frictions go all the way to the end of the sacrum; you have to be careful not to hit the sacrum when you reach the L5-S1 junction.

Three times for three seconds.

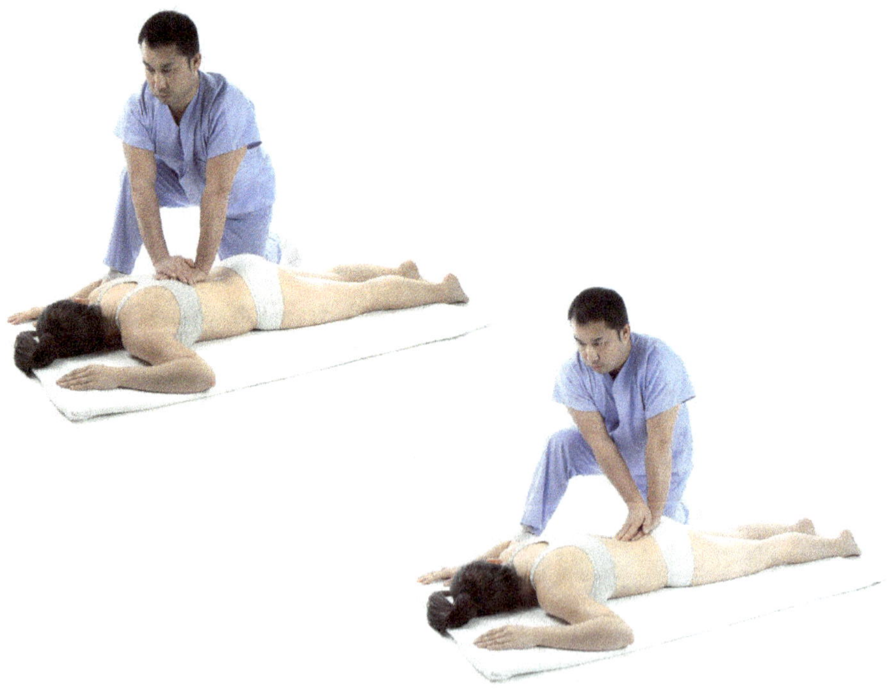

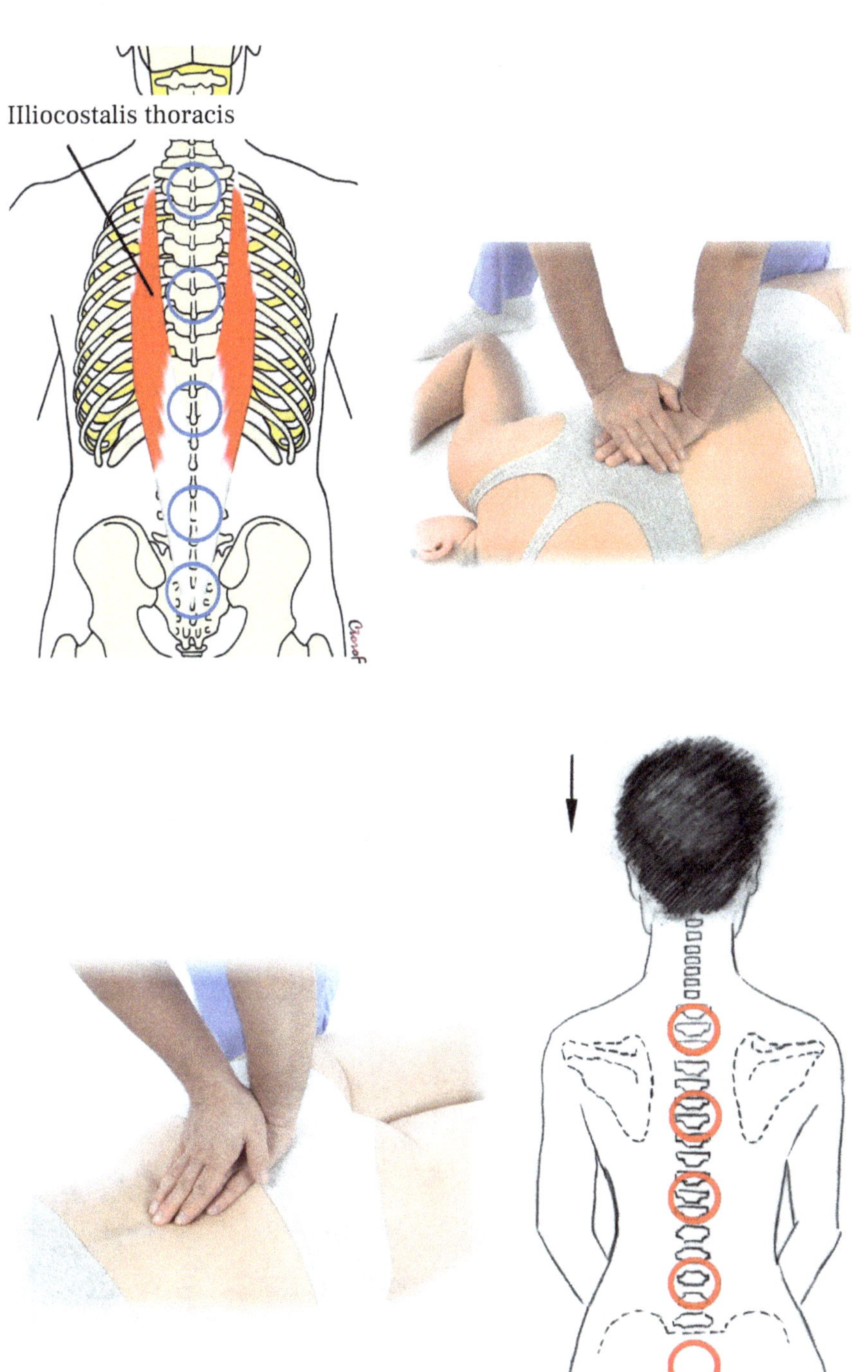

143

Aze Shiatsu

2. Basic treatment in supine decubitus

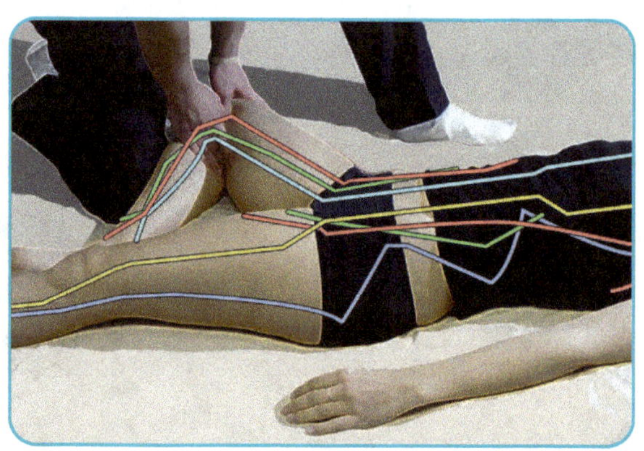

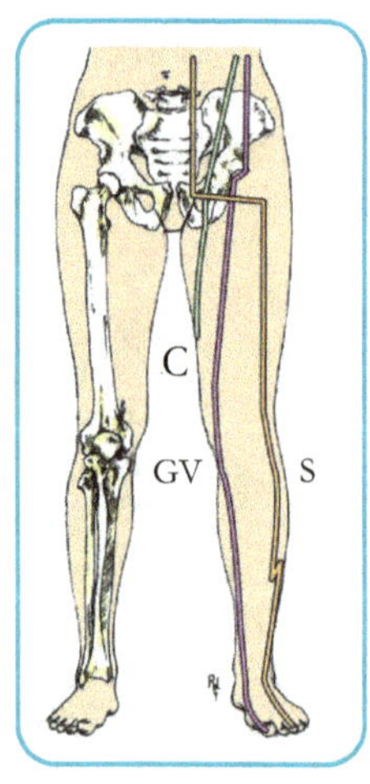

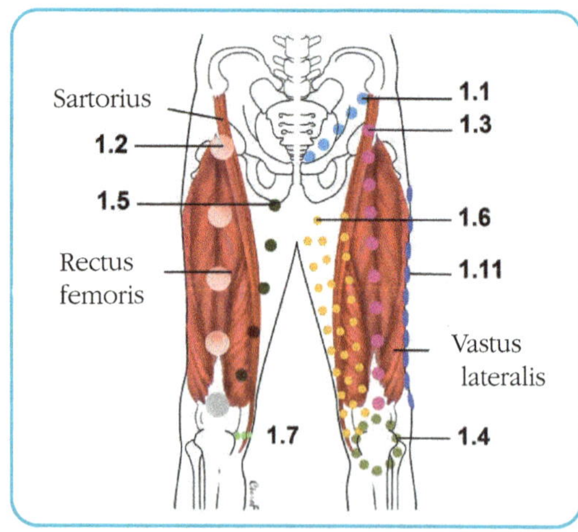

1. Lower limbs

1.1. Inguinal region.
1.2. Anterior femoral region.
    Palm pressure.
1.3. Anterior femoral region.
    Thumb pressure.
1.4. Patellar region.
1.5. Medial femoral region.
    Palm pressure
1.6. Medial femoral region.
    Thumb pressure.
1.7. Medial patellar region.
1.8. Medial sural region.
1.9. K3 Region.
1.10. Medial calcaneal region.
1.11. Lateral femoral region.
1.12. Lateral tibia region.
1.13. Lateral fibula region.
1.14. Tarsal region.
1.15. Dorsal region of the foot.
1.16. Rotating and extending the toes.
1.17. Digital region of the foot.
1.18. Rocking movement.
1.19. Elongating the Achilles tendon.
1.20. Leg stretch with vibration.

Shiatsu in the lower limbs helps maintain good muscle tone, decongests circulation and helps the heart work more comfortably.

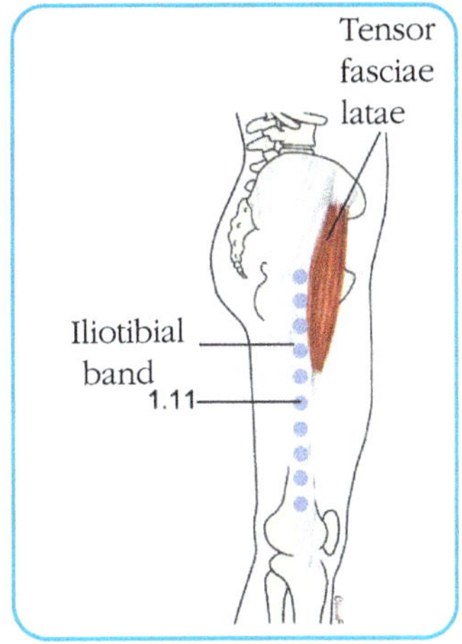

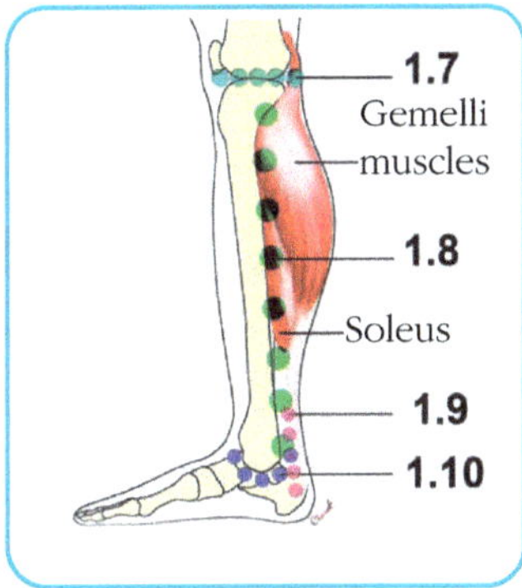

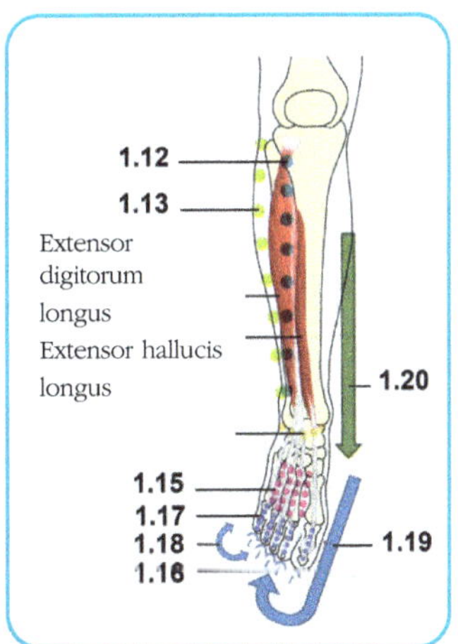

1.1. INGUINAL REGION.

PATIENT'S POSTURE: Supine. Arms straight along the body or crossed over the chest.

THERAPIST'S POSITION: Basic, on the left side of the patient. Left knee at the level of the patient's knee.

TYPE OF PRESSURE: Palm. The far hand from the patient applies gentle pressure on the inguinal region with the thenar eminence. The closer hand rests gently above the knee of the same leg.

N°. OF POINTS: Apply pressure five times. The central point is worked three times for five seconds after the first repetitions.

DIRECTION OF THE LINE: From the PSIS to the pubic symphysis.

OBSERVATIONS: The third point is located on the femoral artery; you can feel its pulse. Work slowly and accurately. It helps to improve blood circulation, especially of the lower limbs.

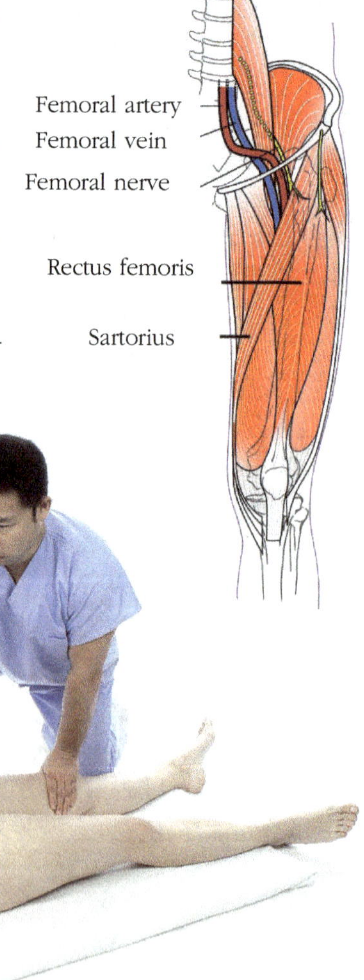

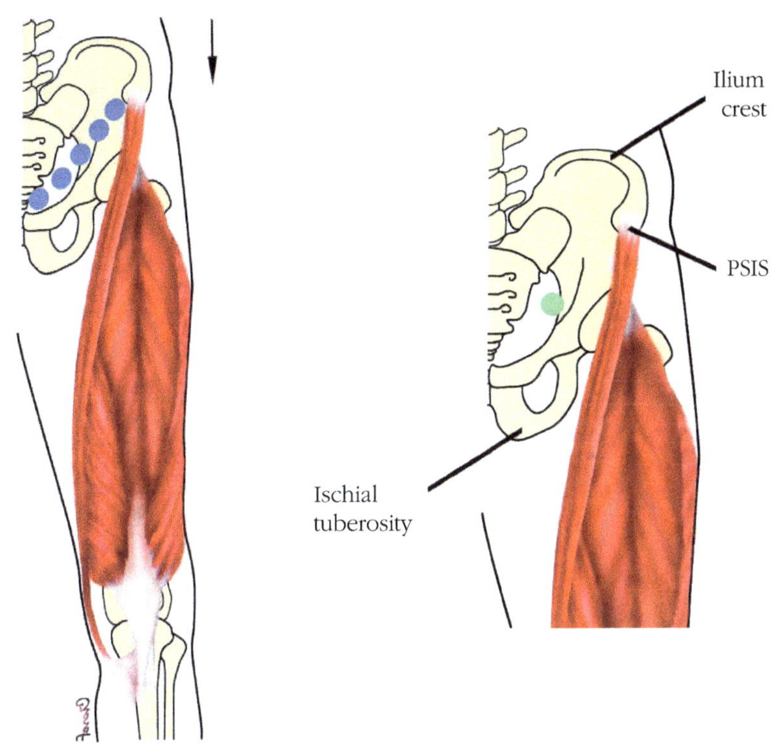
Ilium
crest
PSIS
Ischial
tuberosity

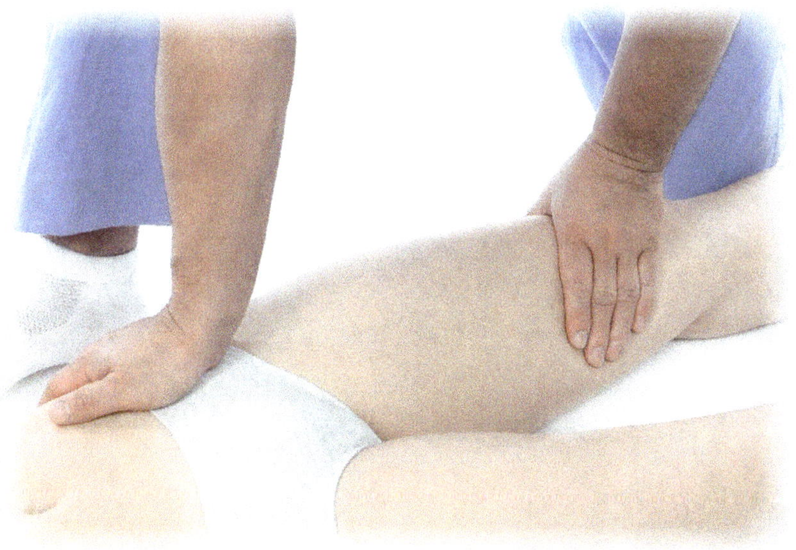

1.2. ANTERIOR FEMORAL REGION. PALM PRESSURE

PATIENT'S POSTURE: Supine. Arms straight along the body or crossed over the chest.

THERAPIST'S POSITION: Basic, maintaining the previous position.

TYPE OF PRESSURE: Palm, with both hands in the logo shape.

Nº. OF POINTS: One line, pressure applied five times.

DIRECTION OF THE LINE: From the inguinal region to the knee. The first point is below the ASIS (anterior superior iliac spine).

Three times for three seconds.

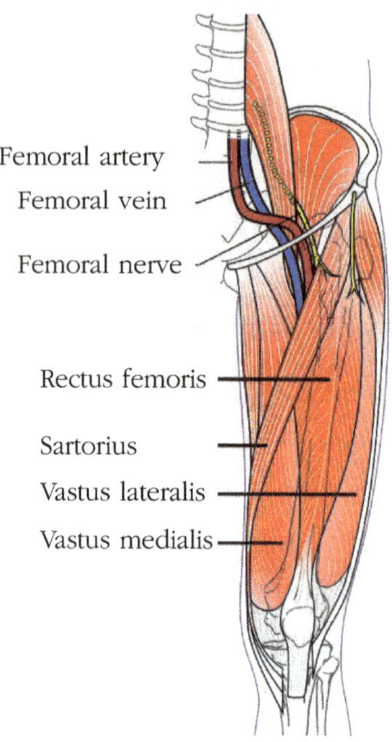

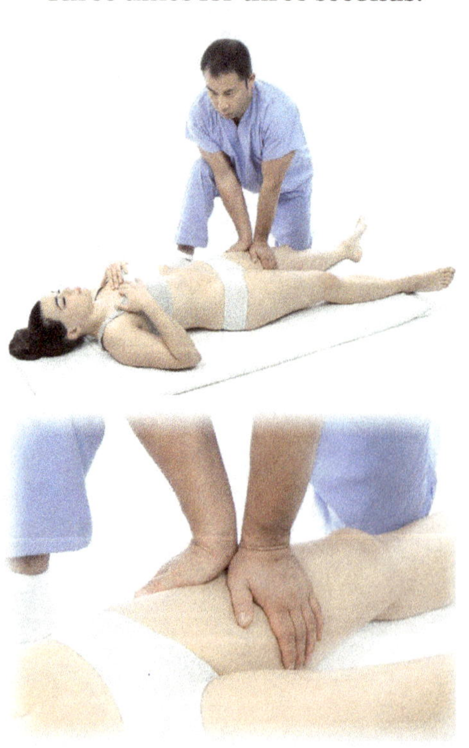

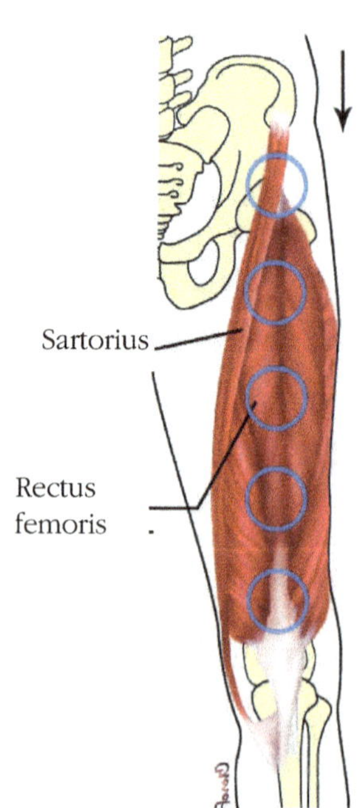

1.3. ANTERIOR FEMORAL REGION. THUMB PRESSURE

PATIENT'S POSTURE: Supine. Arms straight along the body or crossed over the chest.

THERAPIST'S POSITION: Basic, maintaining the previous position.

TYPE OF PRESSURE: 1st and 2nd repetitions: Logo.
3rd repetition: Thumb over thumb (aspa).

Nº. OF POINTS: A ten-point line.

DIRECTION OF THE LINE: From the inguinal region to the knee. The first point is below the ASIS (anterior superior iliac spine).

OBSERVATIONS: Work on this region helps improve heart function. It is suitable for obese people with excessive strain on their heart muscles.

Three times for three seconds.

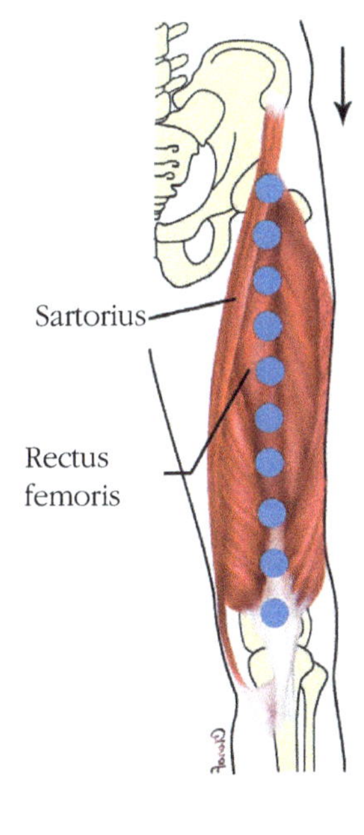

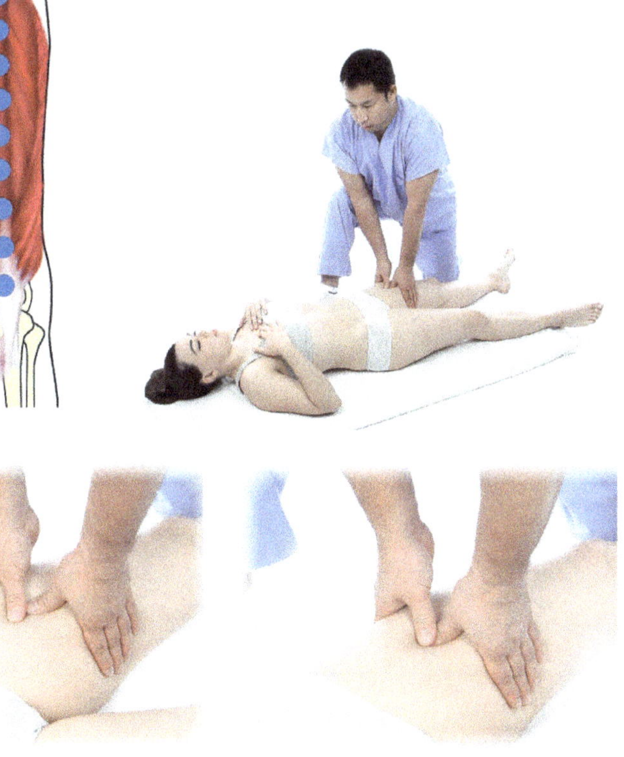

1.4. PATELLAR REGION

PATIENT'S POSTURE: Supine. Arms straight along the body or crossed over the chest.

THERAPIST'S POSITION: Seiza/Kneeling.

TYPE OF PRESSURE: Both thumbs. The other fingers hold the knee on the opposite side to prevent it moving.

N°. OF POINTS: Two five-point lines.

DIRECTION OF THE LINE: First the external line is worked inwardly with both thumbs simultaneously; then the internal line with the thumbs outwardly.

OBSERVATIONS: The work is completed with the following exercises:

Rotations in both directions: Five on each side.

Vibration: Five seconds.

The hand closest to the hip does the exercise, placing it perpendicularly to the leg, while the other rests on the patient's tibia.

Three times for three seconds.

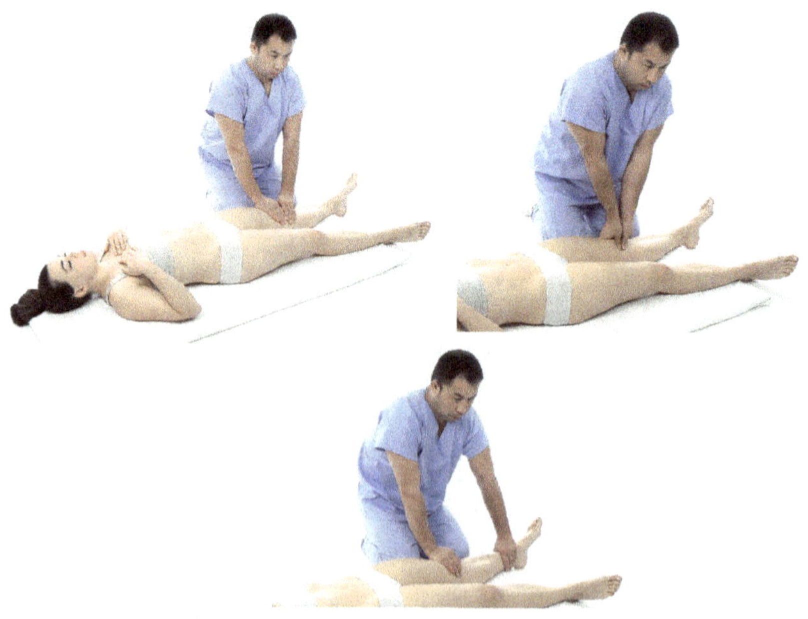

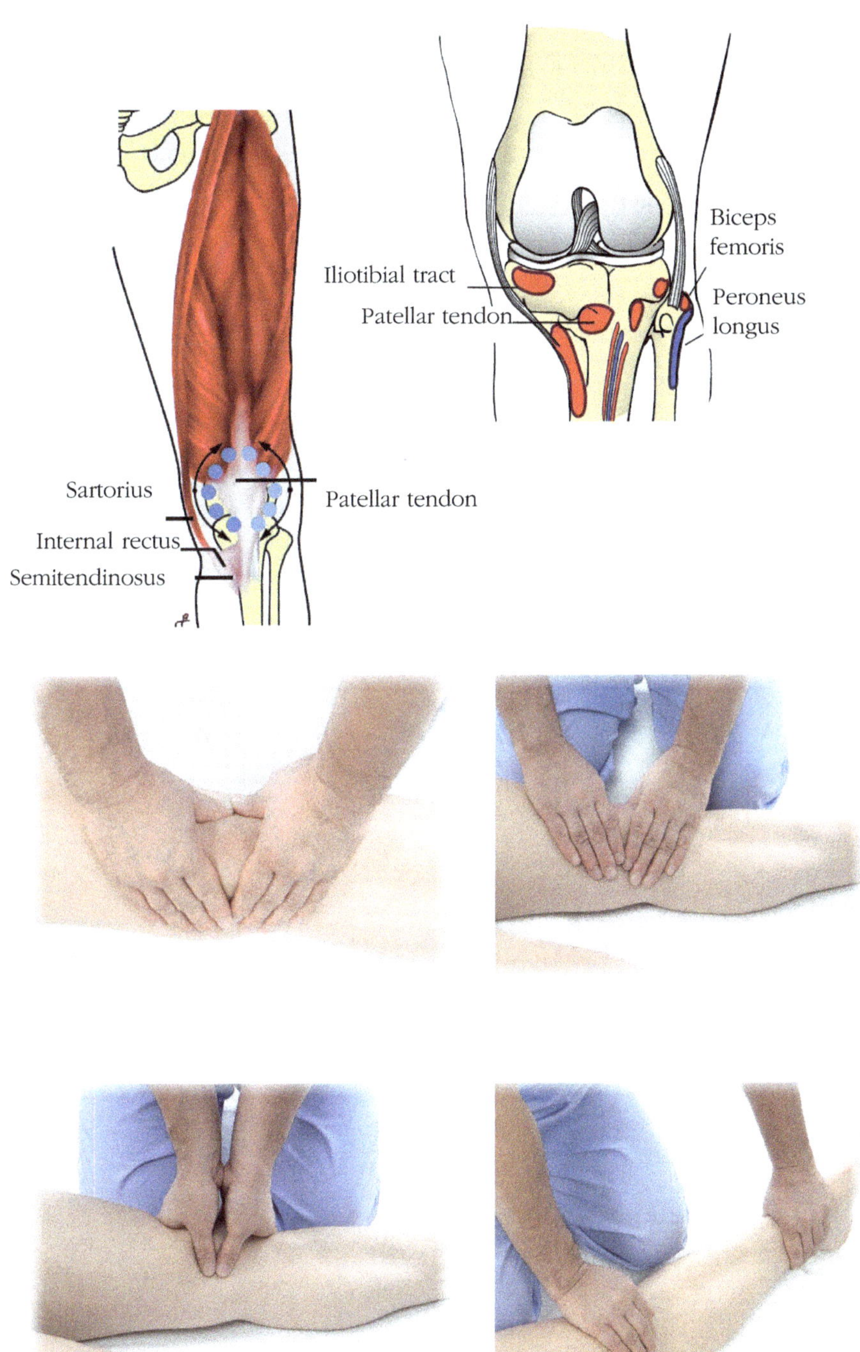

Sartorius
Internal rectus
Semitendinosus
Patellar tendon
Iliotibial tract
Patellar tendon
Biceps femoris
Peroneus longus

1.5. MEDIAL FEMORAL REGION. PALM PRESSURE

PATIENT'S POSTURE: Supine, knees bent and hip rotated externally. The sole of the foot next to the opposite knee.

THERAPIST'S POSITION: Basic, facing the treatment area.

TYPE OF PRESSURE: Palm. The closer hand applies pressure with both eminences, while the far hand holds the knee to protect the area and helps the pressure to penetrate.

Nº. OF POINTS: One line, pressure applied five times.

DIRECTION OF THE LINE: Along the midline of the inner thigh, from the insertion of the adductor longus to the knee.

OBSERVATIONS: Light palm pressure. In Japan the inner part of women's legs is called the "blood path". This area is useful for treating women's cycle disorders. Avoid with pregnant women.

Three times for three seconds.

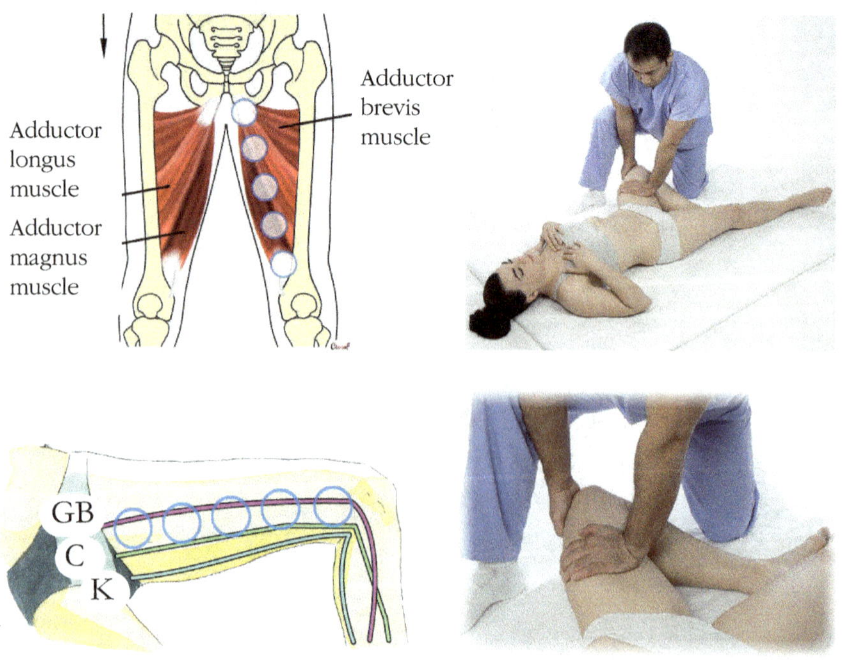

1.6. MEDIAL FEMORAL REGION. THUMB PRESSURE

PATIENT'S POSTURE: Supine, knees bent and hip rotated externally. The sole of the foot next to the opposite knee.

THERAPIST'S POSITION: Basic, maintaining the previous position.

TYPE OF PRESSURE: 1st and 2nd repetitions: Logo.
3rd repetition: Thumb over thumb (right one below on the left side).

N°. OF POINTS: Three ten-point lines.

Central line: From on top of the tendon of the adductor longus and towards the medial face of the knee.

Medial line: Two fingers below the tendon of the adductor longus and towards the medial face of the knee.

Lateral line: Two fingers above the tendon of the adductor longus and towards the medial face of the knee.

DIRECTION OF THE LINE: From the base of the pelvis to the medial face of the knee (goose foot). Repeat alternately in this order: central line, medial line and lateral line.

OBSERVATIONS: Generally, this is a very sensitive area. The central line works on liver conditions; and the eighth, ninth and tenth points especially work on eye problems. The lateral line works on the Spleen-Pancreatic meridian; around the eighth and ninth points is located key point SP10 (*Kekkai*, Sea of Blood).

Three times for three seconds.

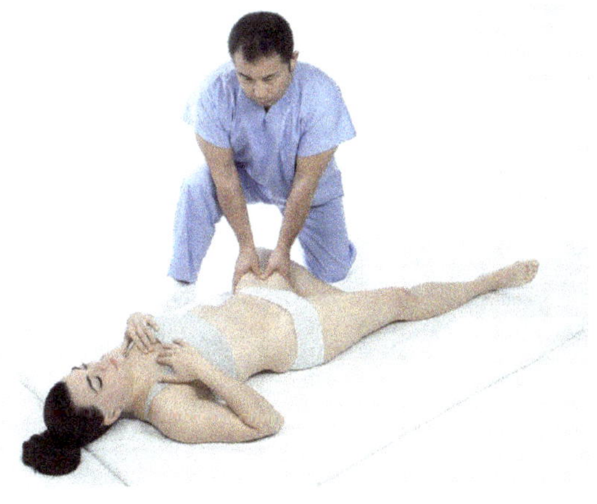

Adductor longus
muscle
Sartorius
Adductor
magnus
muscle
Vastus
medialis
Internal rectus
GB10
Ocular problems

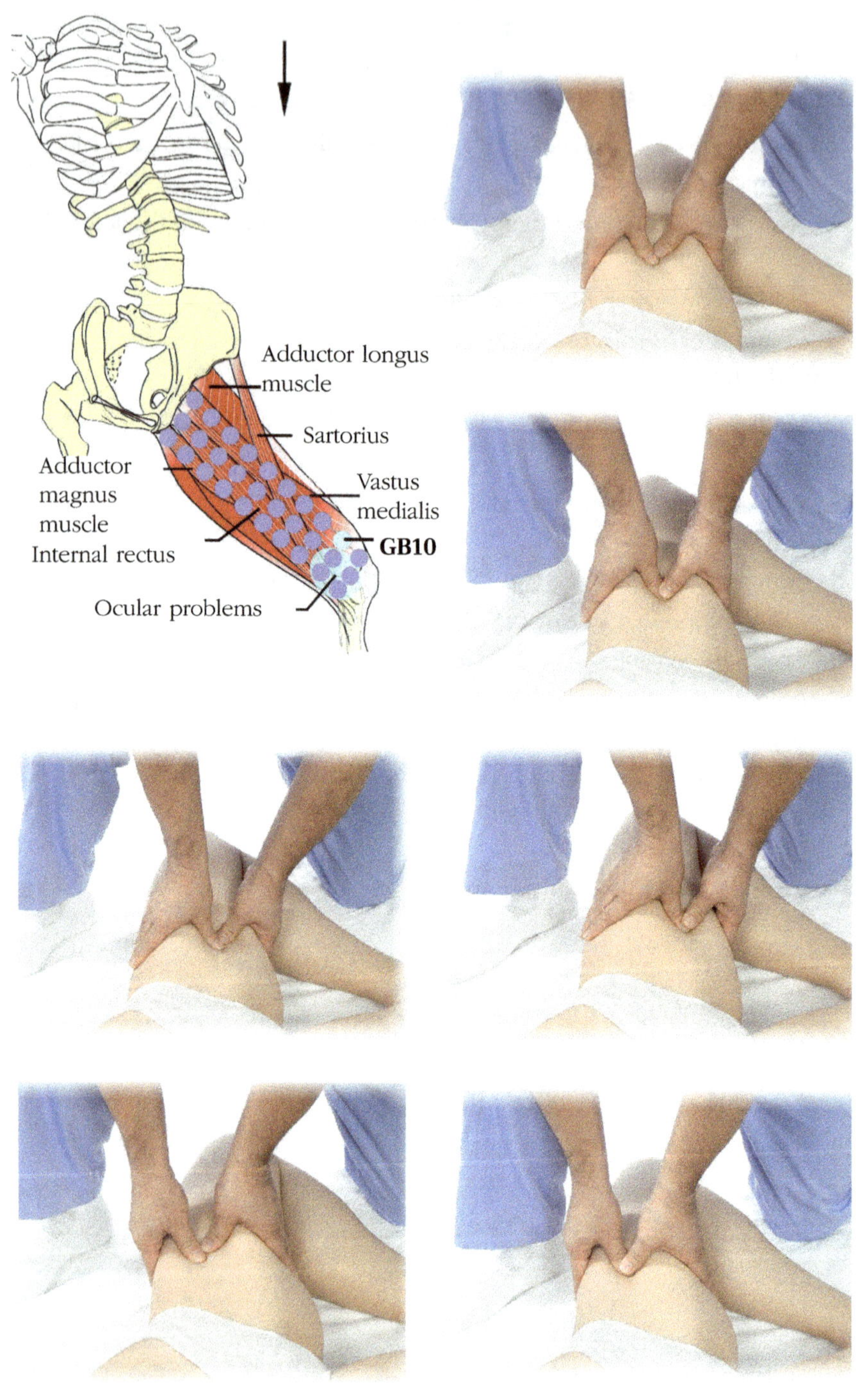

154

1.7. MEDIAL PATELLAR REGION

PATIENT'S POSTURE: Supine, knees bent and hip rotated externally. The sole of the foot next to the opposite knee.

THERAPIST'S POSITION: Basic, maintaining the previous position.

TYPE OF PRESSURE: One thumb (right on the left side). The other hand rests on the patient's ankle.

N°. OF POINTS: A five-point line.

DIRECTION OF THE LINE: Towards the patella along the medial knee joint.

OBSERVATIONS: The first point **K10 (Inkoku)**, is mainly indicated for male sexual function disorders. The second point corresponds to key point **L8 (Kyokusen)**.

Three times for three seconds.

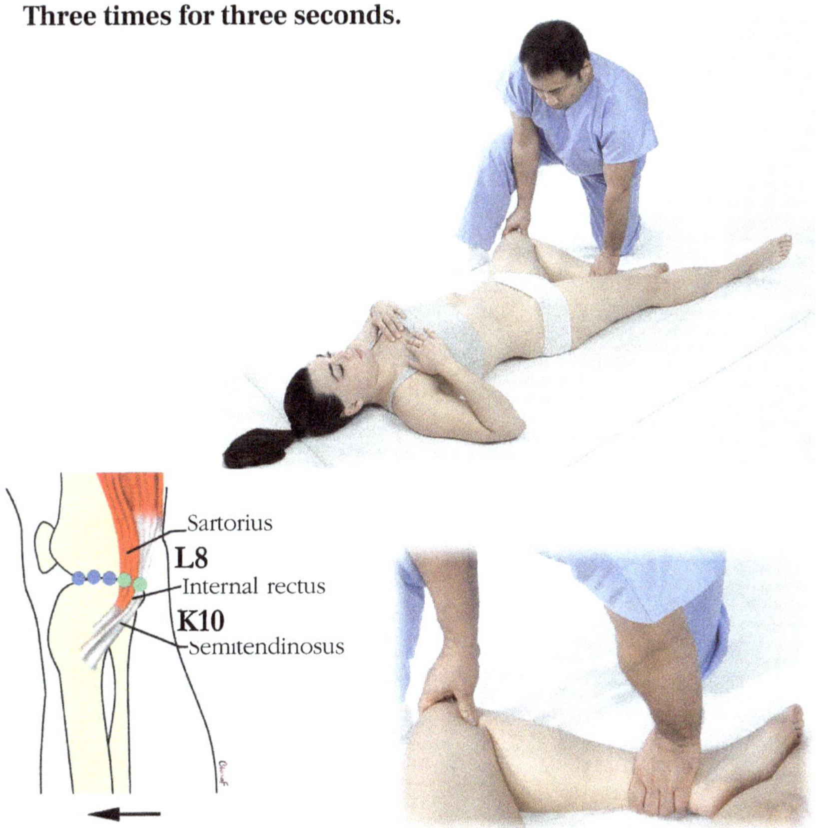

1.8. MEDIAL SURAL REGION

PATIENT'S POSTURE: Supine, knee bent and hip rotated externally.

THERAPIST'S POSITION: Basic, moving a little back.

TYPE OF PRESSURE: One thumb (right on the left side). The other hand holds the patient's foot.

Nº. OF POINTS: A eight-point line.

DIRECTION OF THE LINE: From the medial condyle of the knee to the ankle along the posterior edge of the tibia.

OBSERVATIONS: It's a very painful but effective area to treat menstrual/hormonal disorders and fluid retention (kidney problems).

The first point corresponds to key point *S9 (Inryousen)*; the seventh to key point *S6 (Saninkou)*.

Three times for three seconds.

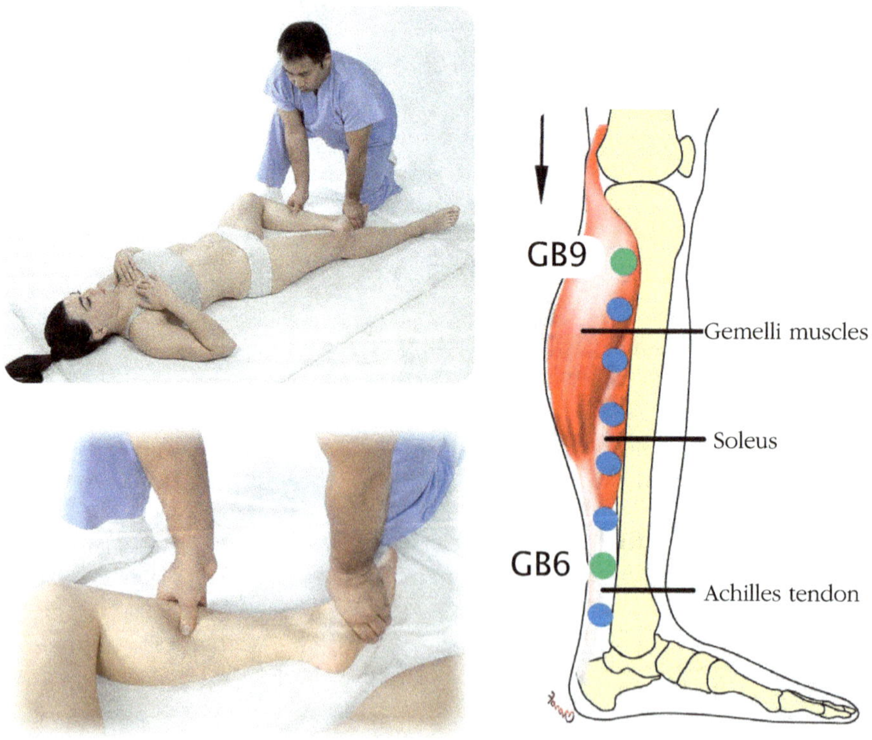

1.9. K3 REGION

PATIENT'S POSTURE: Supine, knee bent and hip rotated externally.

THERAPIST'S POSITION: Basic, maintaining the previous position.

TYPE OF PRESSURE: One thumb (right on the left side). The other hand holds the patient's foot.

Nº. OF POINTS: A five-point line.

DIRECTION OF THE LINE: Towards the heel, between the medial malleolus and the calcaneal tendon. The third point corresponds to key point *K3 (Taikei)*. The first and last points are located three fingers above and below the previous one, respectively.

Three times for three seconds.

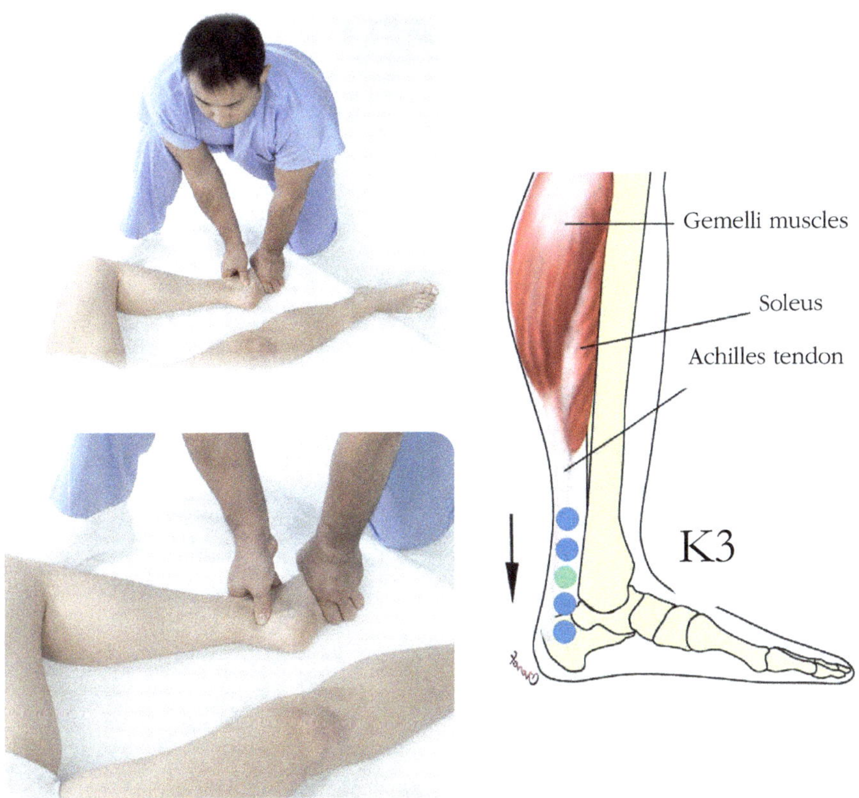

1.10. MEDIAL CALCANEAL REGION

PATIENT'S POSTURE: Supine, knee bent and hip rotated externally.

THERAPIST'S POSITION: Basic, maintaining the previous position.

TYPE OF PRESSURE: One thumb (right on the left side). The other hand holds the patient's foot.

N°. OF POINTS: A five-point line.

DIRECTION OF THE LINE: Circling the medial malleolus, from the calcaneal tendon to the arch.

OBSERVACIONES: The first point corresponds to key point *K3 (Taikei)*, the third with the *K6 (Syoukai)*, the fourth with *SP5 (Syoukyuu)* and the fifth to *L4 (Chuuhou)*.

Three times for three seconds.

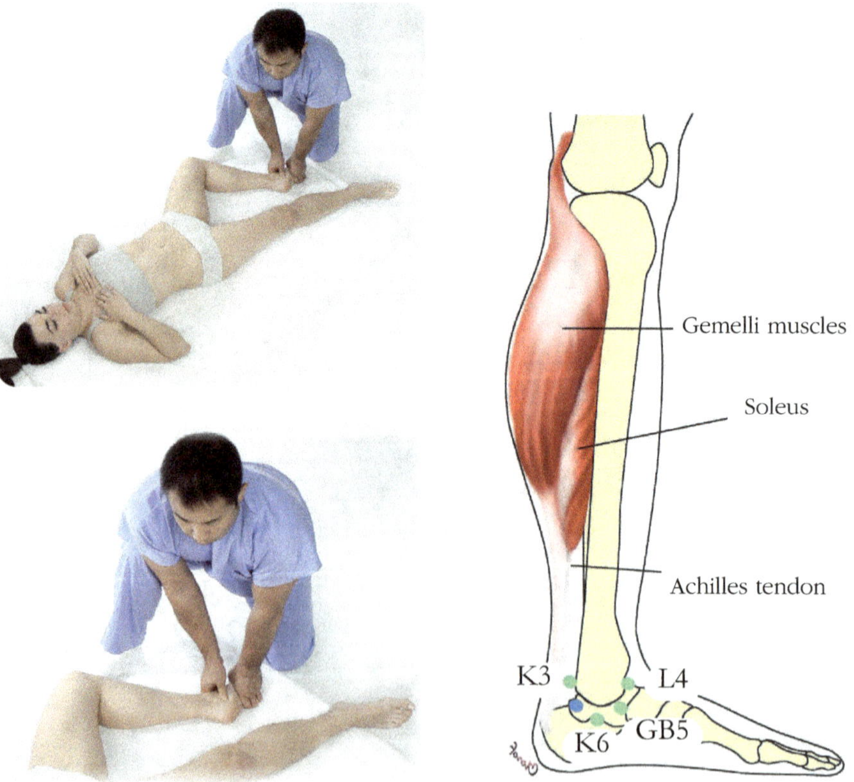

1.11. LATERAL FEMORAL REGION

PATIENT'S POSTURE: Supine. Arms straight along the body or crossed over the chest.

THERAPIST'S POSITION: Seiza, perpendicular to the area.

TYPE OF PRESSURE: Thumbs in V.

N°. OF POINTS: A ten-point line.

DIRECTION OF THE LINE: From the greater trochanter to the lateral edge of the knee.

OBSERVATIONS: The fifth point corresponds to key point *GS31 (Fu-ushi)* and is used in treating hypertension.

Three times for three seconds.

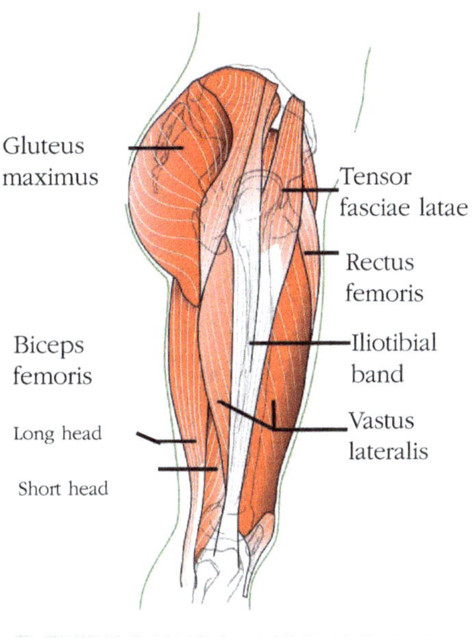

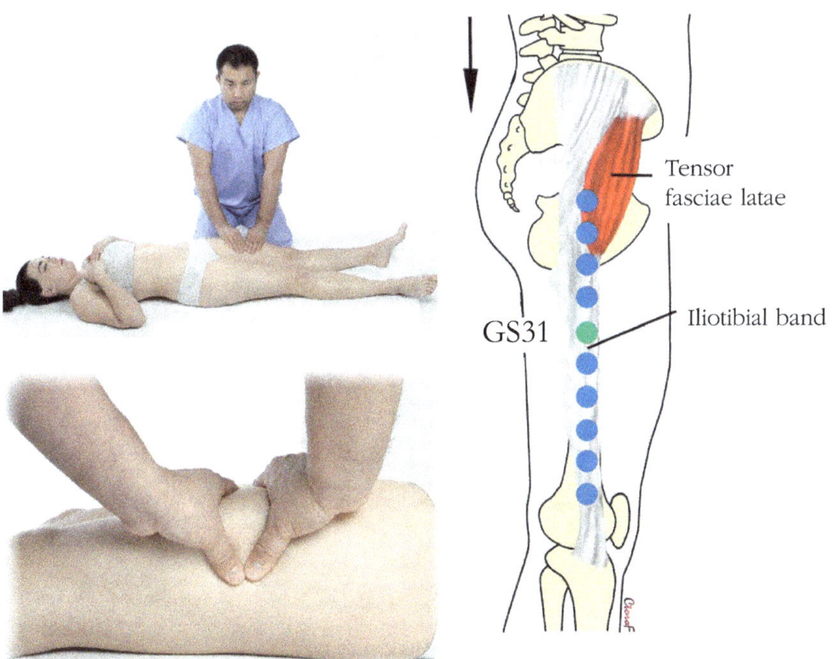

1.12. LATERAL TIBIA REGION

PATIENT'S POSTURE: Supine. Arms straight along the body or crossed over the chest.

THERAPIST'S POSITION: Seiza, perpendicular to the area.

TYPE OF PRESSURE: Thumb over thumb in a V shape (left below on the left side).

Nº. OF POINTS: An eight-point line.

DIRECTION OF THE LINE: Along the anterior tibial muscle; from the lateral condyle of the knee to the ankle.

OBSERVATIONS: The first point corresponds to key point S36 (Sanri) and is located about three centimetres diagonally below the tibial tuberosity and below the lateral condyle of the tibia. It is called Sanri, and is used to relieve general pain or discomfort in the body. With this point we stimulate endorphin secretion, producing a sense of well-being.

First point: Three times for five seconds.
Remaining points: Three times for three seconds.

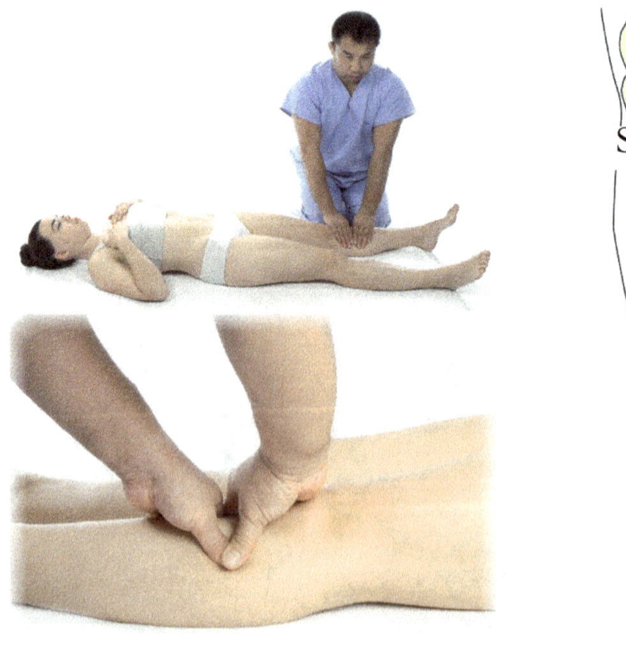

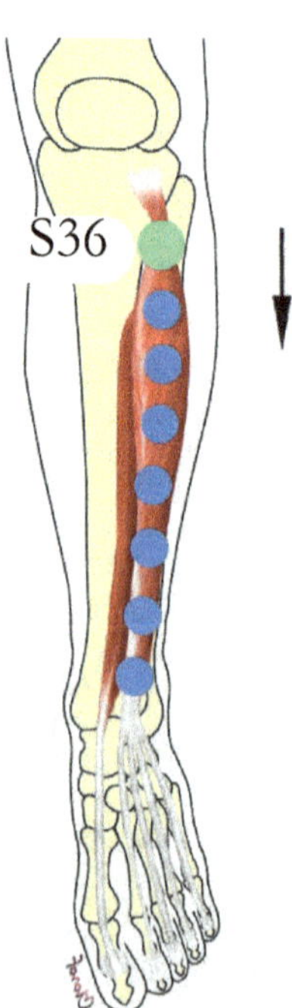

1.13. LATERAL FIBULA REGION

PATIENT'S POSTURE: Supine. Arms straight along the body or crossed over the chest.

THERAPIST'S POSITION: Seiza, perpendicular to the area.

TYPE OF PRESSURE: Thumb over thumb in a V shape (left below on the left side).

Nº. OF POINTS: An eight-point line.

DIRECTION OF THE LINE: From the postero-inferior depression of the fibula head to the lateral malleolus along the posterior edge of the peroneus.

OBSERVATIONS: Working on the peroneal muscles works the gall-bladder meridian which runs along it. Although traditional medicine locates key point **GB34 (Youryousen)** in the antero-inferior depression of the fibula head, Aze Shiatsu locates it at the first point of this region. It's a suitable point for tendon problems.

Three times for three seconds.

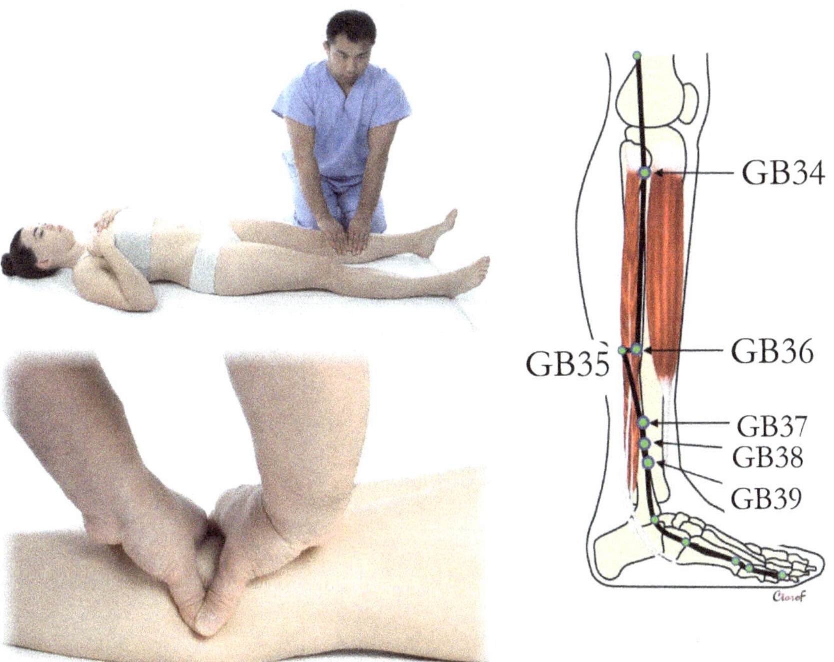

1.14. TARSAL REGION

PATIENT'S POSTURE: Supine. Arms straight along the body or crossed over the chest.

THERAPIST'S POSITION: Seiza, perpendicular to the area.

TYPE OF PRESSURE: One thumb (right on the left side). The other hand flexes the foot and rotates the ankle internally to ease the work.

Nº. OF POINTS: A five-point line.

DIRECTION OF THE LINE: From the lateral to medial malleolus.

OBSERVATIONS: The central point is a very important point for various treatments such as ankle sprain. It corresponds to key point S41 (Kaikei).

Three times for three seconds.

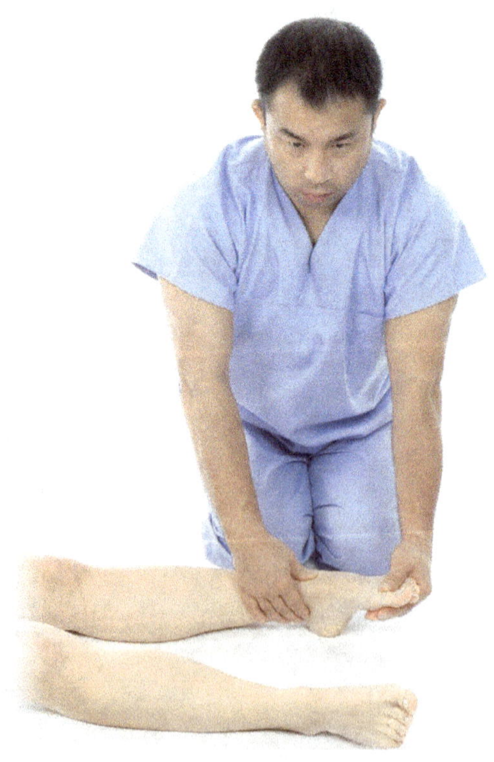

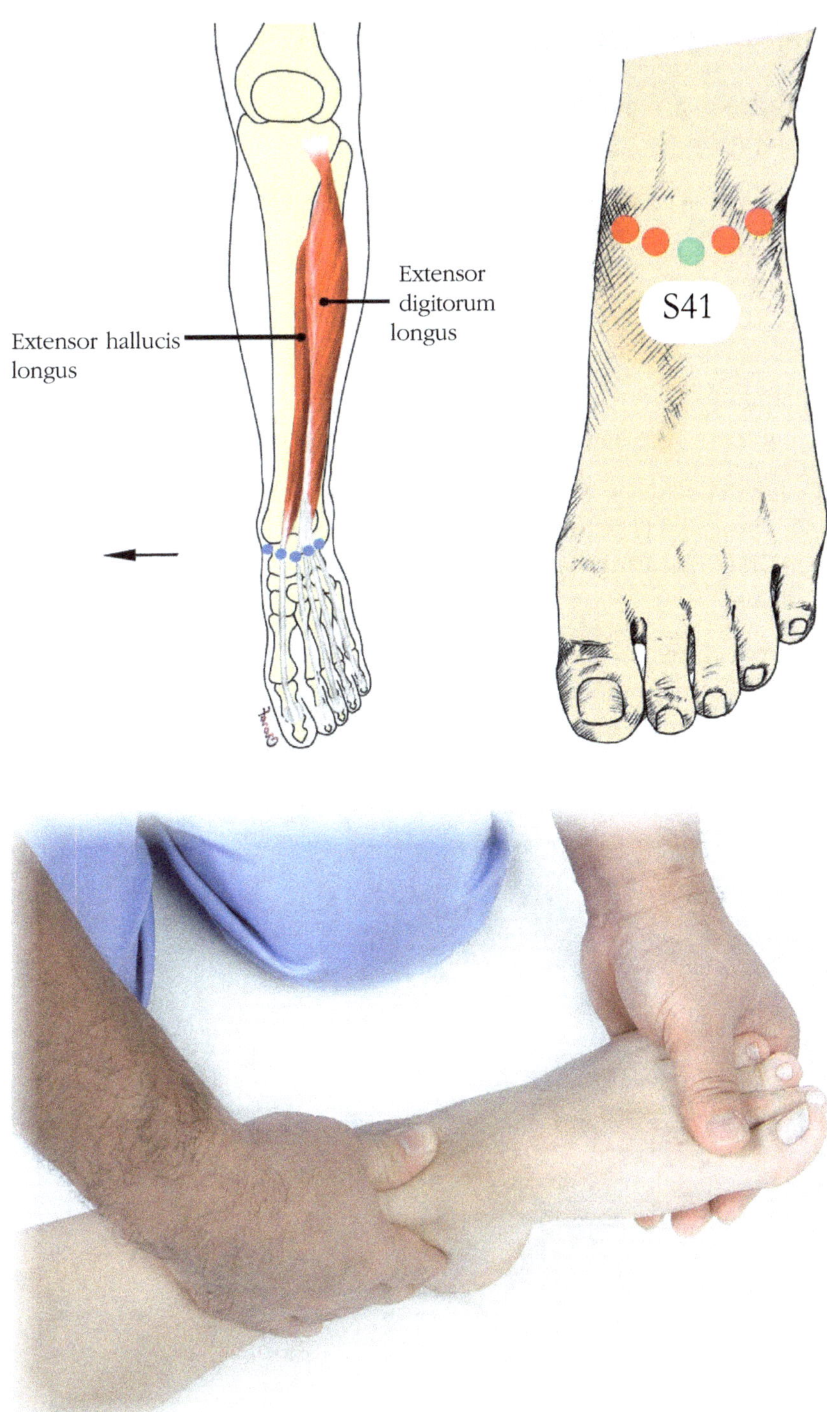

Extensor hallucis longus
Extensor digitorum longus
S41

1.15. DORSAL REGION OF THE FOOT

PATIENT'S POSTURE: Supine. Arms straight along the body or crossed over the chest.

THERAPIST'S POSITION: Seiza, perpendicular to the area.

TYPE OF PRESSURE: One thumb (right on the left side). The other hand flexes the foot and rotates the ankle internally to ease the work.

N°. OF POINTS: Four five-point lines.

DIRECTION OF THE LINE: Between the metatarsal channels; from the big toe to the little one and from the toes to the tarsal bones.

OBSERVATIONS: The fourth point of the first channel corresponds to key point L3 (Taishou). And the fourth of the fourth channel to key point GB41 (Ashirinkyuu). Both are very important for treating lumbar problems.

Three times for three seconds.

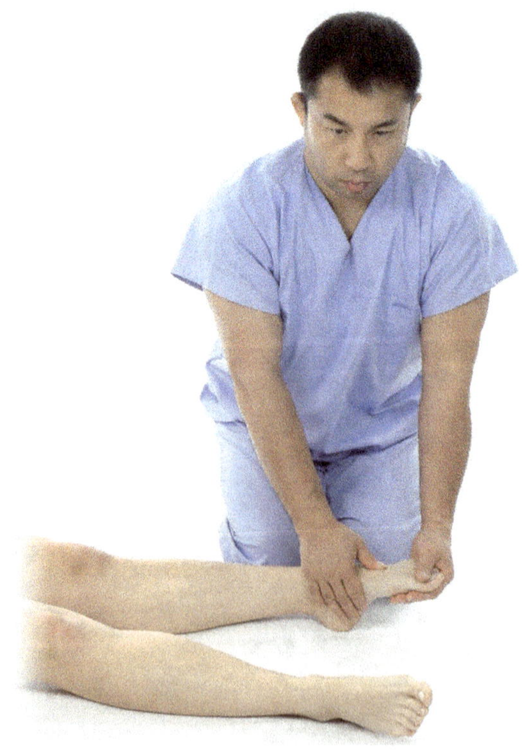

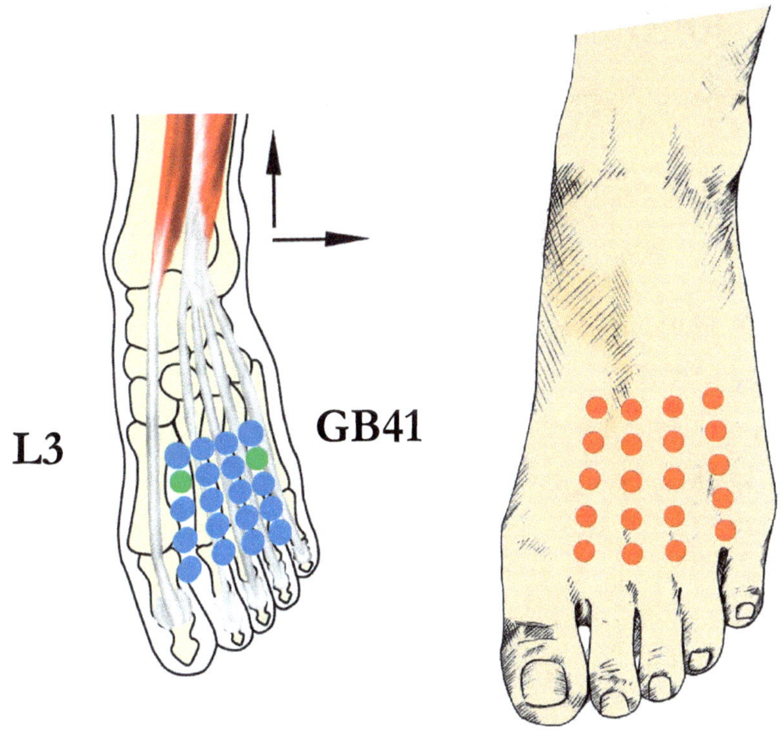
L3
GB41

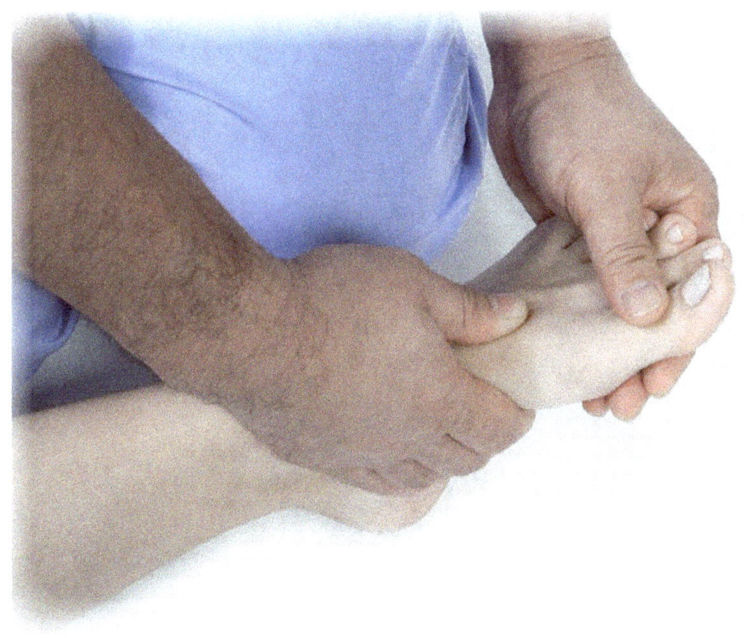

1.16. ROTATING AND EXTENDING THE TOES

PATIENT'S POSTURE: Supine. Arms straight along the body or crossed over the chest.

THERAPIST'S POSITION: Seiza, perpendicular to the area.

TYPE OF PRESSURE: Rotating and light extension. The left hand (on the left side) does the work. The other hand holds the foot to concentrate the movement on the toes.

DIRECTION OF THE LINE: From the big to the little toe.

OBSERVATIONS: After each toe rotation, they are extended.

Five rotations per direction and toe.

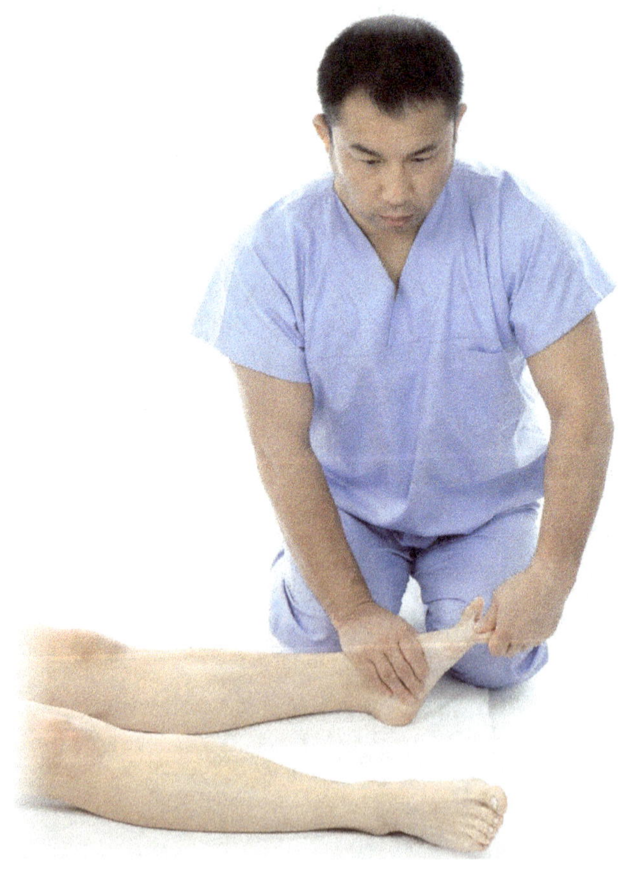

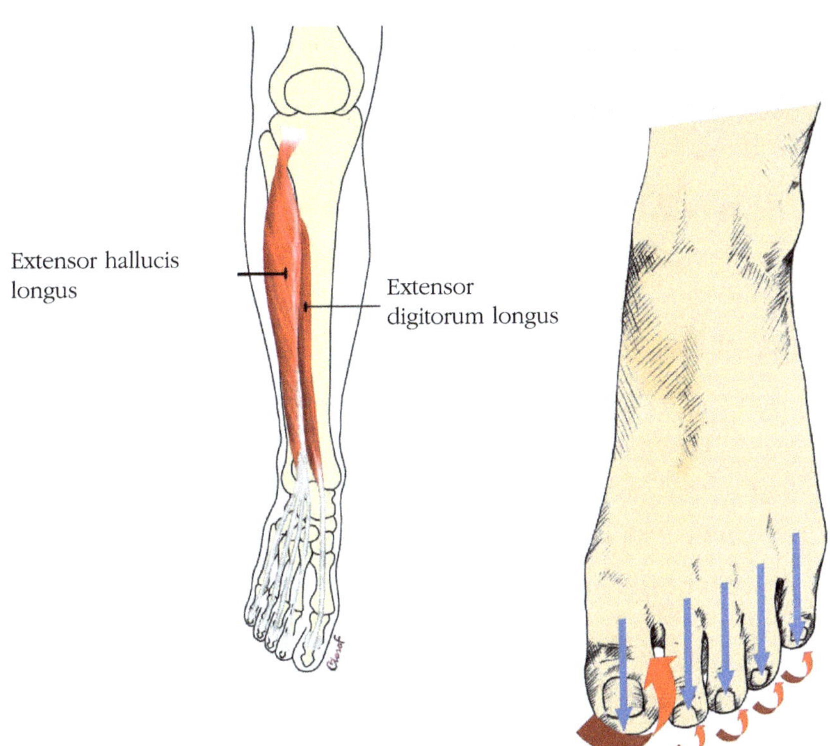

Extensor hallucis
longus
Extensor
digitorum longus

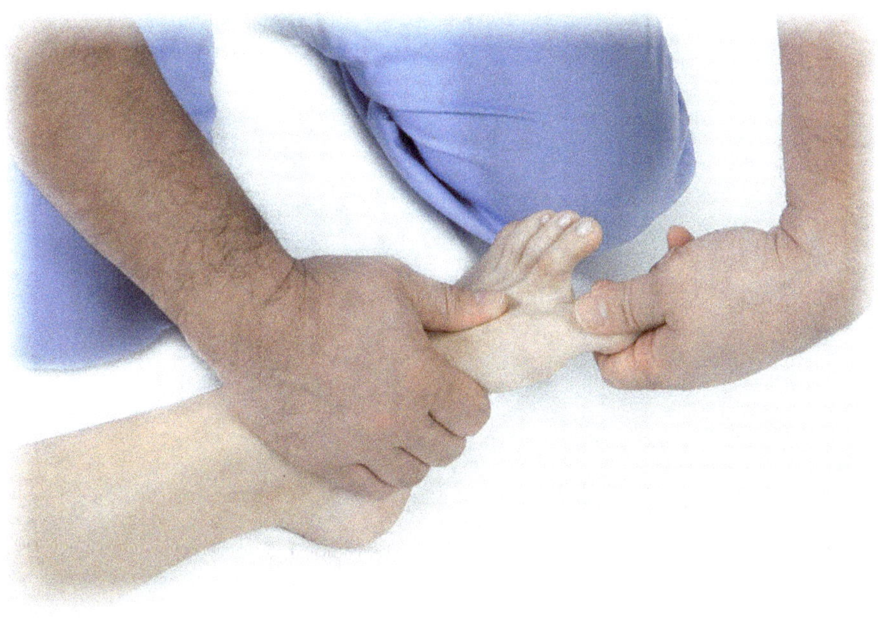

1.17. DIGITAL REGION OF THE FOOT

PATIENT'S POSTURE: Supine. Arms straight along the body or crossed over the chest.

THERAPIST'S POSITION: Seiza, perpendicular to the area.

TYPE OF PRESSURE: The far hand does the work while the other holds the patient's foot.

Nº. OF POINTS: Five five-point lines.

DIRECTION OF THE LINE: From the big to the little toe. From the metatarsus to the nails.

OBSERVATIONS: Apply pressure on the first four points of each toe. Pressure and light traction on the last.

Once for three seconds.

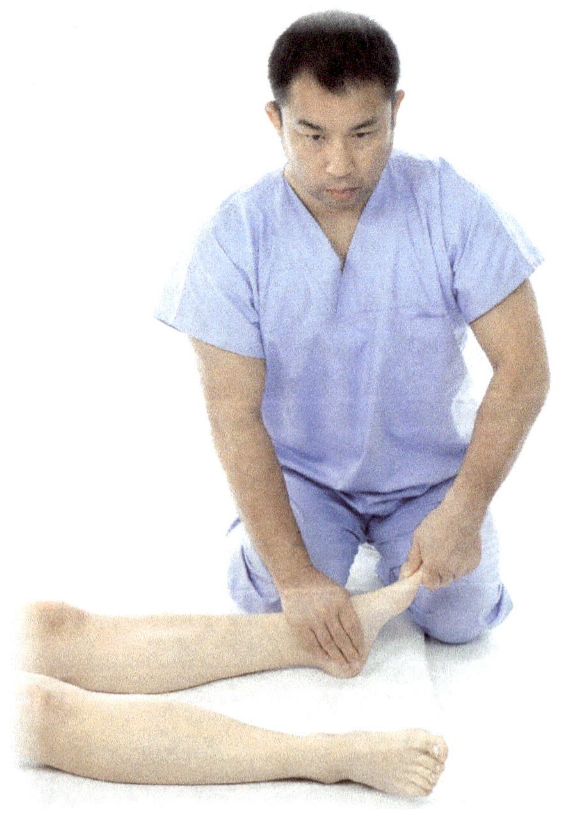

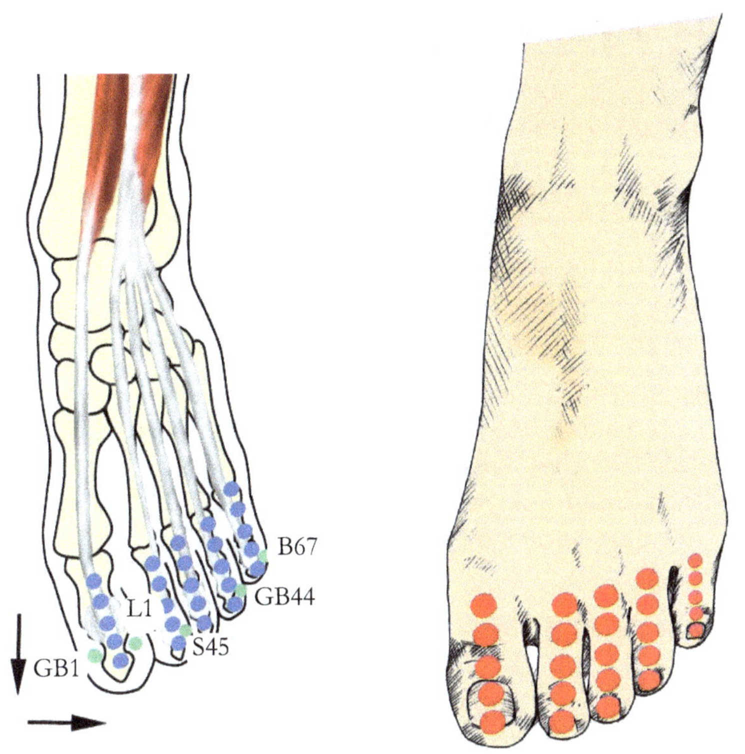

B67
GB44
L1
S45
GB1

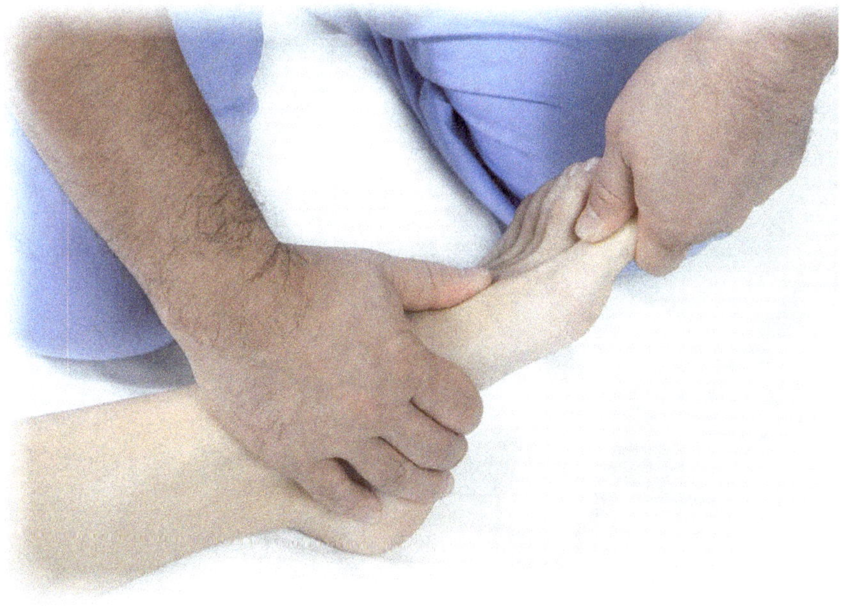

1.18. ROCKING MOVEMENTS

PATIENT'S POSTURE: Supine. Arms straight along the body or crossed over the chest.

THERAPIST'S POSITION: Seiza, perpendicular to the area.

TYPE OF PRESSURE: Rocking back and forth. The right hand (on the left side) locks the ankle, while the other hand is placed cap-shaped over the toes and performs a fast and rhythmic dorsiflexion movement.

OBSERVATIONS: This exercise stimulates the key points located at the top end of the toes. They are as follows: *B67* (Shiin, external nail angle of the little toe), *GB44* (Ashikyouin, external angle of the fourth toenail), *S45* (Reida, external angle of the second toenail), *L1* (Daiton, external angle of the first toenail) and *GB1* (Inpaku, internal angle of the big toenail).

Ten seconds.

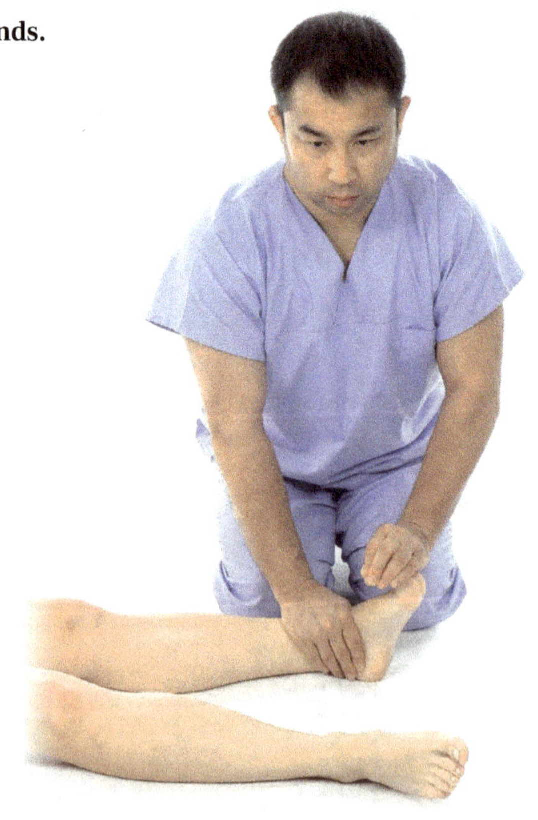

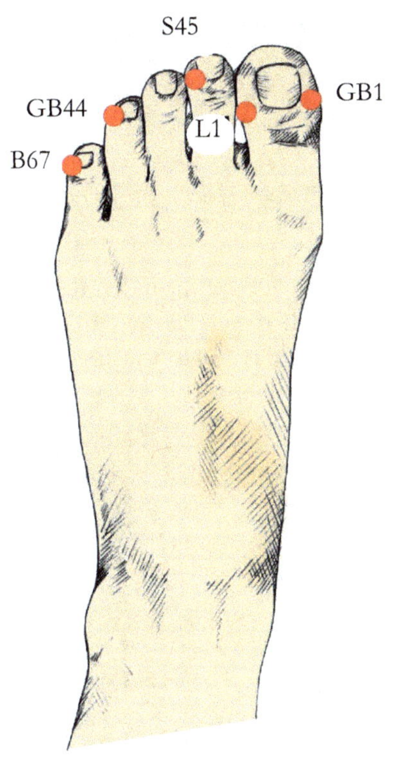

S45
GB44
B67
L1
GB1

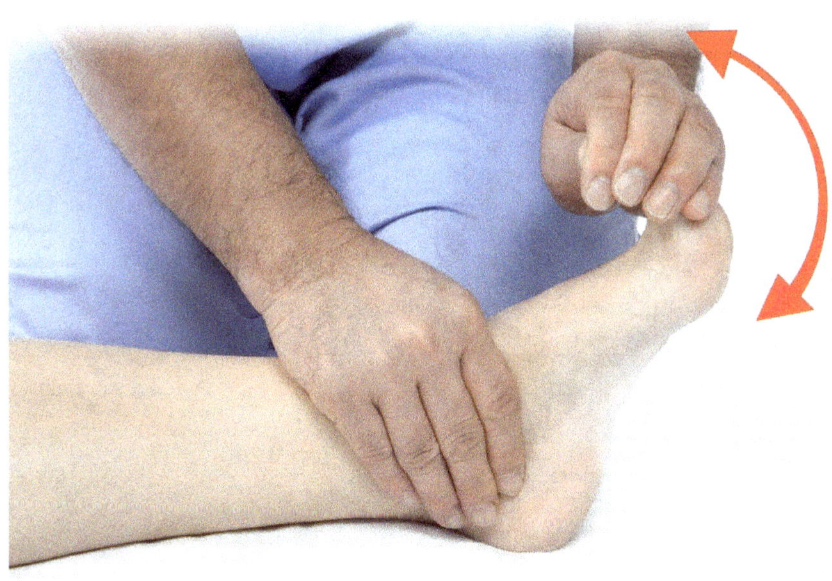

1.19. ELONGATING THE ACHILLES TENDON

PATIENT'S POSTURE: Supine. Arms straight along the body or crossed over the chest.

THERAPIST'S POSITION: Seiza or kneeling, perpendicular to the area.

TYPE OF PRESSURE: The left arm (on the left side) performs a dorsiflexion of the foot with the forearm while holding by the calcaneal bone. The other hand holds the leg to prevent it from rising in order to focus the work on the calcaneal tendon.

Three times for five

seconds.

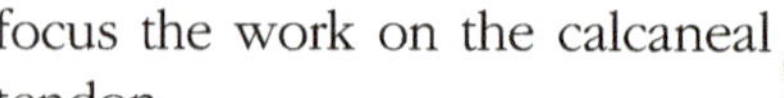

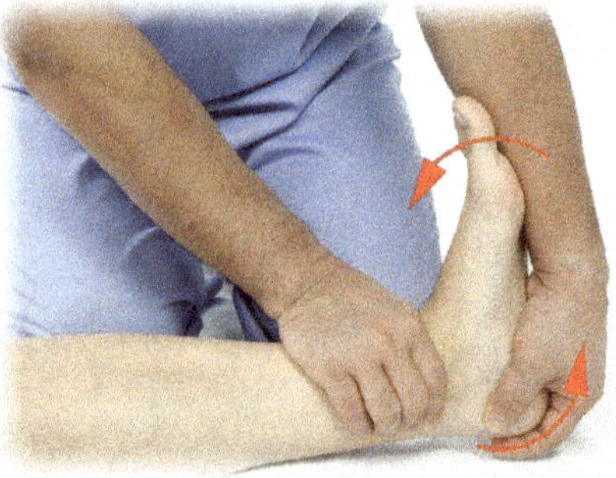

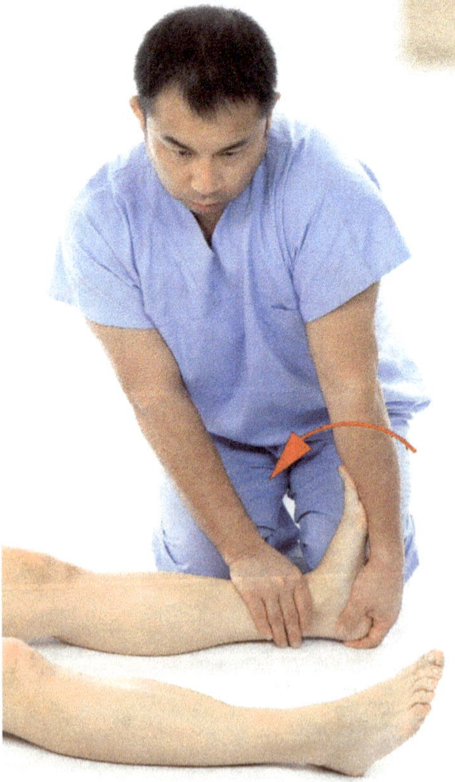

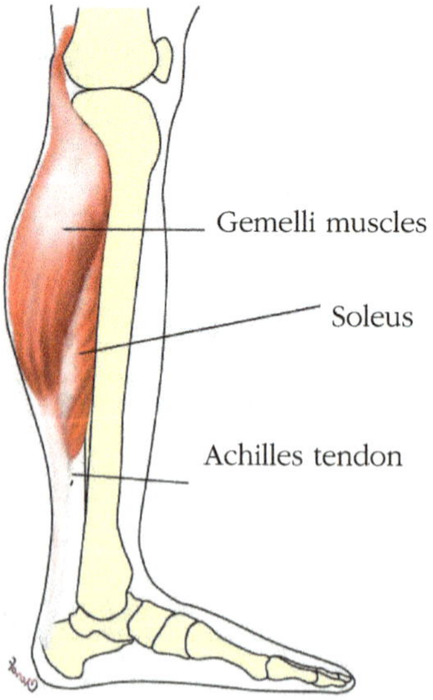

1.20. LEG STRETCH WITH VIBRATION

PATIENT'S POSTURE: Supine. Arms straight along the body or crossed over the chest.

THERAPIST'S POSITION: Seiza, facing the patient's feet.

TYPE OF HANDLING: Perform traction from the patient's foot, concentrating the action on the hand holding the heel. This helps the exercise be carried better to the rest of the leg joints. When performing the third repetition, combine the traction with a slight vibration.

OBSERVATIONS: This exercise can be performed in two different directions by varying the angle the leg is opened. First, directing the exercise towards the opposite shoulder in aspa form. Second, directing the exercise towards the lumbar muscle on the same side.

Three times.
Stretch, first and second time.
Third time, vibration.

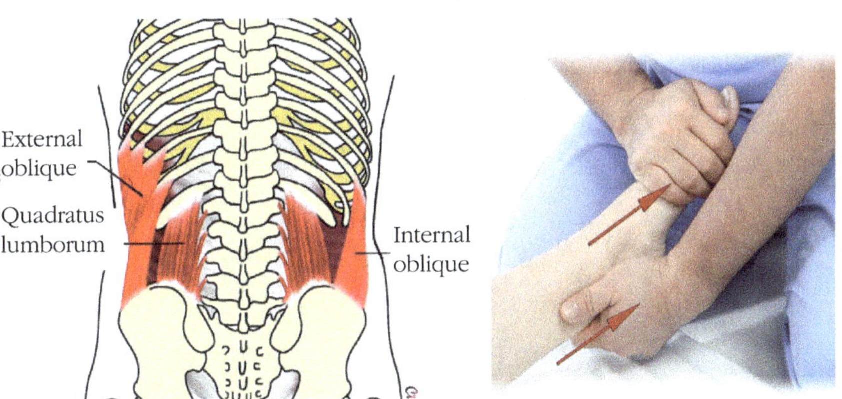

Repeat the lower limb routine on the RIGHT LEG.

2. Head and face

2.1. Parietal region. Central line.

2.2. Parietal region. Lateral lines.

2.3. GV20.

2.4. Frontal region.

2.5. Superior orbital region.

2.6. Inferior orbital region.

2.7. Nasal region.

2.8. Zygomatic region.

2.9. Superior maxillary region.

2.10. Inferior maxillary region.

2.11. Three important points.

2.12. Temple Region. One side.

2.13. Ear region. One side.

2.14. Covering the eyes.

2.15. Covering the face.

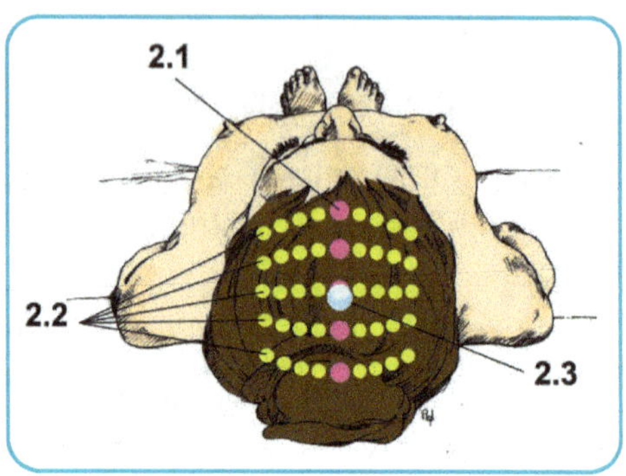

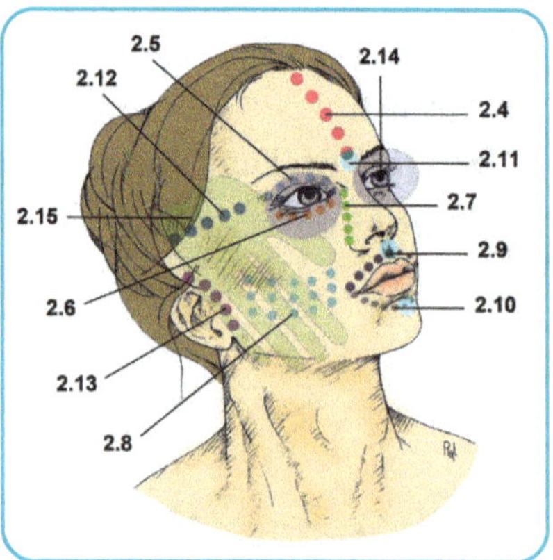

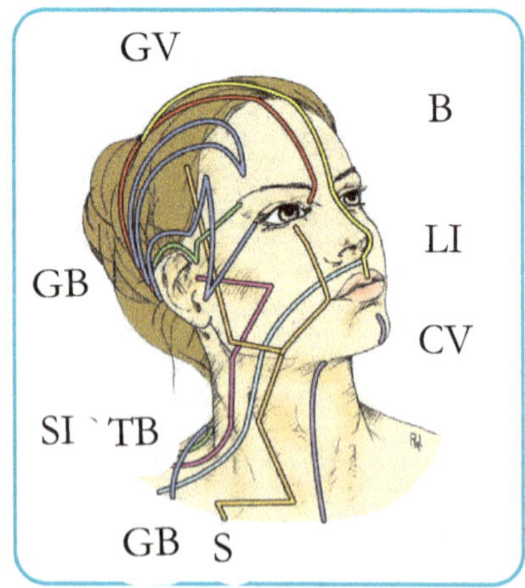

2. TO KEEP IN MIND, HEAD AND FACE

PATIENT'S POSTURE: Supine. Ideally arms straight along the body or crossed over the chest.

THERAPIST'S POSITION: Seiza. Facing the area, above the head.

This position will be the same for all regions.

OBSERVATIONS: The head and face are one of the areas that reflects more tension more clearly. Shiatsu can help relieve stress and relax the patient's expression.

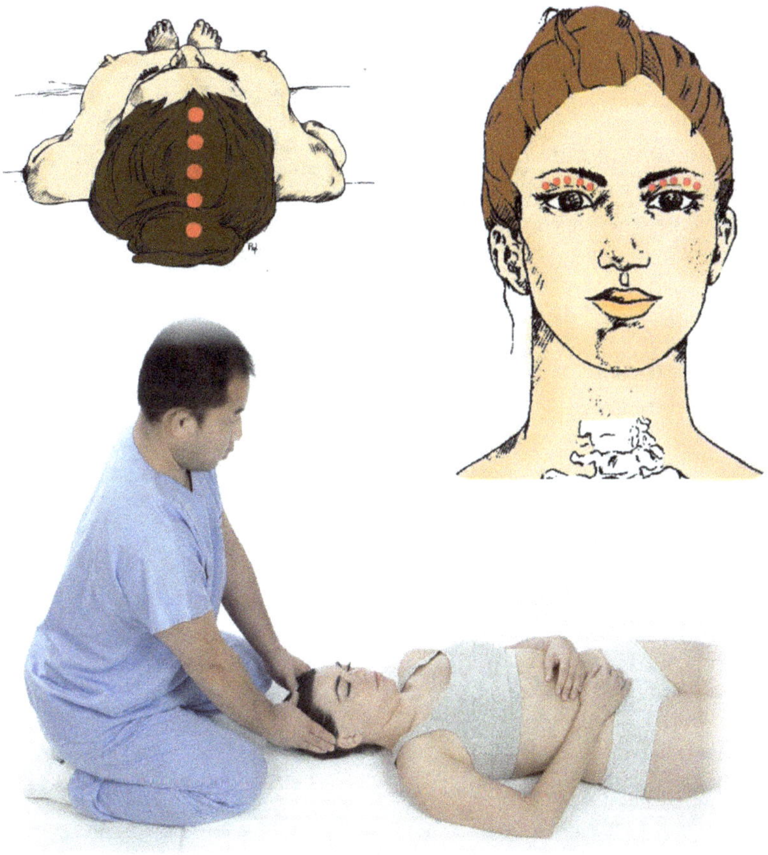

2.1. PARIETAL REGION. CENTRAL LINE

PATIENT'S POSTURE: Supine.

THERAPIST'S POSITION: Seiza.

TYPE OF PRESSURE: Thumb over thumb (right one below). The rest of the fingers hold the head by the temporal area.

Nº. OF POINTS: A five-point line.

DIRECTION OF THE LINE: From the hair line to the crown.

OBSERVATIONS: The head must be held by the hands while pressure is applied by the fingers; it is a fan movement with the middle fingers as a pivot point. On the tatami it is better not to get too low so as to mainatin the therapist's position of balance.

The central parietal region in turn coincides with the passage of the GV meridian.

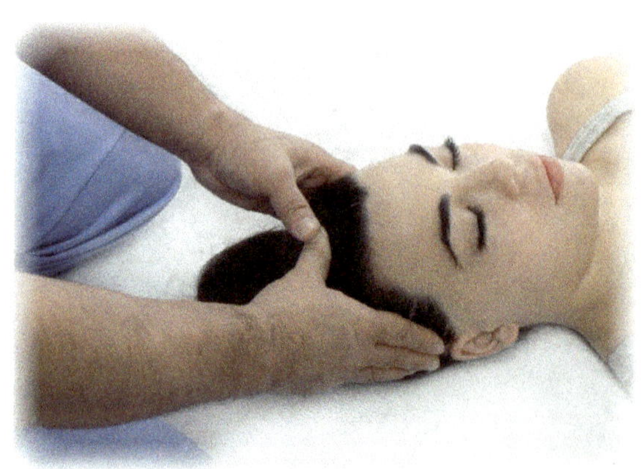

Three times for three seconds.

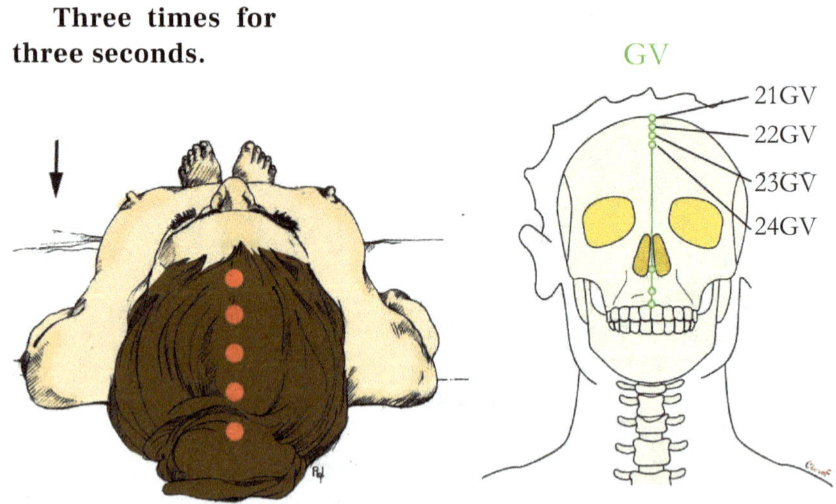

176

2.2. PARIETAL REGION. LATERAL LINES

PATIENT'S POSTURE: Supine.

THERAPIST'S POSITION: Seiza.

TYPE OF PRESSURE: With both thumbs running along both parietals laterally.

Nº. OF POINTS: Five five-point lines.

DIRECTION OF THE LINE: From the hair line to the crown. Always starting from the central line laterally.

Three times for two seconds.

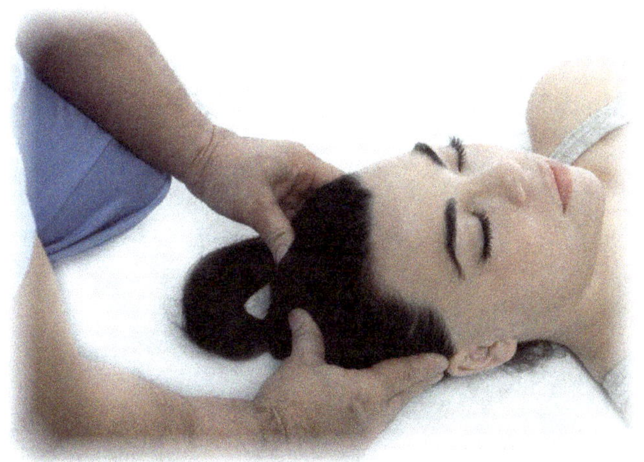

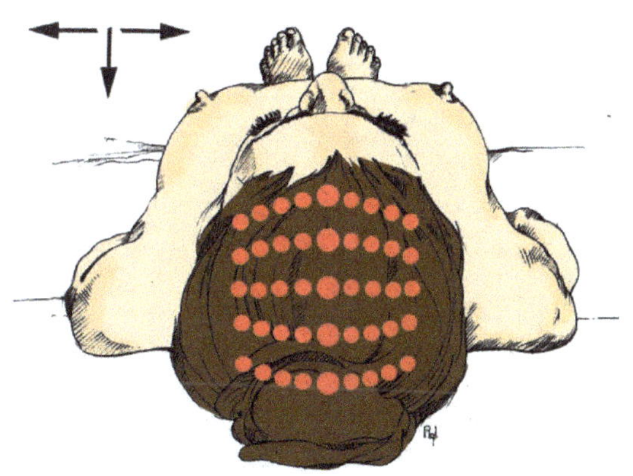

2.3. GV20

PATIENT'S POSTURE: Supine.

THERAPIST'S POSITION: Seiza.

TYPE OF PRESSURE: Thumb over thumb (right one below).

Nº. OF POINTS: One.

LOCATION OF THE POINT: Approximately between the third and fourth points of the parietal region central line. Pressure is applied towards the patient's feet.

OBSERVATIONS: If properly worked, this point *GV20 (Hyakue)* is very effective in treating hemorrhoids and acute lumbalgia.

Three times for five seconds.

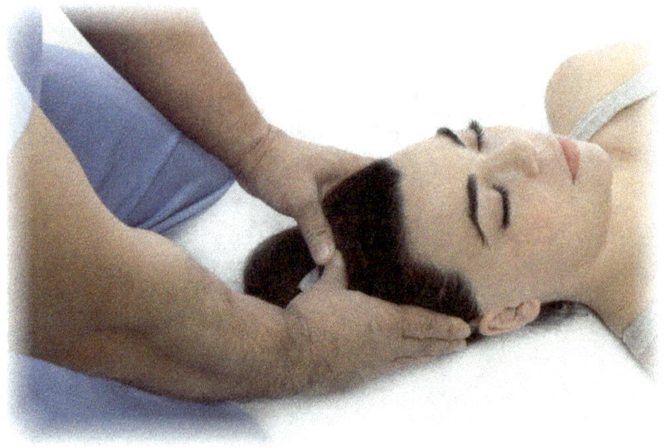

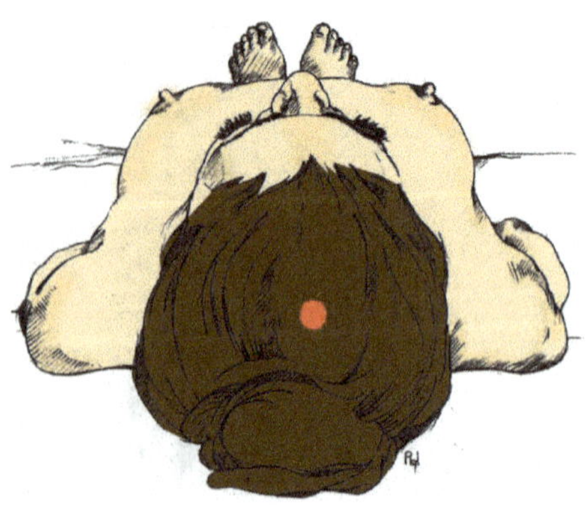

2.4. FRONTAL REGION

PATIENT'S POSTURE: Supine.

THERAPIST'S POSITION: Seiza.

TYPE OF PRESSURE: Thumb over thumb (right one below).

Nº. OF POINTS: A five-point line.

DIRECTION OF THE LINE: From between the eyebrows to the hair line.

Three times for three seconds.

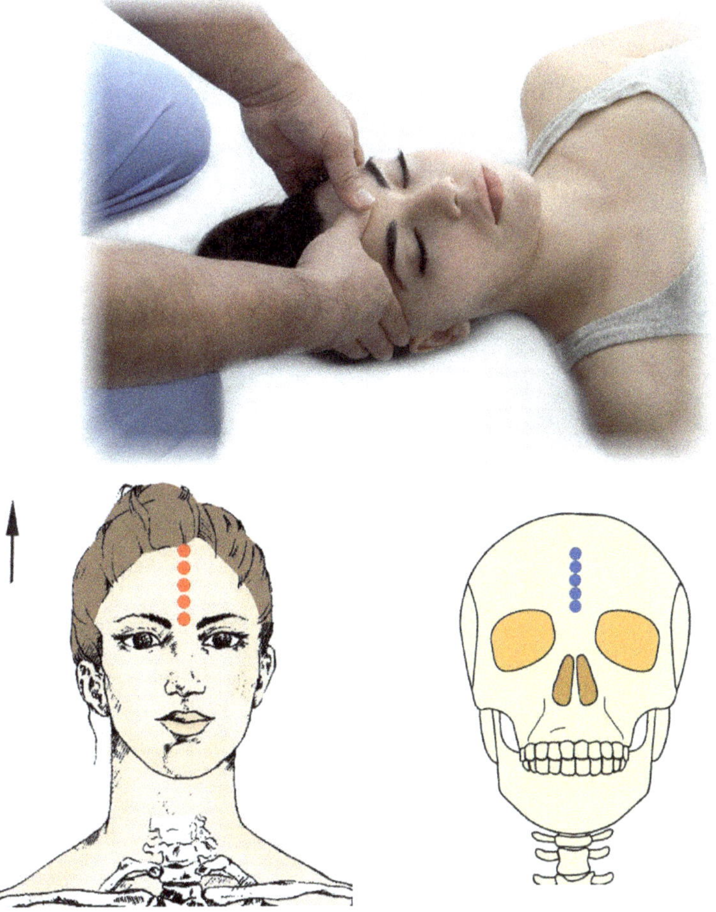

2.5. SUPERIOR ORBITAL REGION

PATIENT'S POSTURE: Supine.

THERAPIST'S POSITION: Seiza.

TYPE OF PRESSURE: Pressure with the index, middle and ring fingers of each hand. The index finger applies pressure to the first point.

N°. OF POINTS: Two five-point lines.

DIRECTION OF THE LINE: Along the supraorbital edge from the nasal region to the ears. Be careful not to press the eyeball. The direction of the pressure will be towards point **GB20 (Fuuchi)**, located on the occipital edge.

OBSERVATIONS: The first point coincides with **B2 (Sanchiku)** and pressure is applied longer.

First point: Three times for five seconds.

The rest: Three times for three seconds.

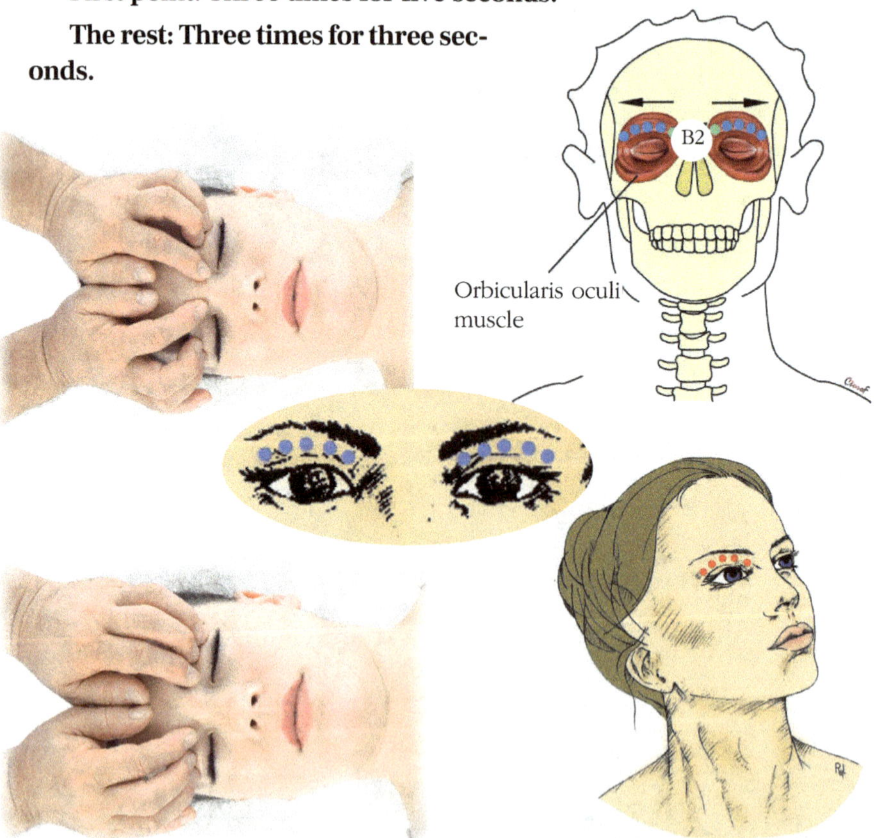

2.6. INFERIOR ORBITAL REGION

PATIENT'S POSTURE: Supine.

THERAPIST'S POSITION: Seiza.

TYPE OF PRESSURE: With both thumbs on each side.

N°. OF POINTS: Two five-point lines.

DIRECTION OF THE LINE: Along the infraorbitary edge from the inside outwards (from the nasal region to the ears).

OBSERVATIONS: The pressure is directed towards the rachidian bulb. Work on this region relieves eye fatigue and helps eliminate dark circles.

Key point S1 (Syoukyuu) is located at the third point.

Three times for three seconds.

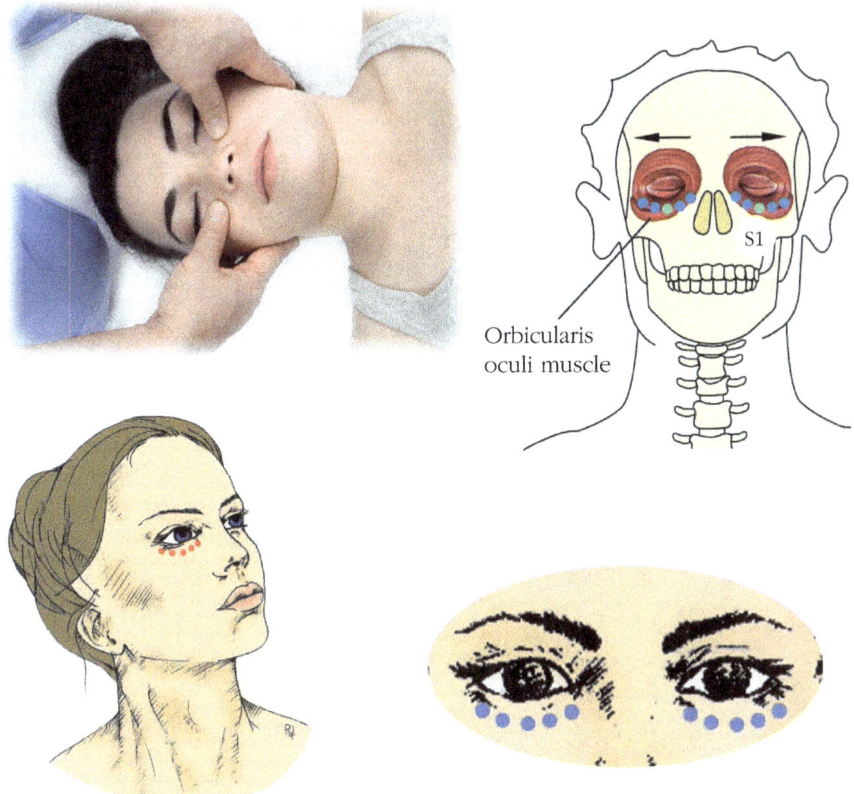

2.7. NASAL REGION

PATIENT'S POSTURE: Supine.

THERAPIST'S POSITION: Seiza.

TYPE OF PRESSURE: Middle finger over the index of each hand.

Nº. OF POINTS: Two five-point lines.

DIRECTION OF THE LINE: From the lower area of the corner of the eyes towards the upper jaw.

OBSERVATIONS: The last point (LI20, Geikou) is indicated for treating sinusitis and nasal congestion. For the gum and upper tooth pain, pressure is applied towards the rachidian bulb.

Three times for three seconds. Last point for five seconds.

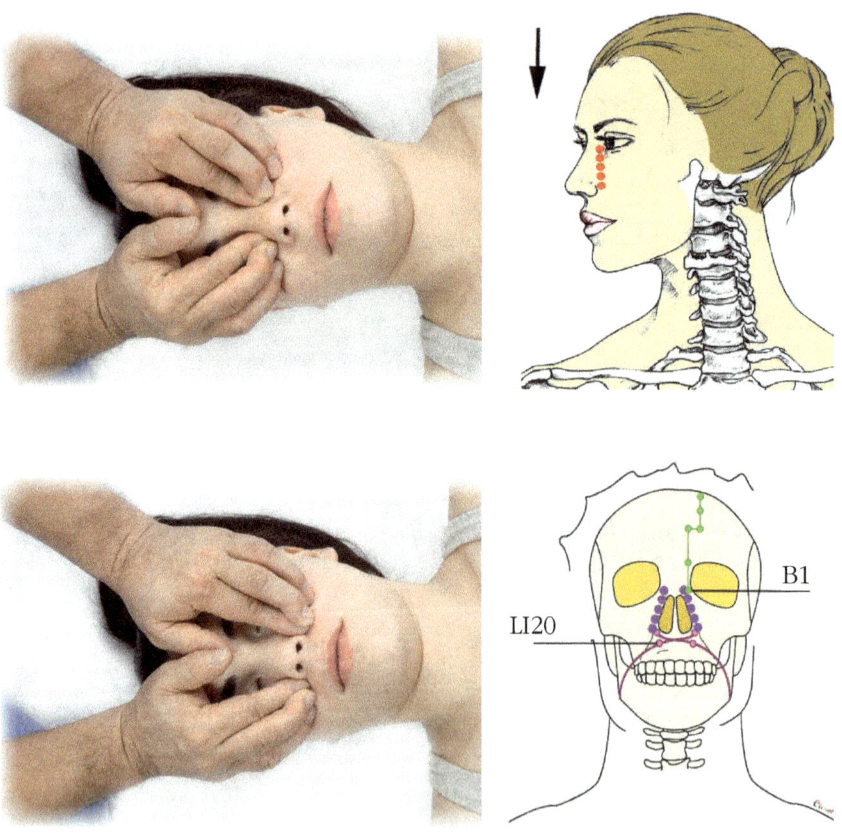

2.8. ZYGOMATIC REGION

PATIENT'S POSTURE: Supine.

THERAPIST'S POSITION: Seiza.

TYPE OF PRESSURE: With the fingertips of the index, middle and ring fingers.

Nº. OF POINTS: Three five-point lines on each side.

DIRECTION OF THE LINE: Pressure is applied towards the therapist, laterally from the nose.

OBSERVATIONS: Traction towards the Atlas (C1). For treating upper tooth pain use points 1 to 3.

For treating the temporomandibular joint and trigeminal neuralgia, use points 4 and 5. In both cases, traction towards the Atlas (C1).

Three times for three seconds.

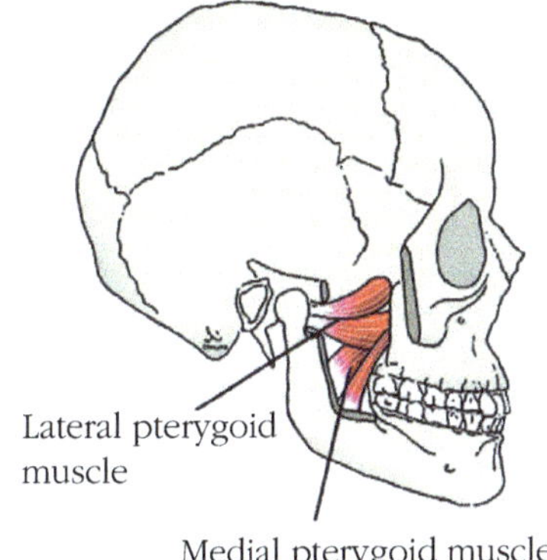

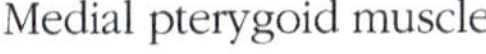

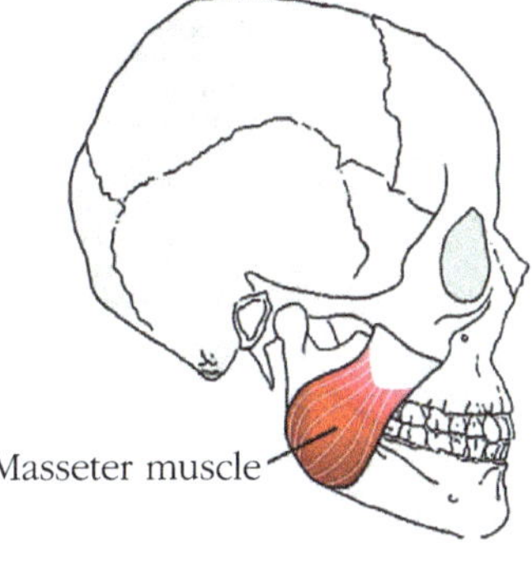

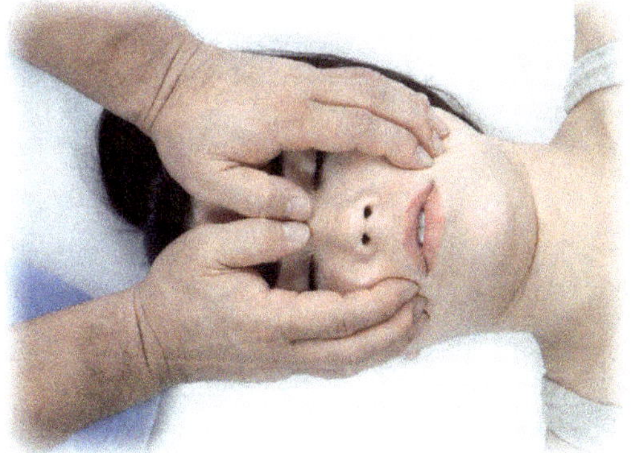

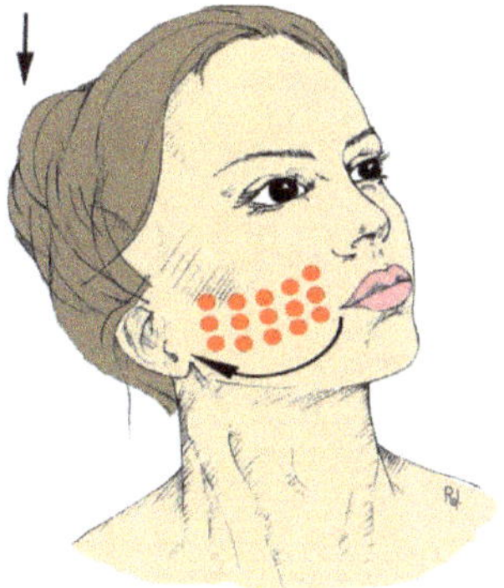

2.9. UPPER MAXILLARY REGION

PATIENT'S POSTURE: Supine.

THERAPIST'S POSITION: Seiza.

TYPE OF PRESSURE: With both thumbs opening laterally.

Nº. OF POINTS: Two five-point lines.

DIRECTION OF THE LINE: From the centre of the upper jaw laterally, perpendicular to the upper gum.

OBSERVATIONS: It is a very effective area for treating inflamed gums.

Three times for three seconds.

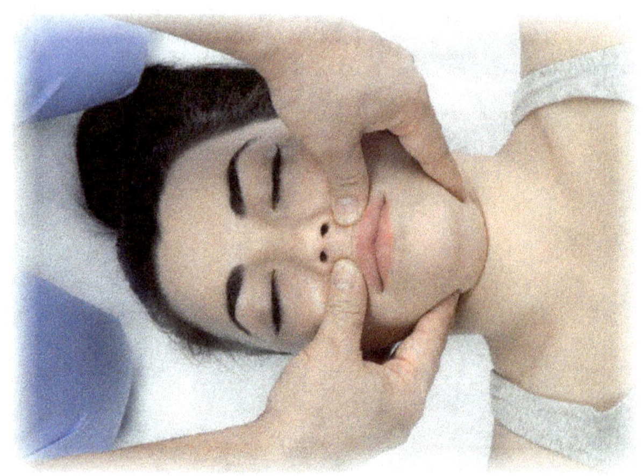

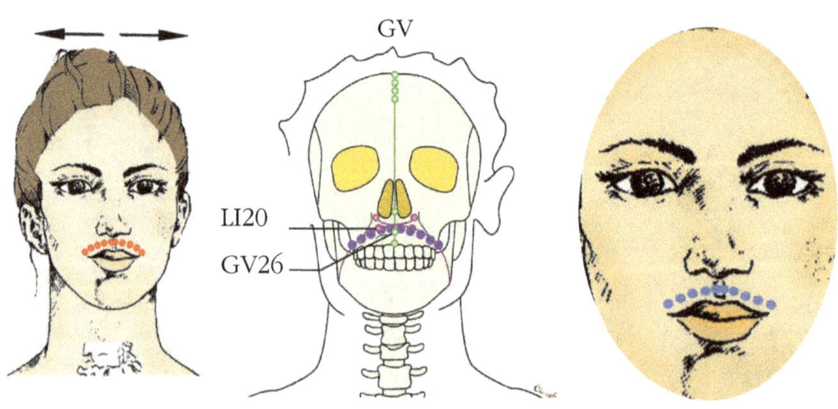

2.10. LOWER MAXILLARY REGION

PATIENT'S POSTURE: Supine.

THERAPIST'S POSITION: Seiza.

TYPE OF PRESSURE: With both thumbs opening laterally.

Nº. OF POINTS: Two five-point lines.

DIRECTION OF THE LINE: From the centre of the lower jaw laterally.

OBSERVATIONS: Work well perpendicularly to the lower gum. The mouth should not open; applying the proper pressure tends to close your mouth.

Three times for three seconds.

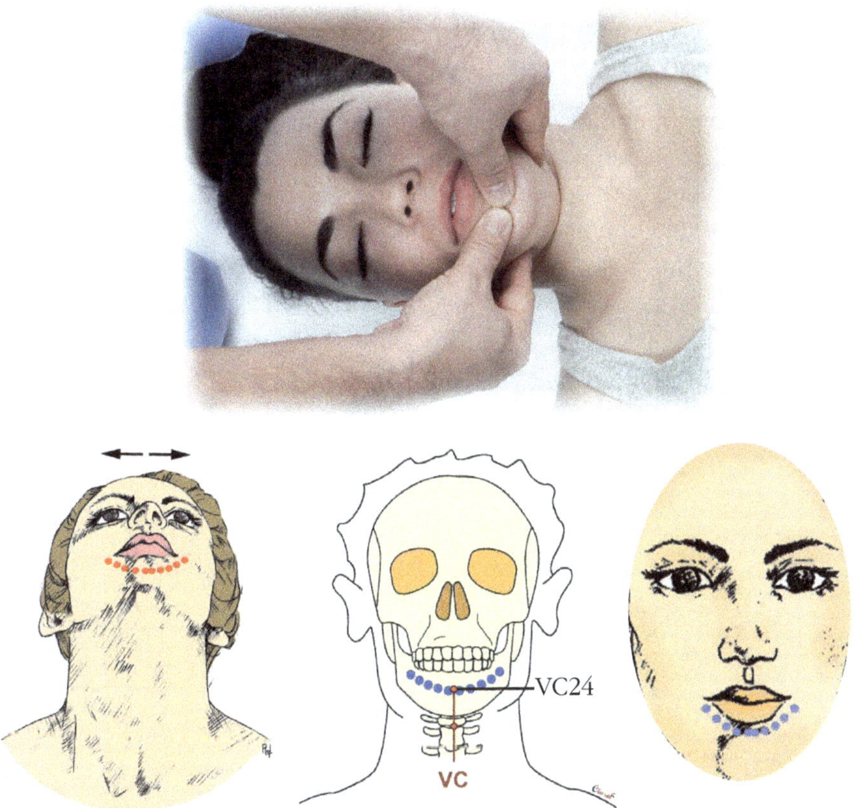

2.11. THREE IMPORTANT POINTS

PATIENT'S POSTURE: Supine.

THERAPIST'S POSITION: Seiza.

TYPE OF PRESSURE: Thumb over thumb (first point) and one single thumb (the rest).

N°. OF POINTS: Three.
1st: Between the eyebrows (Indou).
2nd: Nasolabial groove (GV26, Suikou).
3rd: Chin *(CV24, Syousyou)*.

DIRECTION OF THE PRESSURE: First point: Towards a point between crown and rachidian bulb.

Second point: Towards the rachidian bulb.

Third point: Towards where the C7-D1 vertebras join.

OBSERVATIONS: Point 1 is used for mental stress. Point 2, to recover from fainting. Point 3, to recover from low blood pressure and dizziness.

Keep your thumb on the first point throughout the routine applying light pressure. Highlights include point **GB14 (Youhaku)**, located 2 cun above the centre of the eyebrow. Used to balance the Autonomous Nervous System and eliminate mental stress.

Once for five seconds.

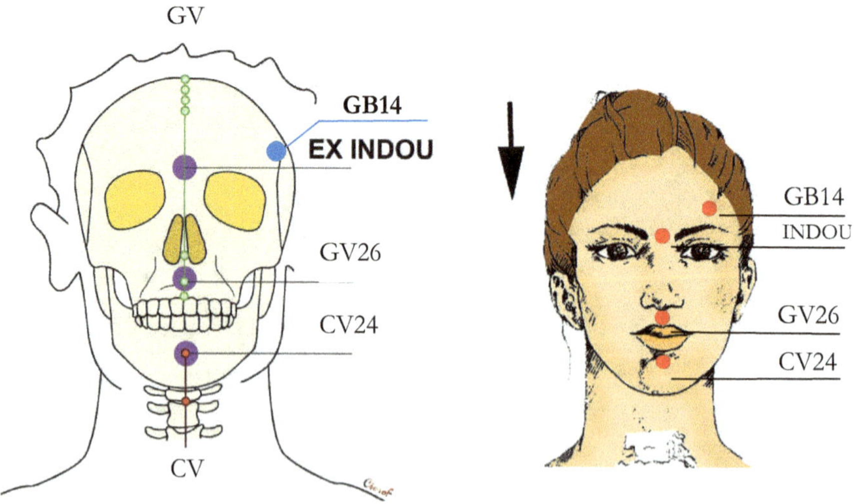

1. Between the eyebrows
   (InDou)

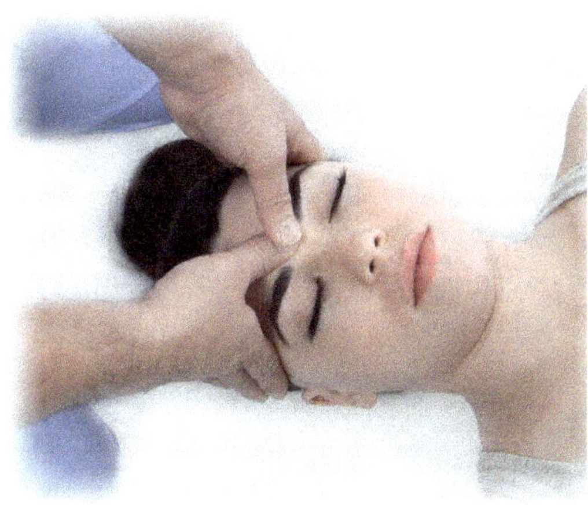

2. Nasolabial groove
(GV26)

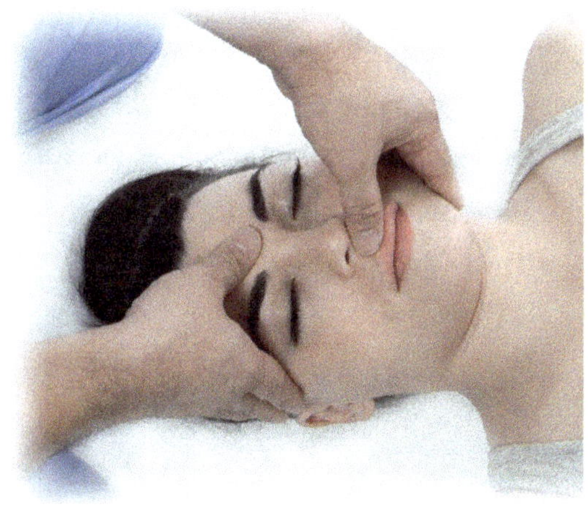

3. Chin (CV24)

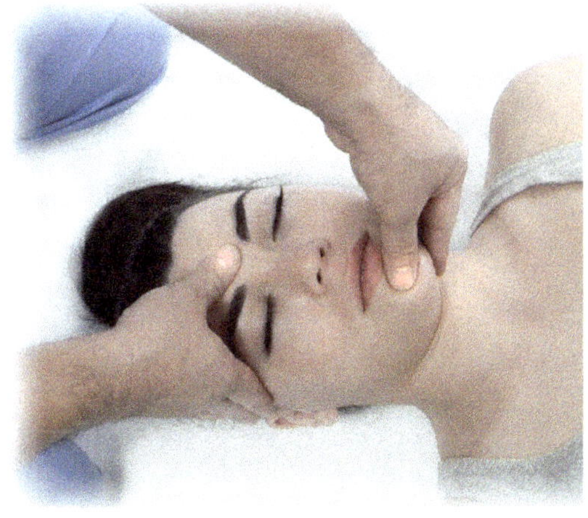

2.12. TEMPLE REGION. ONE SIDE

PATIENT'S POSTURE: Supine, head turned.

THERAPIST'S POSITION: Seiza.

TYPE OF PRESSURE: One thumb (left on the left side). The other hand supports the patient's head from the opposite occipital and temporal regions.

Nº. OF POINTS: A five-point line.

DIRECTION OF THE LINE: The first point is located 1.5 cun from the side angle of the eye and the line is directed towards the ear. Pressure is applied towards the centre of the other hand's palm.

OBSERVATIONS: For treating headaches and mental stress.

Key point TB23 (Shichikukuu) is located at the first point; and the key point **Taiyou (Sun)** in the third. Both points are suitable for treating temporal headaches, eye fatigue, facial pains and nerve disorders.

First point, five seconds.

Three times for three seconds.

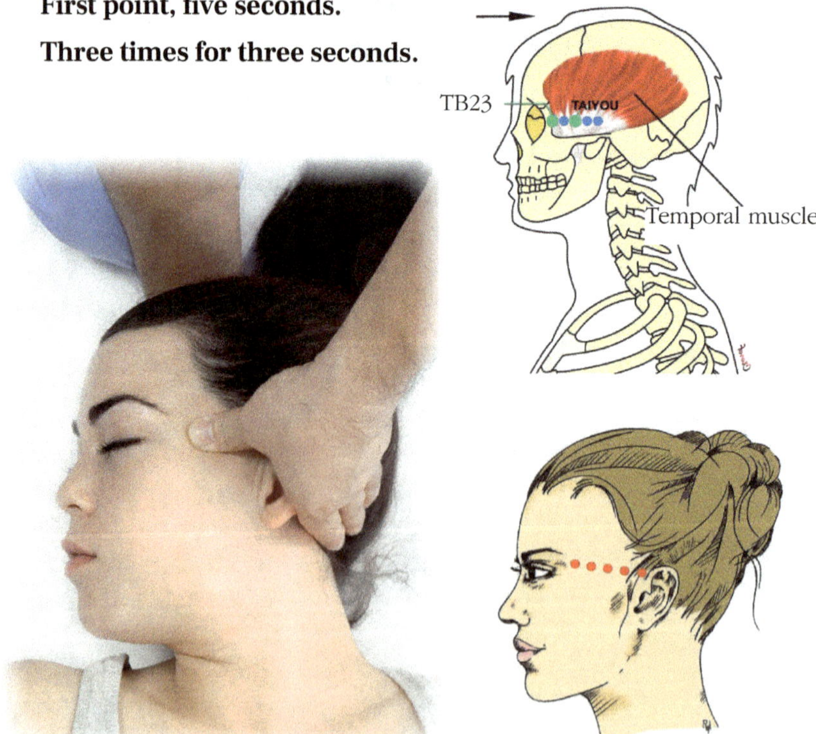

2.13. EAR REGION. ONE SIDE

PATIENT'S POSTURE: Supine, head turned.

THERAPIST'S POSITION: Seiza.

TYPE OF PRESSURE: One thumb (left on the left side). The other hand supports the patient's head.

Nº. OF POINTS: A five-point line.

DIRECTION OF THE LINE: From the ear lobe to the top.

OBSERVATIONS: Locate the hollows and areas of discomfort (Aze points) and work deeply: 2nd point GB2 (Choue), 3rd point SI19 (Choukyuu), 4th point TB21 (Jimon), 5th point TB22 (Waryou).

Three times for three seconds.

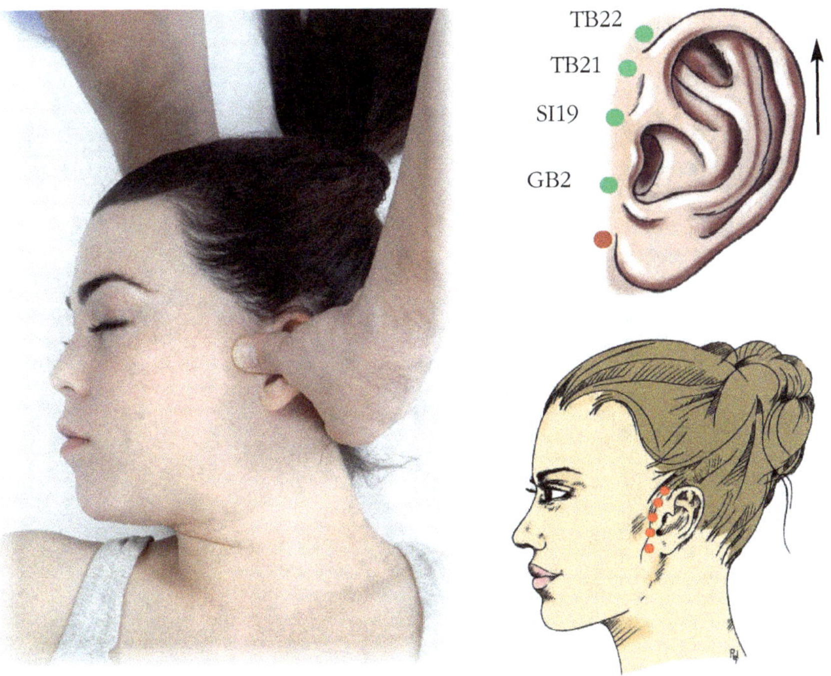

Repeat 2.12 and 2.13 on the RIGHT SIDE before proceeding.

2.14. COVERING THE EYES

PATIENT'S POSTURE: Supine.

THERAPIST'S POSITION: Seiza.

TYPE OF PRESSURE: Both hands rest over the patient's eyeballs.

OBSERVATIONS: Do not exceed the recommended time for this exercise; due to the Aschner phenomenon, it can cause the patient to faint. The gentle and persistent pressure applied to the eyeballs stimulates the endings of the trigeminal nerve, located behind them. This, in turn, through a reflective effect on the vagus nerve's central body causes a vasovagal response that reduces the pulse and decreases blood pressure.

Once for ten seconds.

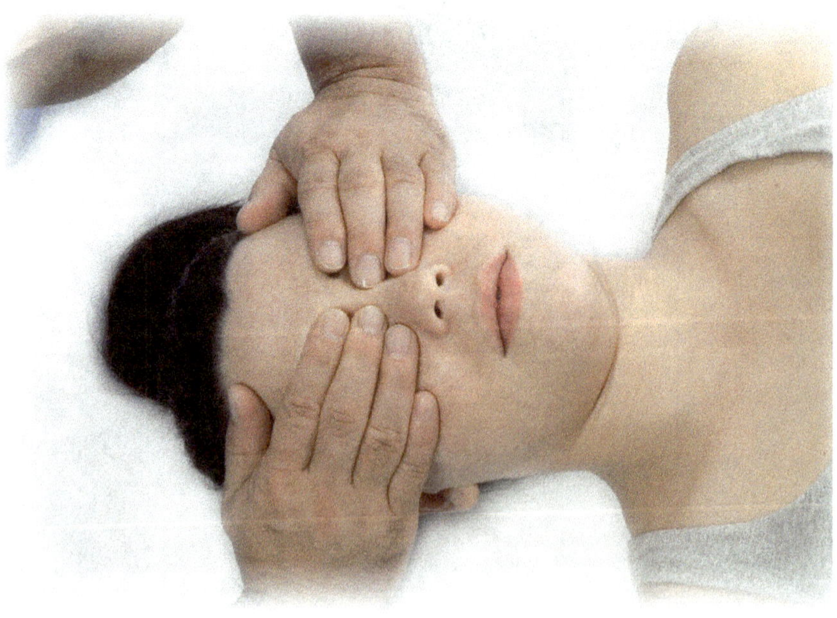

2.15. COVERING THE FACE

PATIENT'S POSTURE: Supine.

THERAPIST'S POSITION: Seiza.

TYPE OF PRESSURE: Both hands rest lightly over the patient's face.

After ten seconds, move them away from the face maintaining posture at the same time.

Once for twenty seconds.

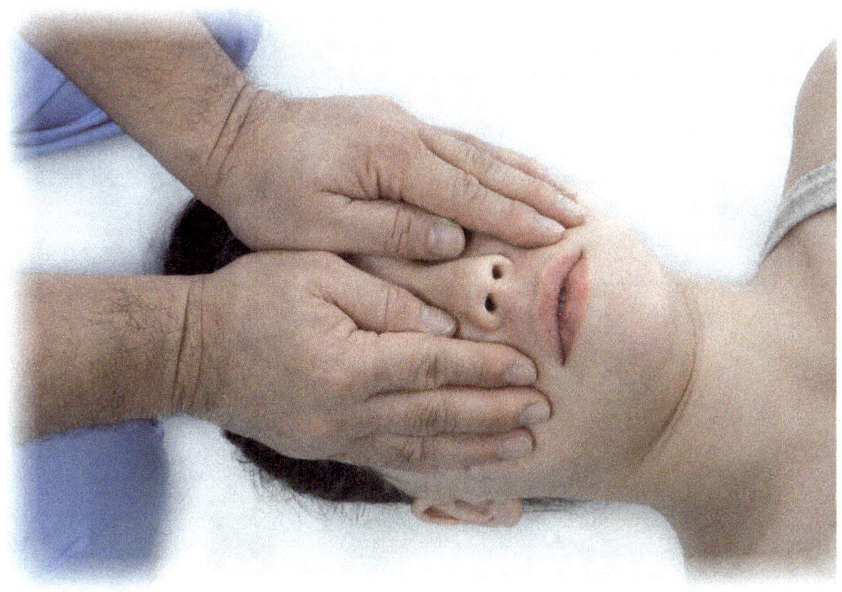

3. The Neck

3.1. Vertebra region. Traction.
3.2. Posterior cervical region. One side.
3.3. Lateral cervical region. One side.
3.4. Anterior cervical region. 1st line.
3.5. Anterior cervical region. 2nd line.
3.6. Occipital Region. One side.
3.7. Rachidian bulb region. Traction.
3.8. Base of neck region.
3.9. Suprascapular Region. Line.
3.10. Suprascapular region. Point.

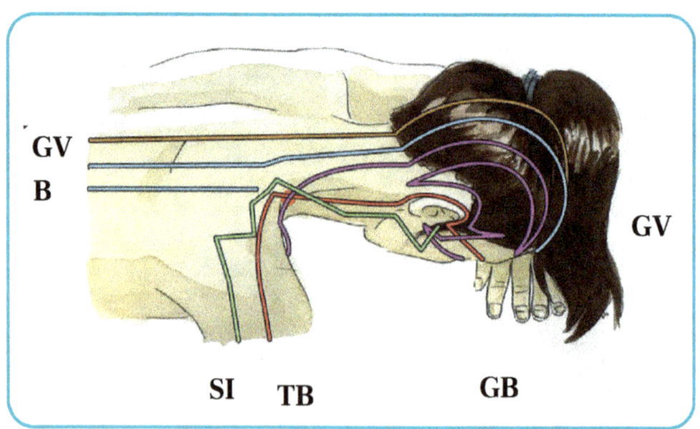

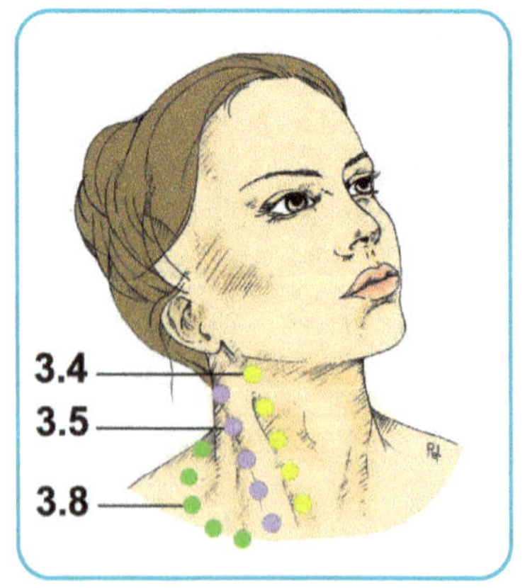

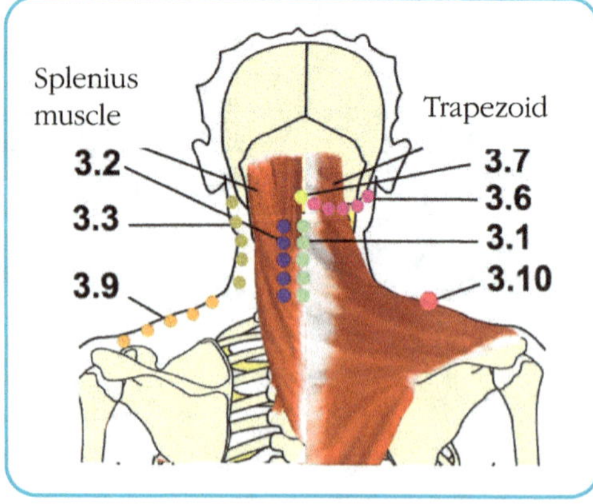

3.1. VERTEBRA REGION. TRACTION

PATIENT'S POSTURE: Supine.

THERAPIST'S POSITION: Seiza.

TYPE OF PRESSURE: Both hands apply pressure on the spinous process while exerting a traction movement toward the therapist. Pressure is concentrated on the third finger.

Nº. OF POINTS: A five-point line.

DIRECTION OF THE LINE: Between the spinous process, from C7-D1 to the rachidian bulb.

OBSERVATIONS: The fifth point (Rachidian bulb) corresponds to key point GV16 (Fuufu).

Three times for three seconds.

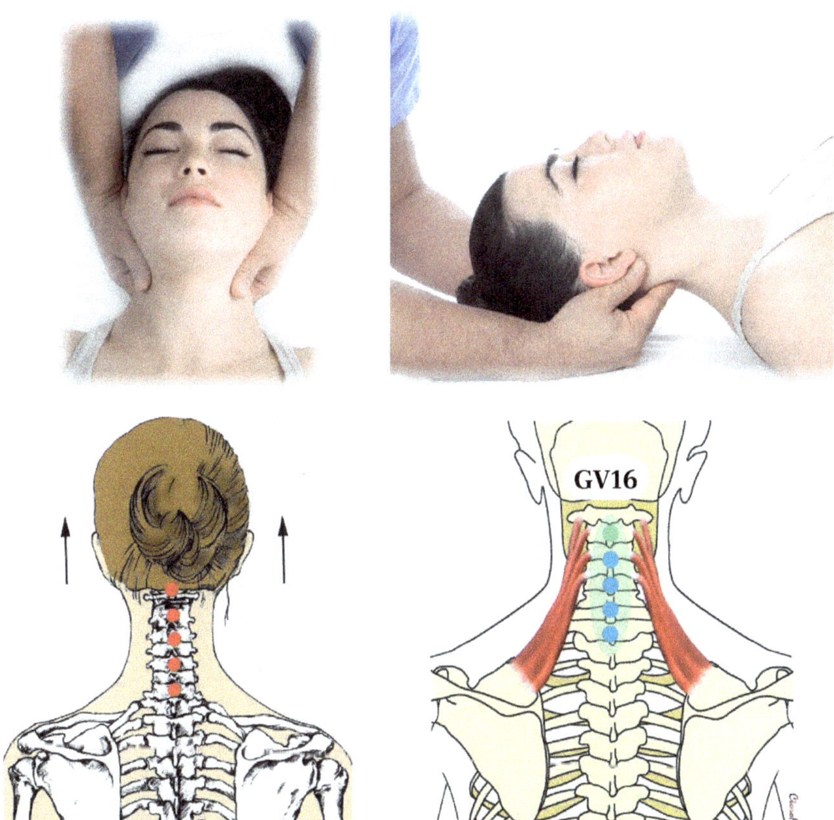

3.2. POSTERIOR CERVICAL REGION. ONE SIDE

PATIENT'S POSTURE: Supine, neck rotated.

THERAPIST'S POSITION: Seiza.

TYPE OF PRESSURE: The fingertips of the second, third and fourth fingers (left hand on the left side). The other hand holds the patient's head.

Nº. OF POINTS: A five-point line.

DIRECTION OF THE LINE: Along the cervical paravertebral musculature. From C7-D1 to the occipital edge.

OBSERVATIONS: The fifth point B10 (Tenchuu) located one finger outside the rachidian bulb coincides with the first point of the posterior cervical line.

The first point of the line is located between C7-D1 and, as the rest of the line, on the vertebrae laminae. Another variant for the posterior cervical region is located above the levator scapula.

Three times for three seconds.

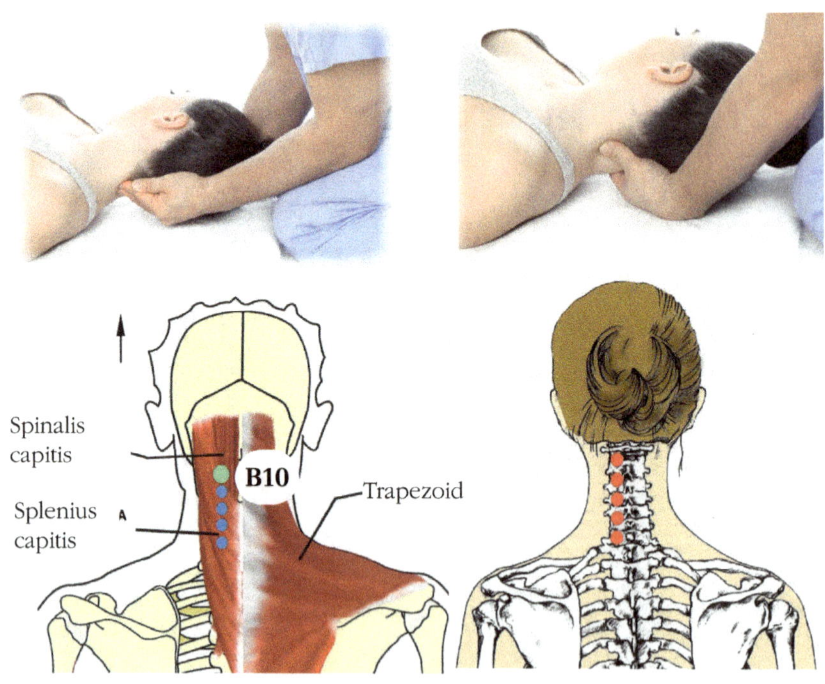

3.3. LATERAL CERVICAL REGION. ONE SIDE

PATIENT'S POSTURE: Supine, neck rotated.

THERAPIST'S POSITION: Seiza.

TYPE OF PRESSURE: The fingertips of the second, third and fourth fingers (left hand on the left side). The other hand holds the patient's head

N°. OF POINTS: A five-point line.

DIRECTION OF THE LINE: Along the lateral musculature of the neck. From the base of the neck to the mastoid process. Pressure is directed towards the centre of the neck.

OBSERVATIONS: The first point coincides with the third point at the base of the neck. The last point **GB12 (Kankotsu)** is located in the mastoid part's posteroinferior depression (insertion of the esternocleido-mastoid muscle). The area between the fourth and fifth points helps to balance the Autonomous Nervous System (insomnia and other sleep disorders) and prevent arteriosclerosis. You can apply pressure with your thumb as shown in the image, when deemed necessary.

Three times for three seconds.

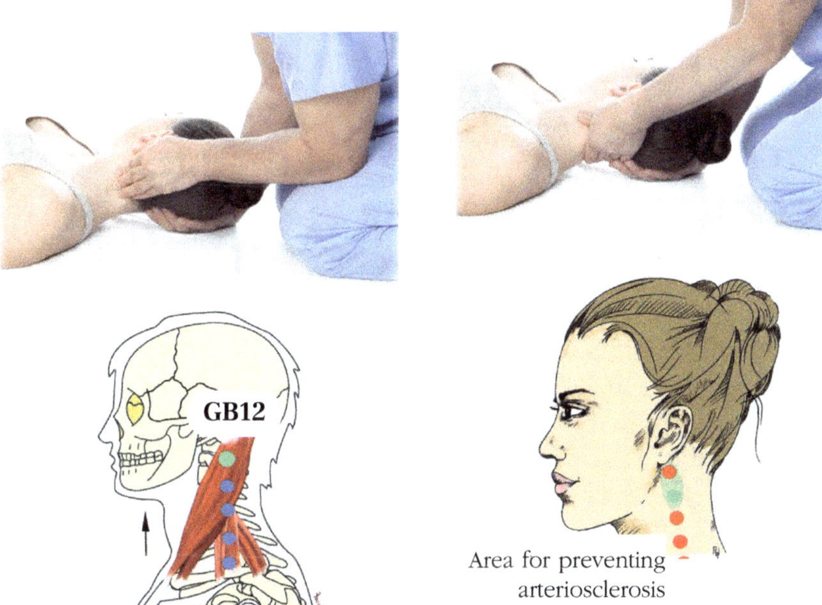

3.4. ANTERIOR CERVICAL REGION. FIRST LINE

PATIENT'S POSTURE: Supine, neck rotated approximately 45°.

THERAPIST'S POSITION: Seiza.

TYPE OF PRESSURE: One thumb (left on the left side). The other hand holds the head. Pressure is applied with the entire thumbpad, the rest of the fingers surround the neck.

N°. OF POINTS: A five-point line.

DIRECTION OF THE LINE: Along the anterior edge of the esternocleido-mastoid muscle. From the muscle belly to the mastoid part of the temporal bone. Pressure is directed to-wards the cervical spinous process.

OBSERVATIONS: The third point corresponds to key point S9 (Jingei) within the carotid triangle area, where you can perfectly touch the pulse (carotid sine).

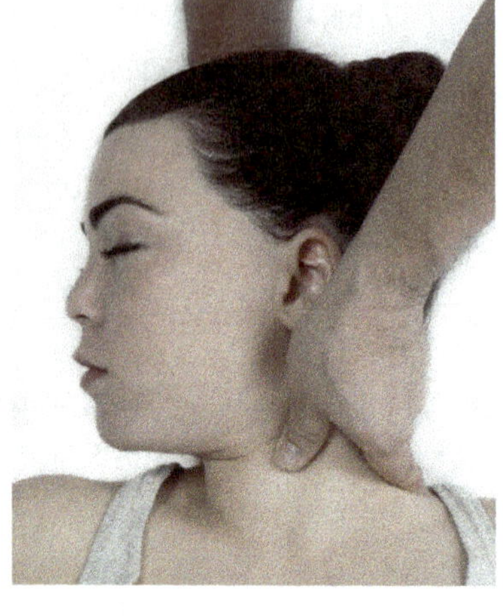

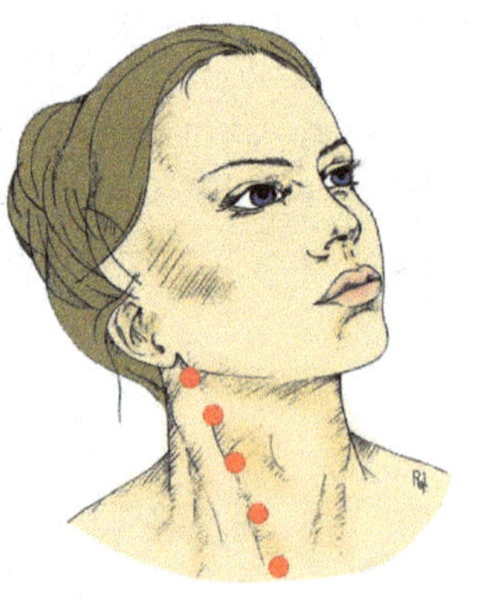

Work carefully. Pressure in the area can cause a drop in blood pres-sure (reflective of the carotid sinus), when working on the vagus nerve we balance the autonomic nervous system.

Three times for three seconds.

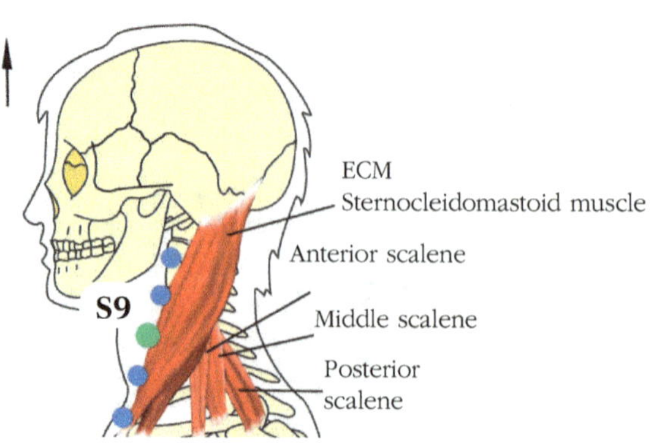

196

3.5. ANTERIOR CERVICAL REGION. SECOND LINE

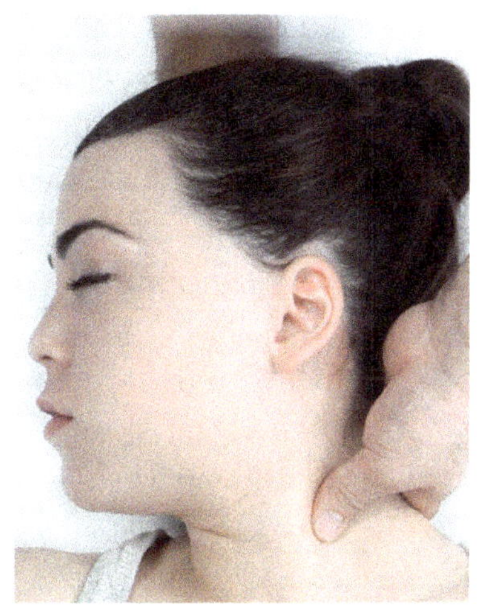

PATIENT'S POSTURE: Supine, neck rotated approximately 45°.

THERAPIST'S POSITION: Seiza.

TYPE OF PRESSURE: One thumb (left on the left side). The other hand holds its head. Pressure is applied with the entire thumbpad, the rest of the fingers surround the neck.

N°. OF POINTS: A five-point line.

DIRECTION OF THE LINE: Along the posterior edge of the esternocleidomastoid muscle to the mastoid part of the temporal bone. The last point in turn coincides with the last point of the occipital line GB12 (kankotsu).

Pressure is directed towards the cervical spinous process. (3rd and 4th point towards the trachea).

OBSERVATIONS: The first line of anterior cervical is to treat the anterior part of the body; digestion, heart (emotion, function) and breathing.

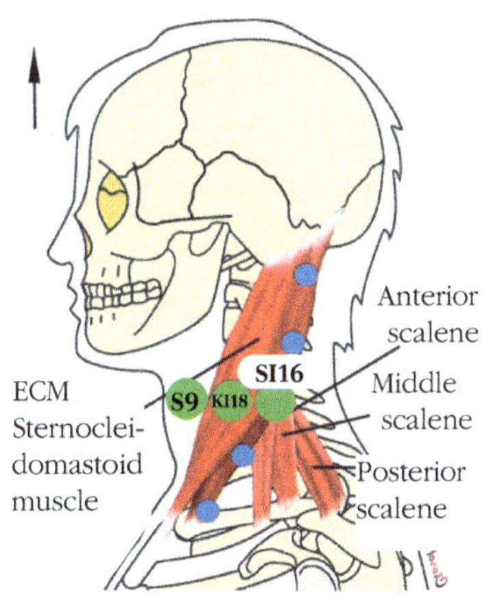

The second line is used for pain and contractures in the shoulder and back.

The first and second points are fundamental for treating physical pain.

The third point coincides with key point SI16 (Tensou). Along the same line are: KI18 (Futotsu, in the muscular belly of the esternocleidomastoid) and S9 (Jingei, on the anterior edge of the same muscle).

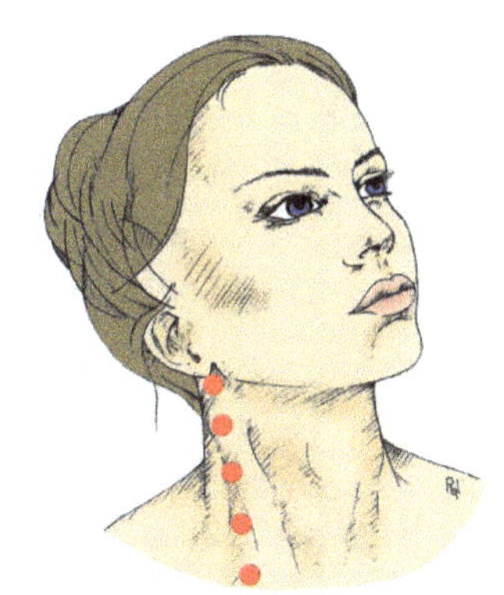

Three times for three seconds.

3.6. OCCIPITAL REGION. ONE SIDE

PATIENT'S POSTURE: Supine, neck rotated.

THERAPIST'S POSITION: Seiza.

TYPE OF PRESSURE: The second, third and fourth fingertips (left hand on the left side). The other hand holds the patient's head.

Nº. OF POINTS: A five-point line.

DIRECTION OF THE LINE: Along the occipital edge, from the mastoid tuberosity to the rachidian bulb. Pressure is applied towards the space between the eyebrows.

OBSERVATIONS: When deemed necessary, you can apply pressure with your thumb as shown in the image.

In the same region we can highlight three key points to avoid menken and control physical pain in the posterior part of the body. To diagnose how the body is we rely on three points of the occipital area: B10 (Tenchuu), GB12 (Kankotsu), GB20 (Fuuchi), which we combine with point GV20 (Hyakue), for a perfect treatment.

For a complete treatment of the area, we work three lines.

Three times for three seconds.

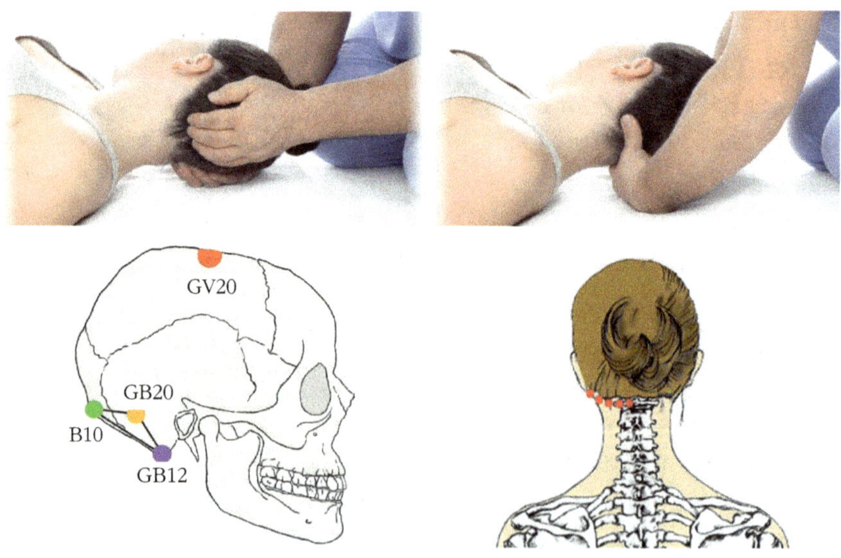

Repeat 3.2 to 3.6 on the RIGHT SIDE before proceeding.

3.7. RACHIDIAN BULB REGION. TRACTION

PATIENT'S POSTURE: Supine.

THERAPIST'S POSITION: Seiza.

TYPE OF PRESSURE: The third fingers of both hands rest on the rachidian bulb. Raise the skull slightly and exert traction backwards towards the therapist.

N°. OF POINTS: One.

OBSERVATIONS: If the work is done correctly, the patient's chin is raised following the cervical extension movement. This point corresponds to key point **GV16 (Fuufu)**.

When performing neck traction, all joints have to be connected and, as proof of this, we can see how the arch of the foot correspondingly flexes and extends.

Three times for five seconds.

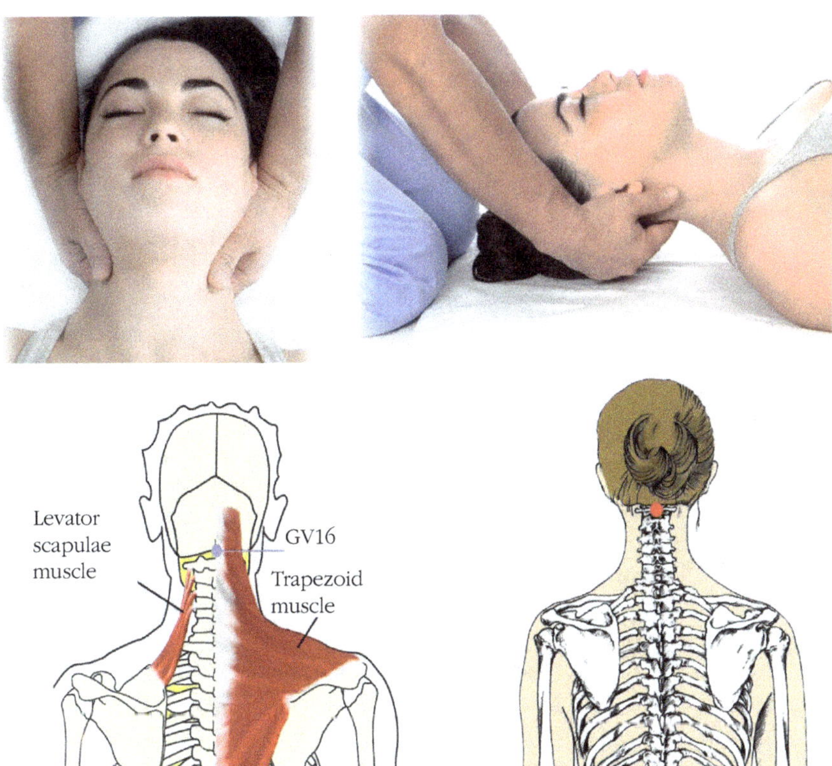

3.8. BASE OF THE NECK REGION

PATIENT'S POSTURE: Supine, neck rotated.

THERAPIST'S POSITION: Seiza.

TYPE OF PRESSURE: A thumb (left on the left side). The other hand holds the patient's head.

Nº. OF POINTS: A five-point line.

DIRECTION OF THE LINE: From the external edge of the levator scapula to the middle third of the collarbone (sternocleidomastoid muscle (ECM), head clavicular).

OBSERVATIONS: When working, stretch the area well to access better, rotating and turning the neck to the side.

The third point is the same as the last point of the lateral cervical region and to the first point of the suprascapular region.

Three times for three seconds.

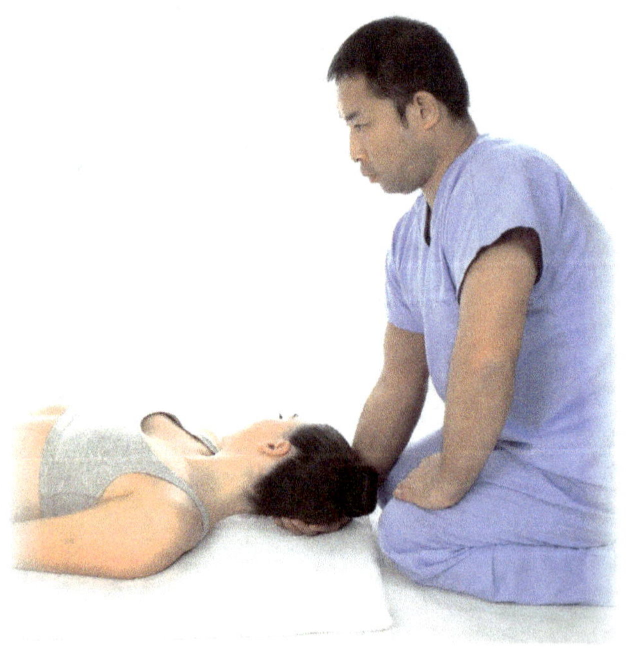

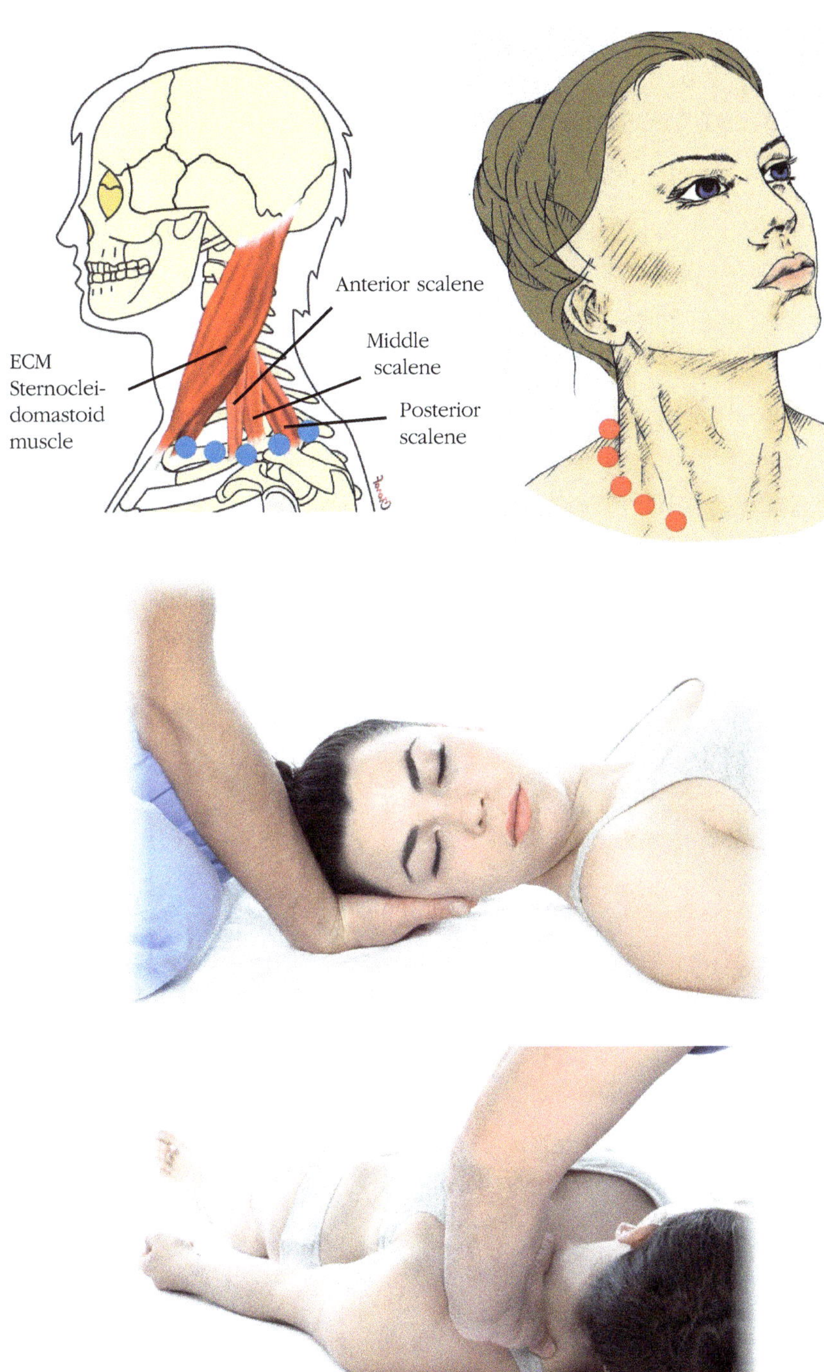

Anterior scalene
Middle
scalene
Posterior
scalene
ECM
Sternoclei-
domastoid
muscle

3.9. SUPRASCAPULAR REGION. LINE

PATIENT'S POSTURE: Supine, neck rotated.

THERAPIST'S POSITION: Seiza.

TYPE OF PRESSURE: One thumb (left on the left side). The other hand holds the patient's head.

Nº. OF POINTS: A five-point line.

DIRECTION OF THE LINE: From the base of the neck (fifth point of the lateral cervical area) towards the acromion, on the superior edge of the trapezium.

OBSERVATIONS: As in the previous case, maintain the neck rotated and turned to the side for better access to the area.

The second point corresponds to key point GB21 (Kensei). Another way to locate it is to find the midpoint between the acromion and the spinous process of the seventh cervical vertebra.

Three times for three seconds.

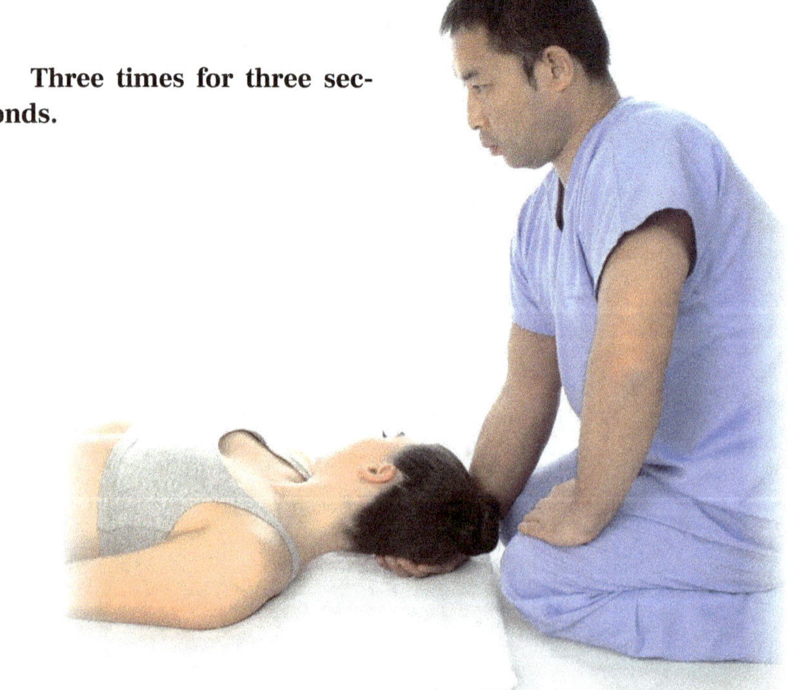

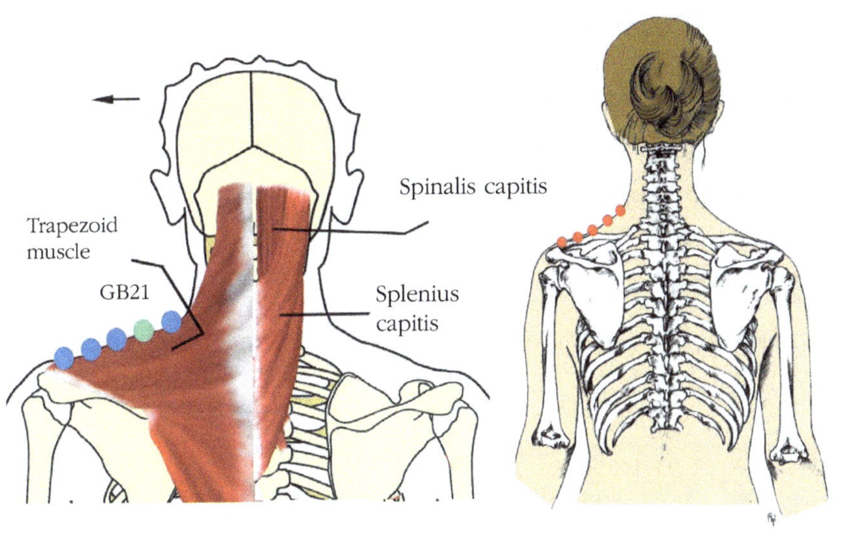

Trapezoid muscle
GB21
Spinalis capitis
Splenius capitis

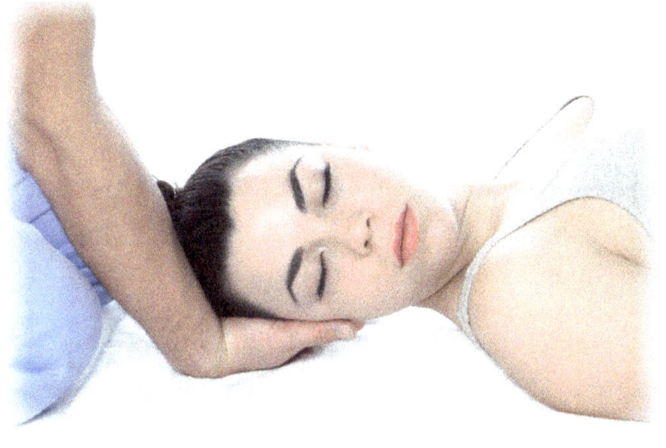

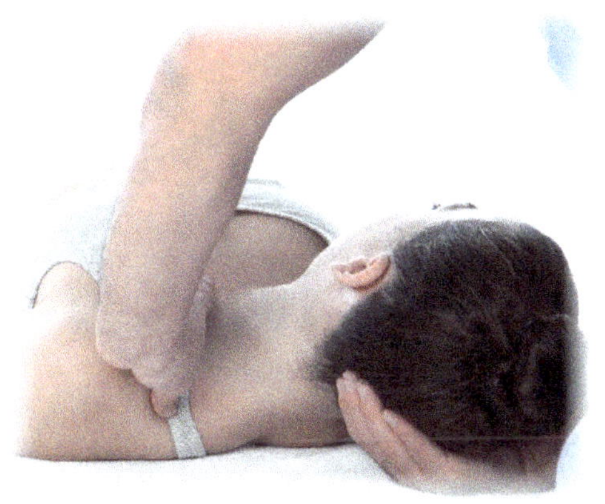

3.10. SUPRASCAPULAR REGION. POINT

PATIENT'S POSTURE: Supine, neck rotated.

THERAPIST'S POSITION: Seiza.

TYPE OF PRESSURE: One thumb (left on the left side). The other hand holds the patient's head.

Nº. OF POINTS: One.

DIRECTION OF THE PRESSURE: Towards the centre line of the body at D7 level.

OBSERVATIONS: Keep the neck rotated and turned to the side for better access to the area.

This point coincides with the second point in the suprascapular region (line) and corresponds to key point GB21 (Kensei).

According to Traditional Chinese Medicine, **GB21 (Kensei)** is discouraged while pregnant, however, with Shiatsu we can work it perpendicularly, slowly and without pulling, using the fingertip and the body's balance.

Three times for five seconds.

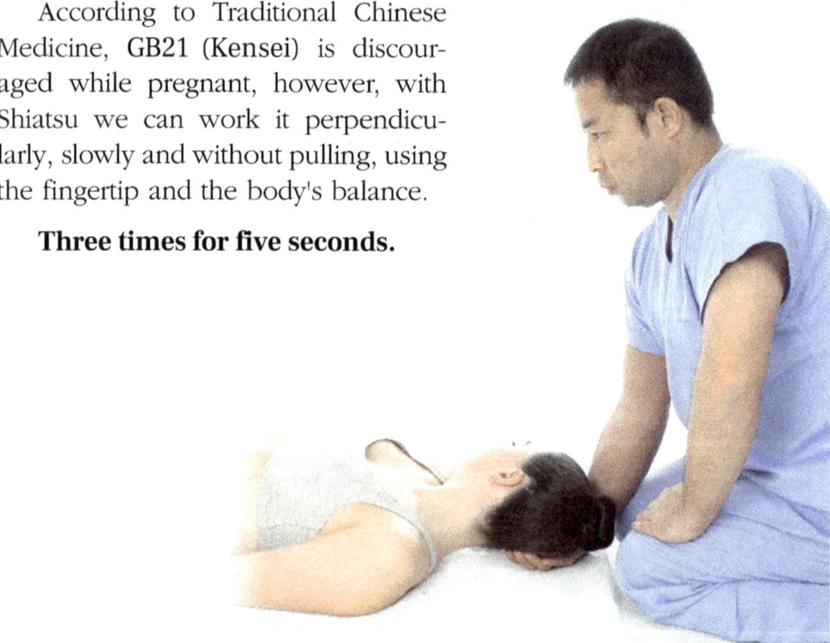

Repeat 3.8 to 3.10 on the RIGHT SIDE before proceeding.

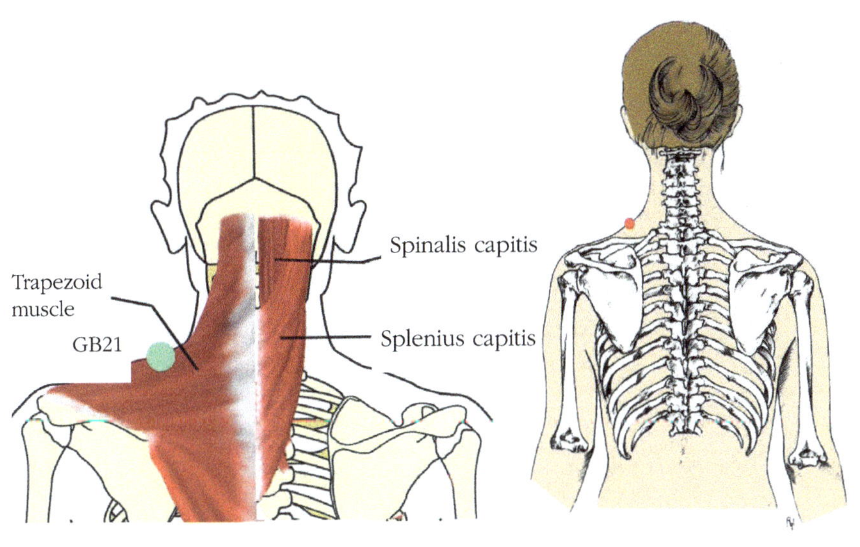

Spinalis capitis
Trapezoid muscle
GB21
Splenius capitis

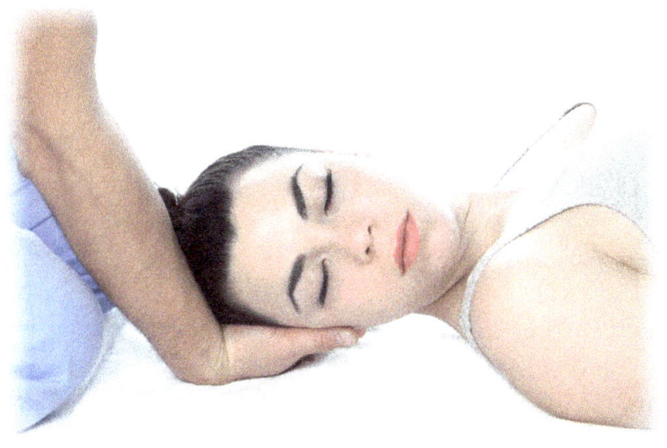

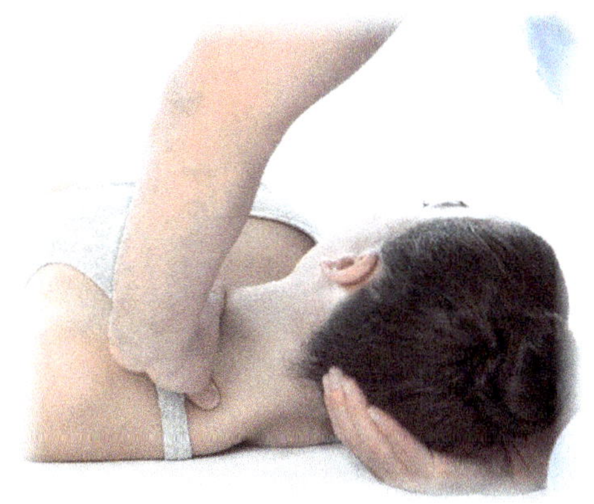

4. The chest

4.1. Sternum region. Line.
4.2. Pectoral region.
4.3. Subclavicular region. Both sides.
4.4. Supraclavicular region.
4.5. Sternum region. Central point.

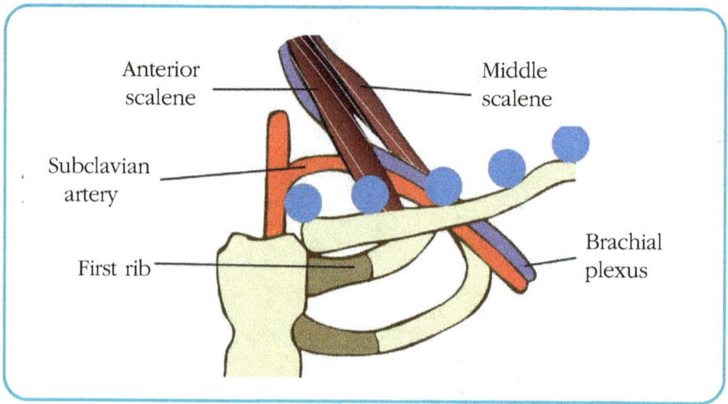

It is a sensitive area for respiratory and circulatory problems, as well as depression and anxiety.

In the case of women, care must be taken with the breasts, so we must keep our hands held backwards in a movement as if folding a fan.

A hunched back posture may result from the tension accumulated in the chest and shoulders.

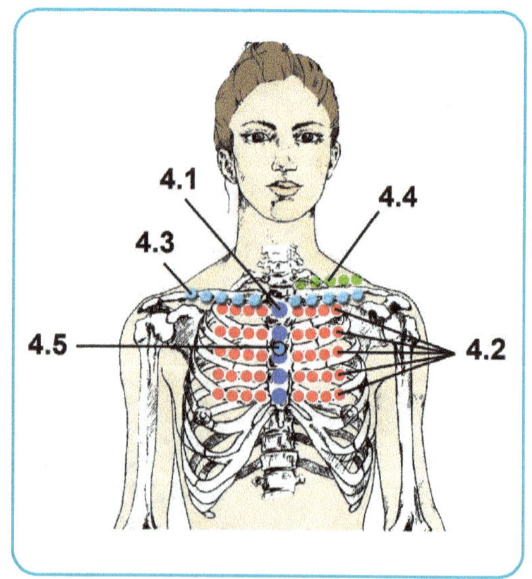

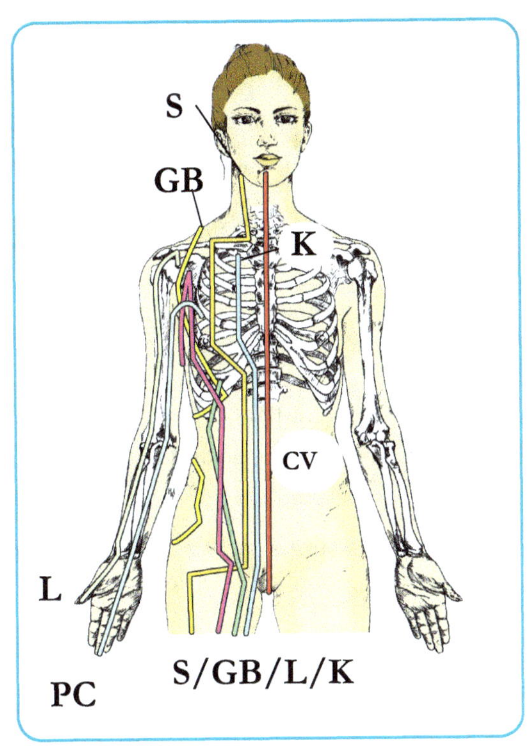

S
GB
K
CV
L
PC
S/GB/L/K

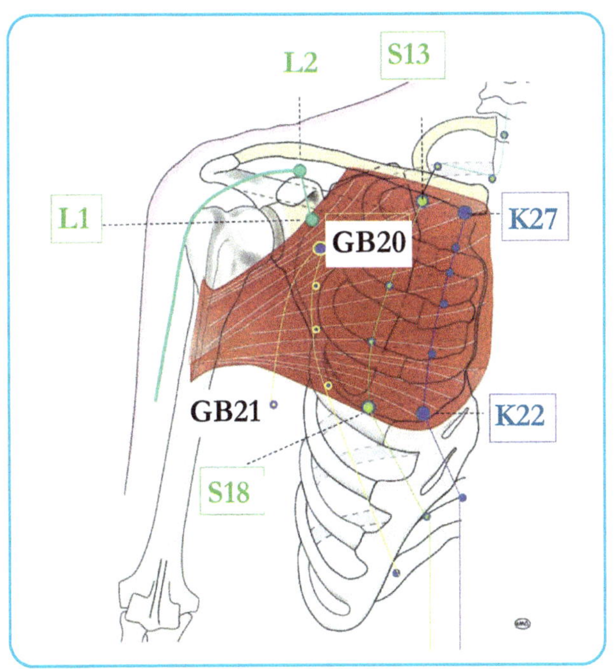

L2
S13
L1
GB20
K27
GB21
K22
S18

4.1. STERNUM REGION

PATIENT'S POSTURE: Supine.

THERAPIST'S POSITION: Kneeling above the patient's head.

TYPE OF PRESSURE: Thumbs in A. The rest of the hand rests on the deltopectoral regions.

N°. OF POINTS: A five-point line.

DIRECTION OF THE LINE: From the manubrium to the xiphoid.

OBSERVATIONS: Apply gentle pressure. The third point coincides with key point CV17 (**Danchuu**), indicated to treat respiratory and emotional problems.

We can also work three lines above the sternum. In this case it is important to work at the patient's breathing rate.

Three times for three seconds.

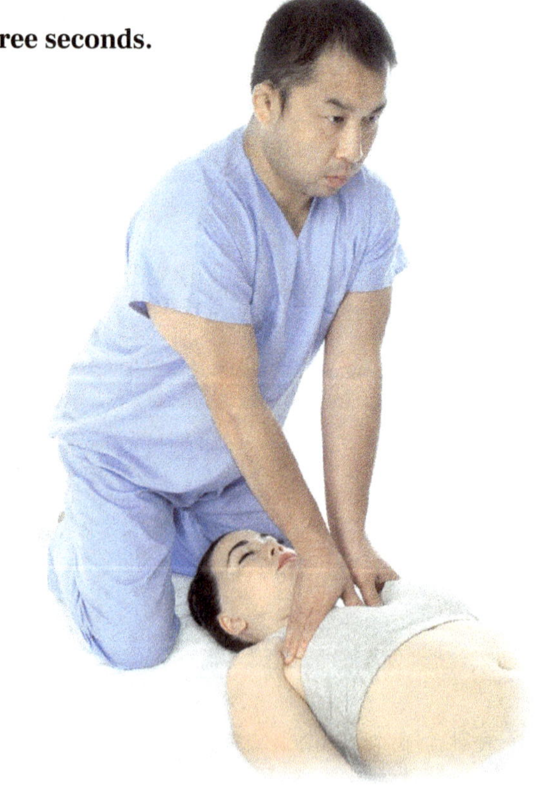

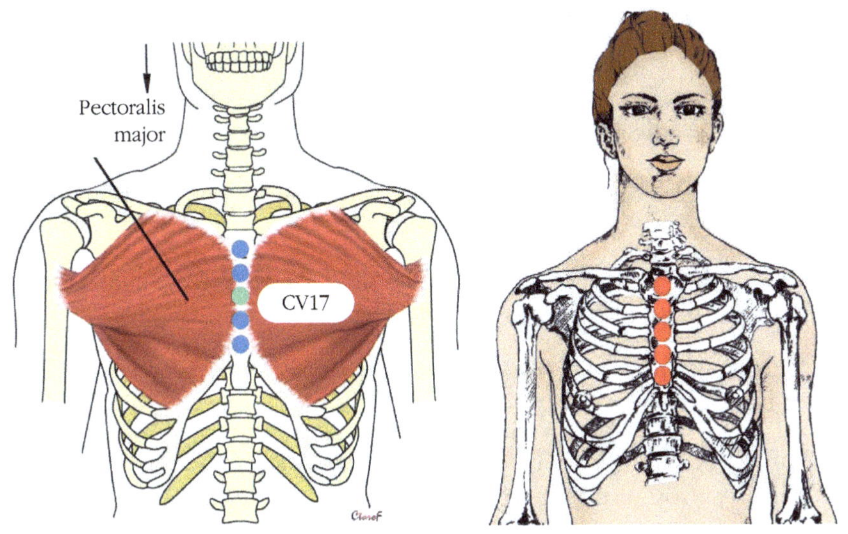

Pectoralis
major
CV17

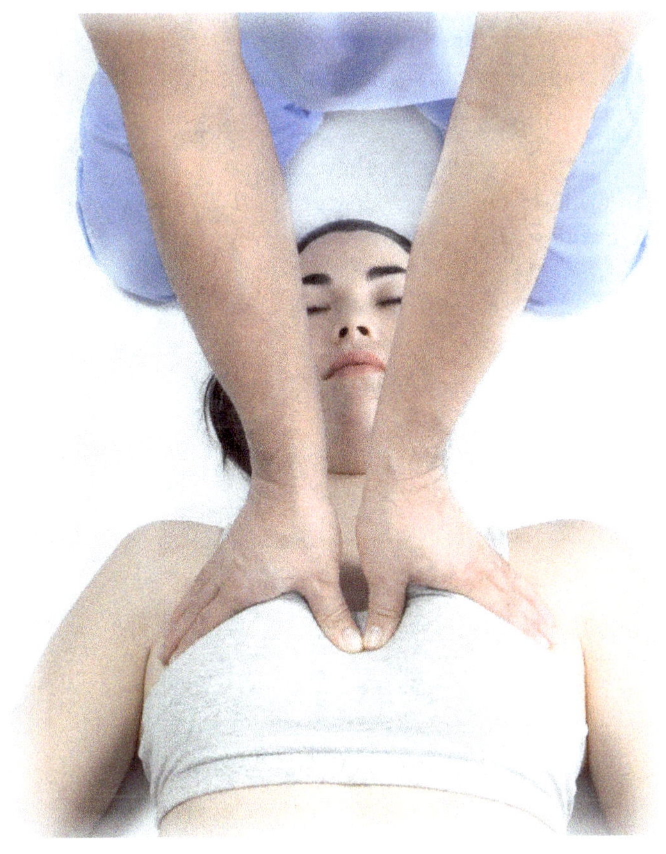

4.2. PECTORAL REGION

PATIENT'S POSTURE: Supine.

THERAPIST'S POSITION: Kneeling, maintaining the previous position.

TYPE OF PRESSURE: Both thumbs at once. The rest of the hand rests on the deltopectoral regions.

Nº. OF POINTS: A five-point line on each side (starting from the centre).

DIRECTION OF THE LINE: Starting from the central line working laterally and from the manubrium towards the xiphoid process.

OBSERVATIONS: In women you can skip some lines so you don't apply pressure on the mammary glands.

This treatment is useful for respiratory and circulatory problems, especially sore throats and colds.

As the pectoral region is worked, the patient's breathing becomes slower and deeper, alleviating back contractures.

**Three times for
three seconds.**

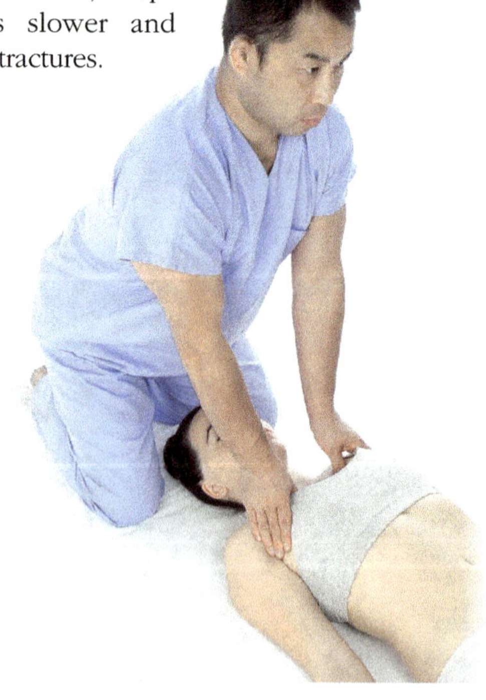

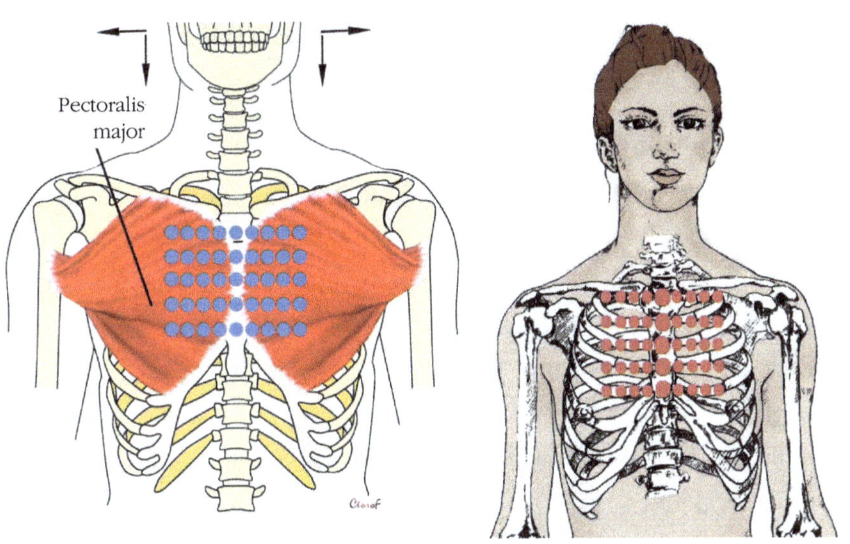

Pectoralis
major

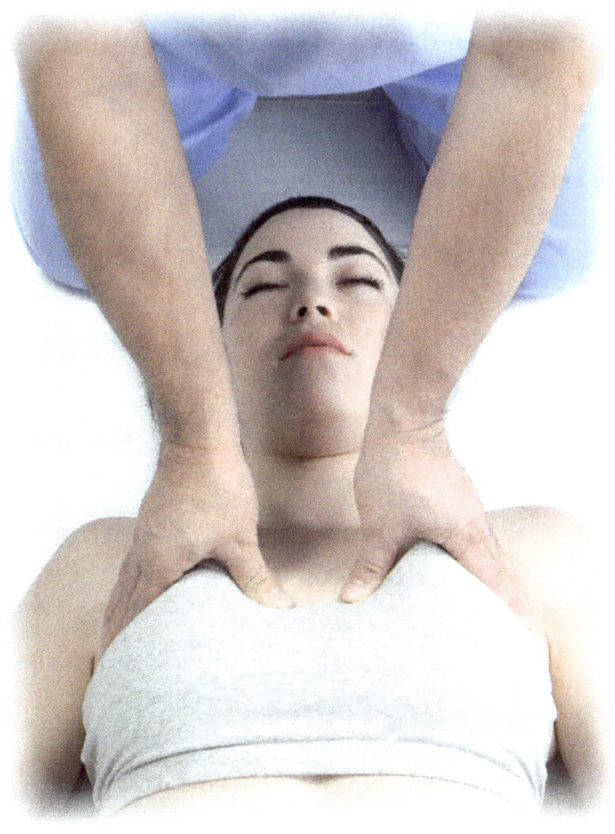

4.3. SUBCLAVICULAR REGION. BOTH SIDES

PATIENT'S POSTURE: Supine.

THERAPIST'S POSITION: Kneeling, maintaining the previous position.

TYPE OF PRESSURE: Both thumbs at once. The rest of the hand rests on the deltopectoral regions.

Nº. OF POINTS: Two five-point lines.

DIRECTION OF THE LINE: Along the inferior edge of the clavicular, from the esternoclavicular joint towards the acromion.

OBSERVATIONS: The first point corresponds to key point K27 (Yufu); and the third with key point S13 (Kiko), located in the subclavian muscle.

While working on the subclavian muscle, we alleviate pathologies such as frozen shoulder, and cervical and back pain.

Three times for three seconds.

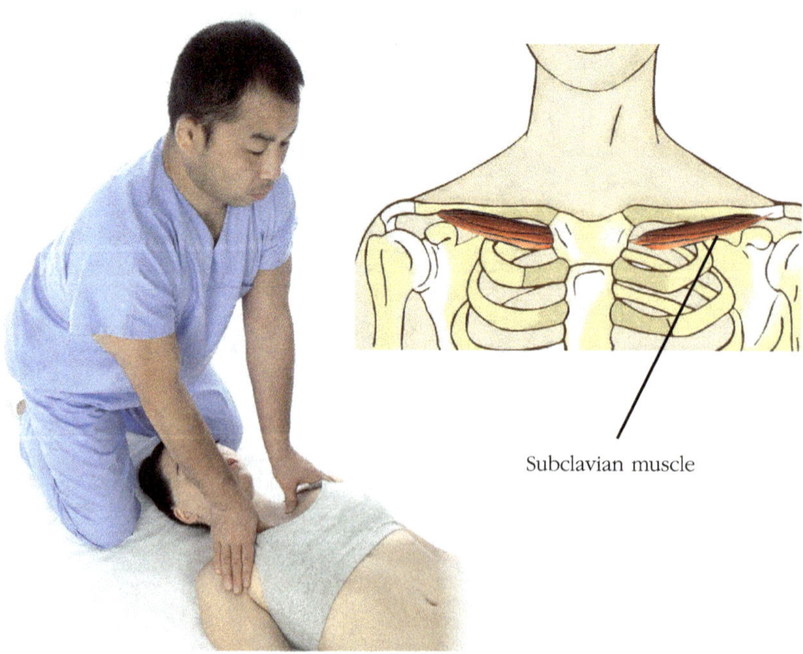

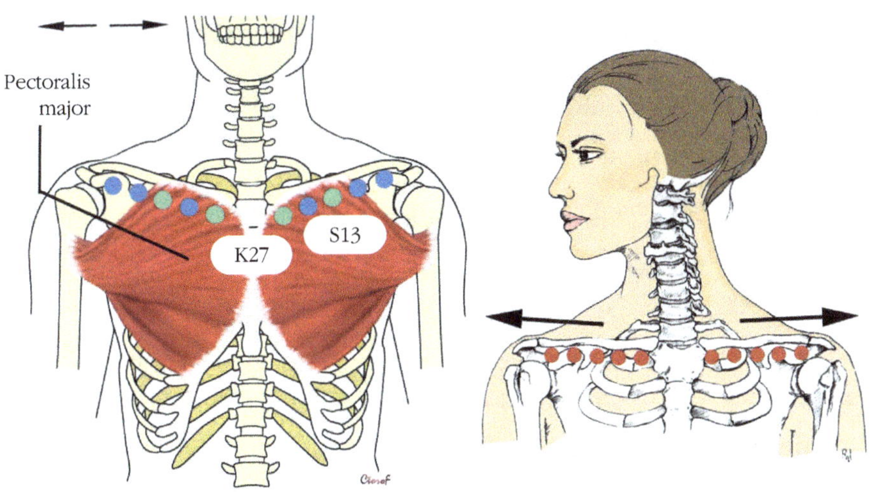

Pectoralis
major
K27
S13

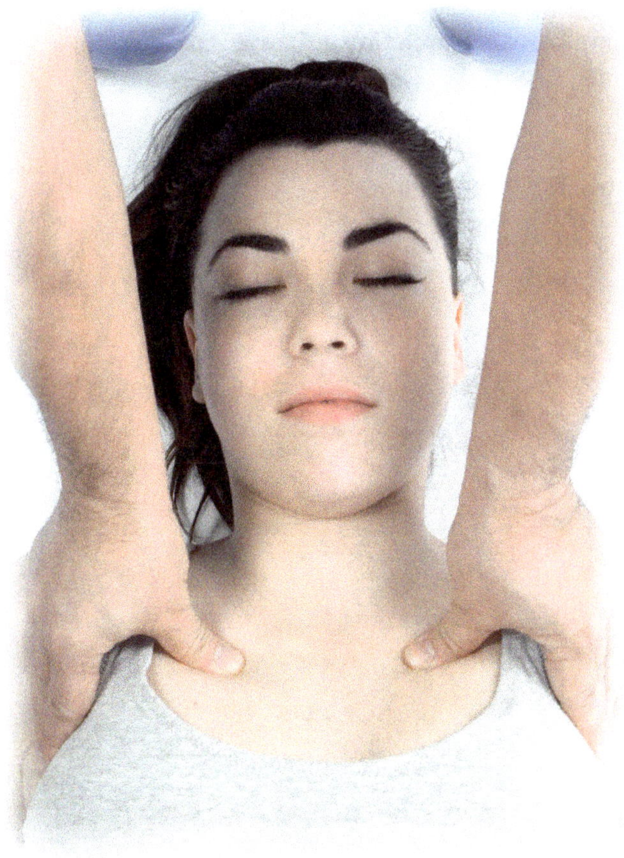

4.4. SUPRACLAVICULAR REGION. ONE SIDE

PATIENT'S POSTURE: Supine, neck rotated.

THERAPIST'S POSITION: Seiza, above the patient's head.

TYPE OF PRESSURE: Index, middle and ring fingertips (left hand on left side). The other hand holds the patient's head.

Nº. OF POINTS: A five-point line.

DIRECTION OF THE LINE: Along the superior edge of the clavicular, from the esternoclavicular joint towards the acromion.

OBSERVATIONS: The first point corresponds to key point **S11** (Kisya) and the third to key point **S12** (Ketsubon).

By applying pressure on the supraclavicular area we can relieve tingling and arm pain. We also improve the patient's breathing and emotional problems.

Three times for three seconds.

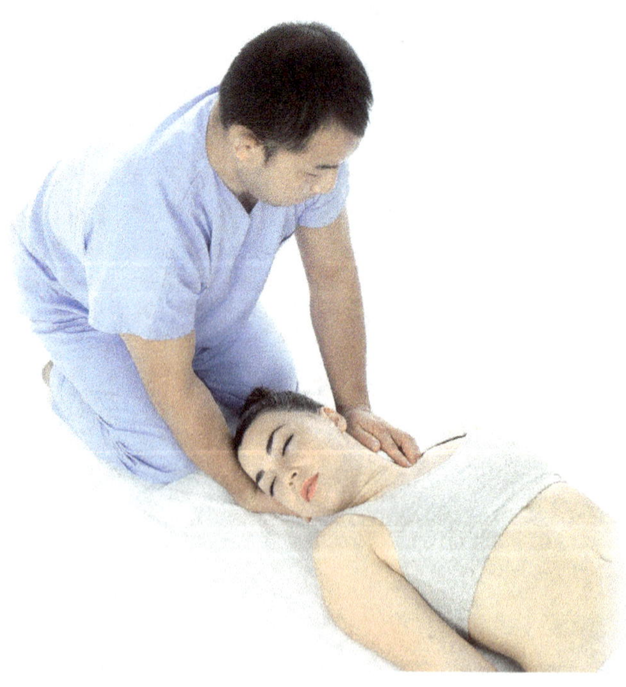

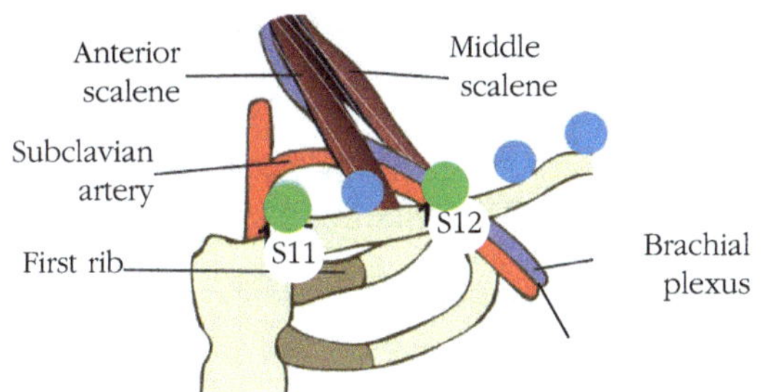

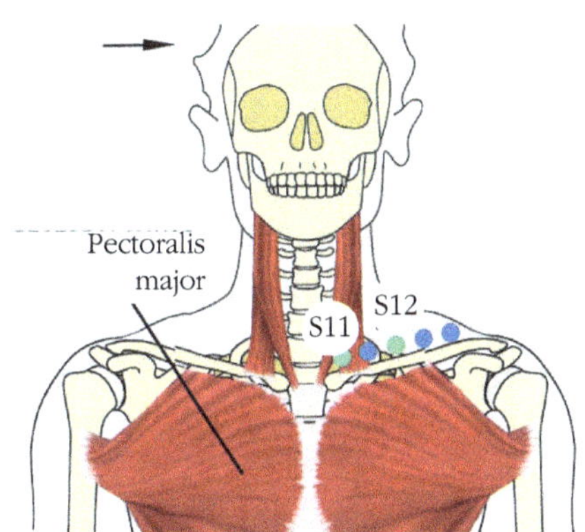

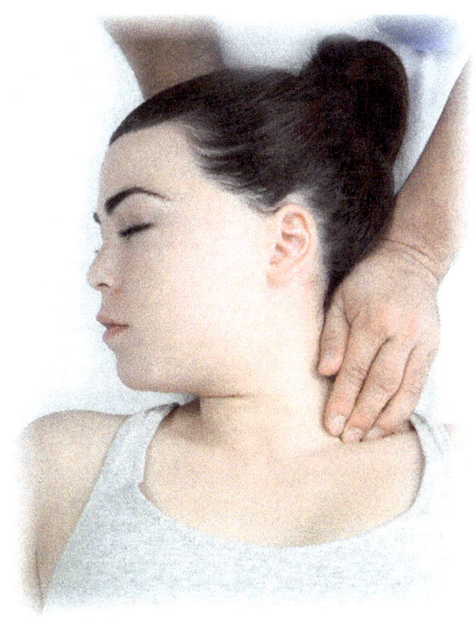

Repeat 4.4 on the RIGHT SIDE before proceeding.

4.5. STERNUM REGION. CENTRAL POINT

PATIENT'S POSTURE: Supine.

THERAPIST'S POSITION: Kneeling above the patient's head.

TYPE OF PRESSURE: Palm over palm. Pressure and vibration applied with the three middle fingers. The phalanges should rest on the patient's chest.

N°. OF POINTS: One.

OBSERVATIONS: Gently apply pressure to the central point of the sternum region.

This point corresponds to key point CV17 (Danchuu).

By applying pressure we release the patient's ribcage which helps breathing and eliminates contractures in the shoulder, neck and diaphragm.

Ten seconds.

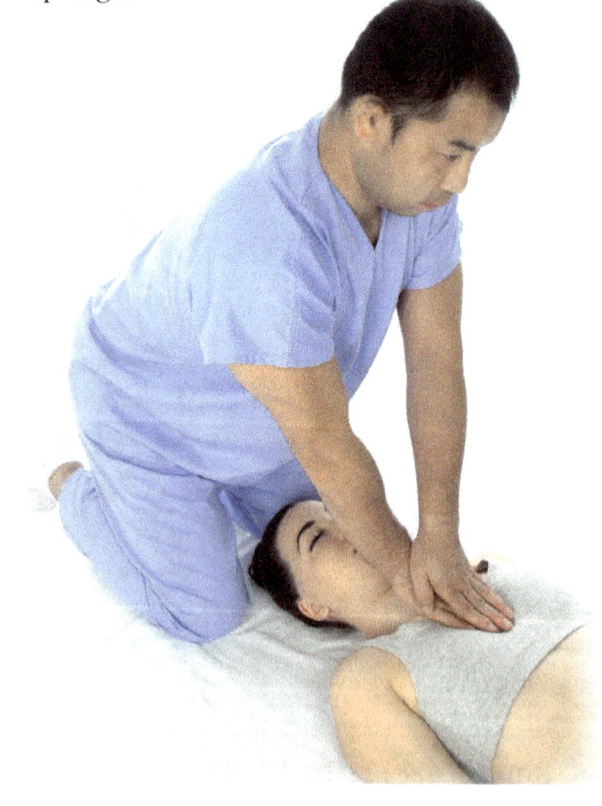

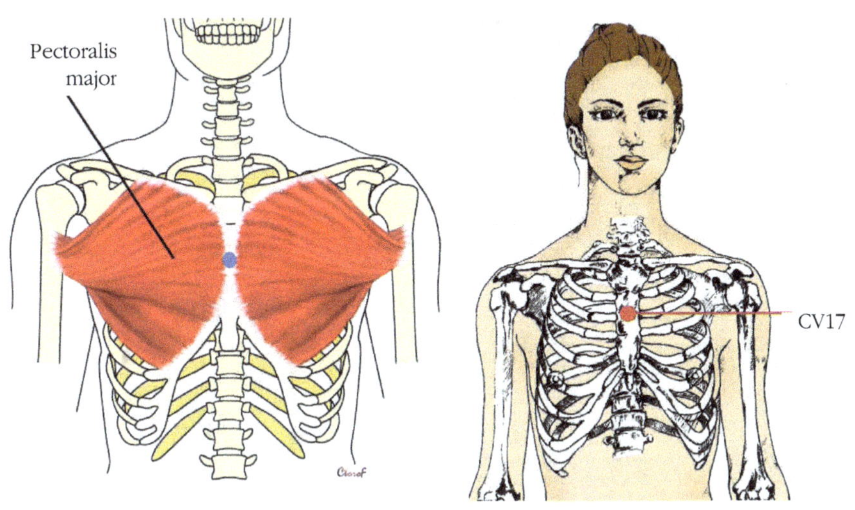

Pectoralis
major
CV17

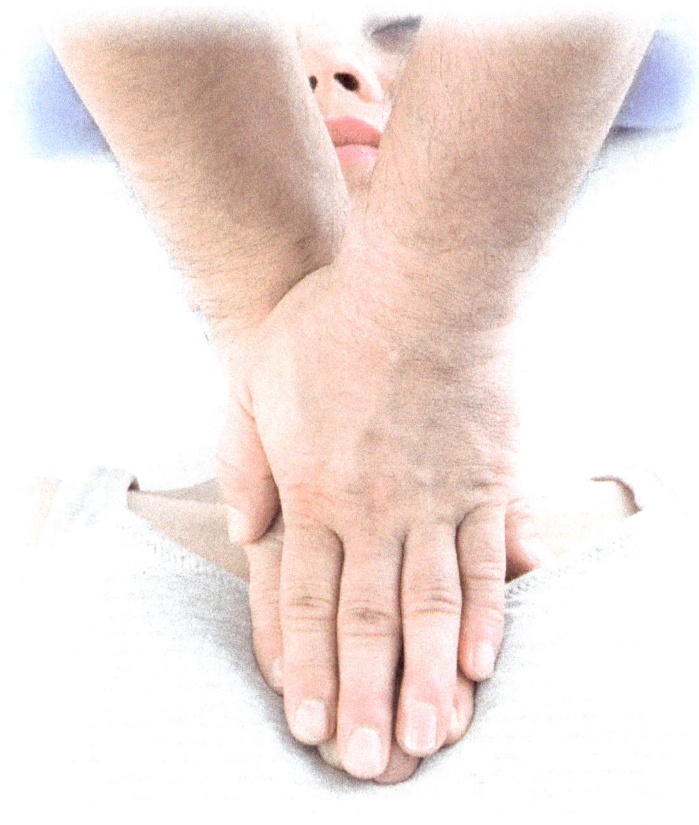

5. Upper limbs

5.1. Axillary region.
5.2. Medial brachial region.
5.3. Region of the ulnar fossa.
5.4. Medial antebrachial region.
5.5. Medial carpal region.
5.6. Palmar region. Central line.
5.7. Palmar region. Lateral lines.
5.8. Palmar region. Eminences.
5.9. Palmar region. Central point.
5.10. Deltopectoral Region.
5.11. Lateral brachial region.
5.12. Lateral elbow pit region.
5.13. Lateral antebrachial region.
5.14. Lateral carpal region.
5.15. Dorsal region of the hand.
5.16. Dorsal-palm and lateral digital region.

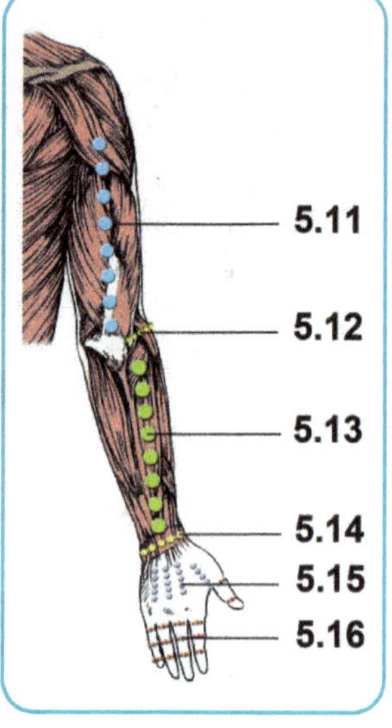

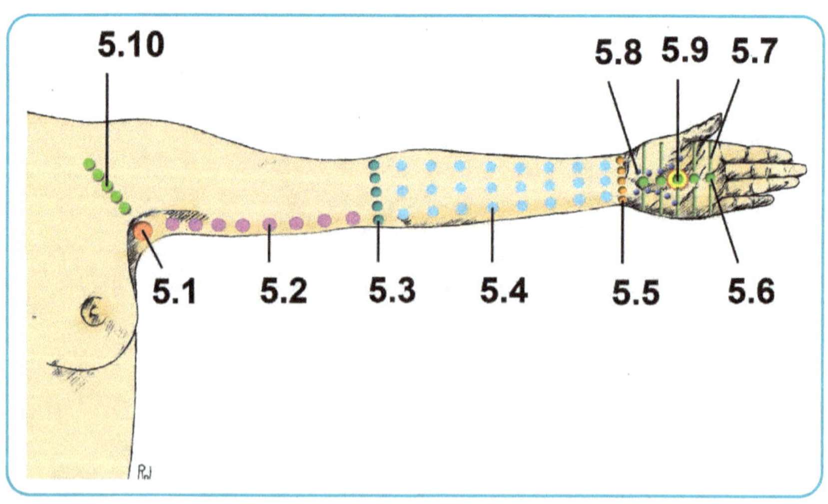

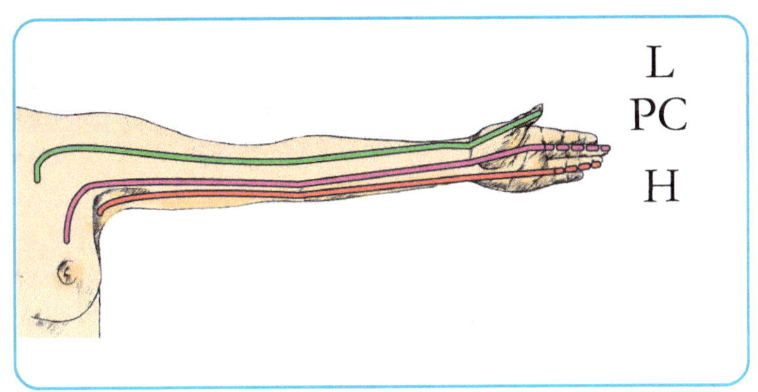

L
PC
H

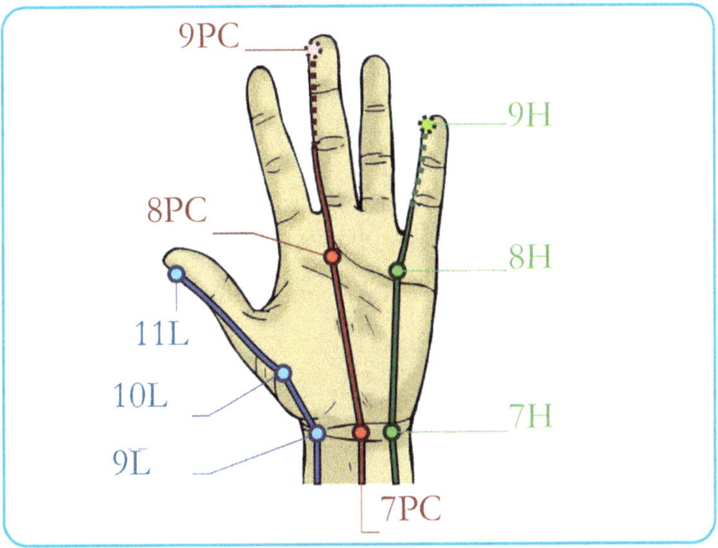

9PC
9H
8PC
8H
11L
7H
10L
9L
7PC

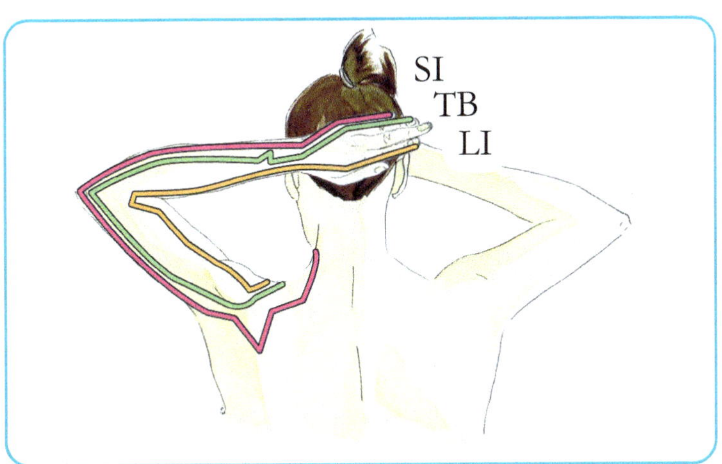

SI
TB
LI

5.1. AXILLARY REGION

PATIENT'S POSTURE: Supine, arm in 90° abduction and forearm in supine.

THERAPIST'S POSITION: Seiza, facing the arm.

TYPE OF PRESSURE: Thumb over thumb (right below on the left side).

Nº. OF POINTS: One.

DIRECTION OF THE PRESSURE: Towards the suprascapular point on the same side. Maintain pressure and perform a slight traction movement in the direction of the elbow.

OBSERVATIONS: Locate the pulse of the radial artery as it passes through the patient's wrist with the right index, middle and ring fingers. The point, in the centre of the armpit, is the one that decreases the arterial pulse when pressure is applied with the left thumb.

This point corresponds to key point H1 (Kyokusen).

Three times for five seconds.

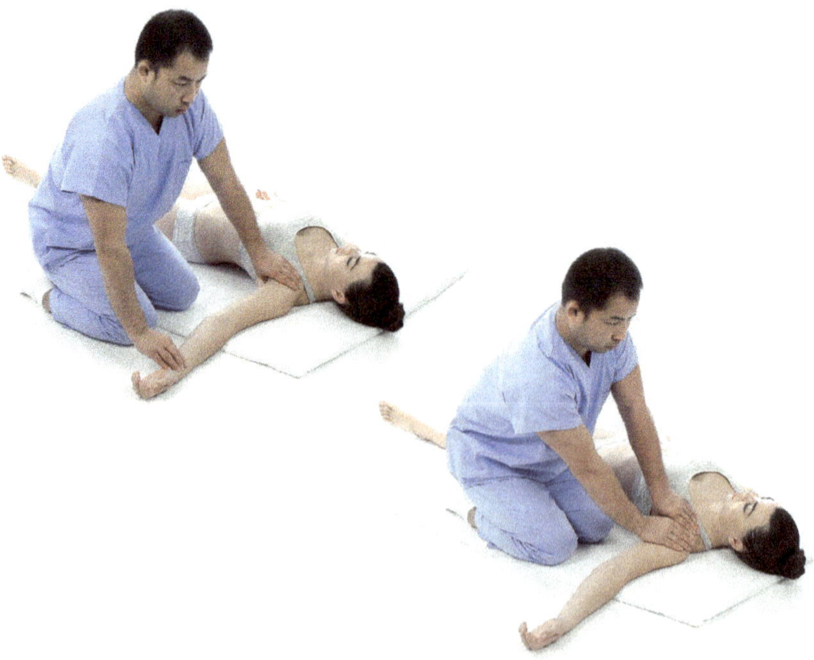

H1

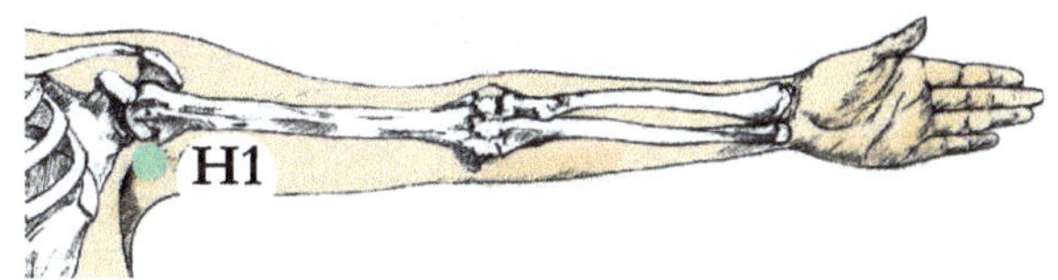

Serratus anterior muscle

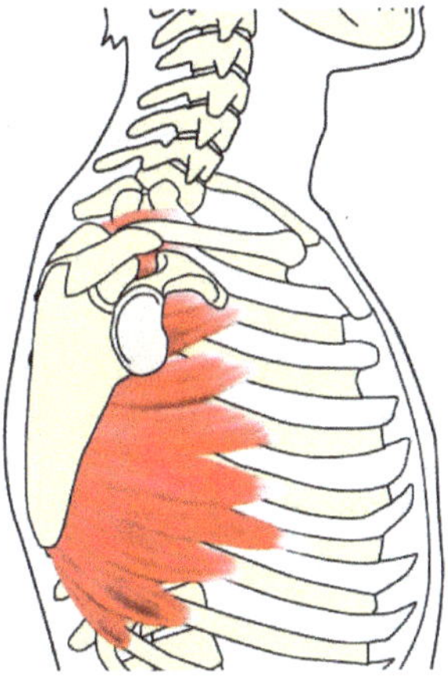

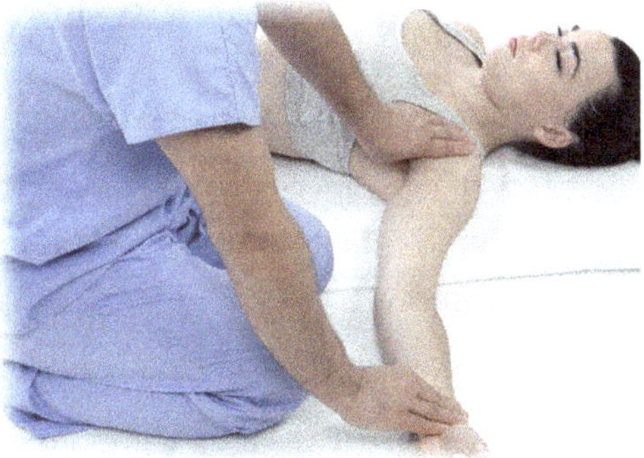

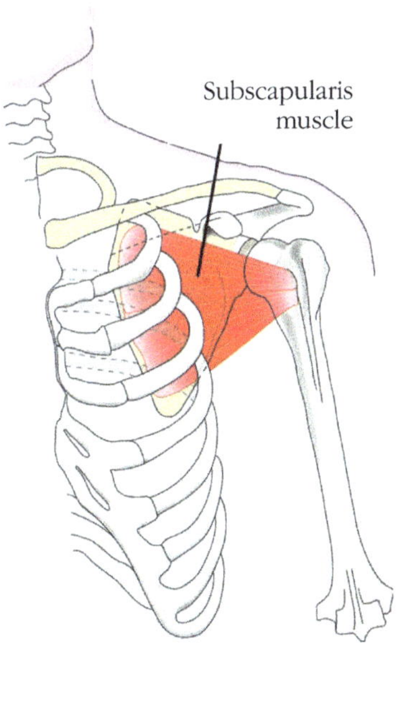

Subscapularis
muscle

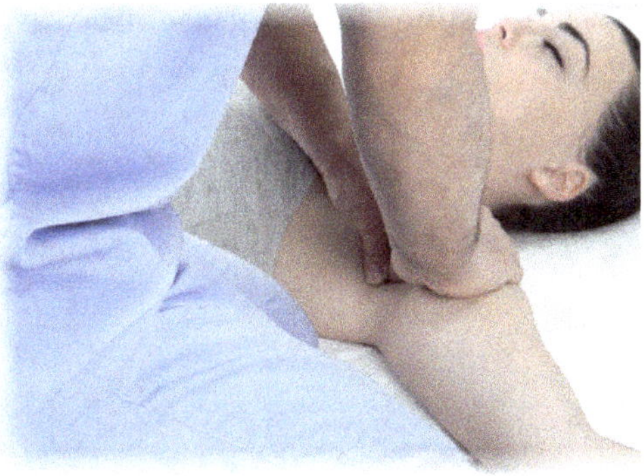

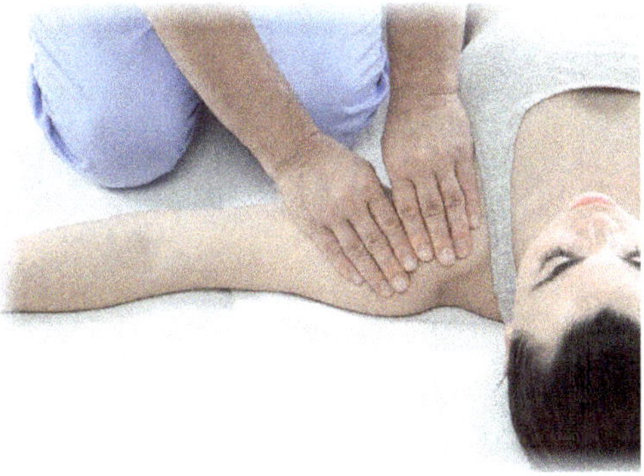

5.2. MEDIAL BRACHIAL REGION

PATIENT'S POSTURE: Supine, arm in 90° abduction and forearm in supine.

THERAPIST'S POSITION: Seiza, facing the patient's arm.

TYPE OF PRESSURE: Thumb over thumb in a V-shape (right below on the left side).

N°. OF POINTS: An eight-point line.

DIRECTION OF THE LINE: From the armpit to the lateral epicondyl of the arm. The first point is the one from the axillar region.

OBSERVATIONS: It is a very useful area to treat a frozen shoulder, tingling in the fingers and heart problems, in particular of the left arm.

The first point coincides with key point H1 (**Kyokusen**); and the last with key point H3 (**Syoukai**).

Three times for three seconds.

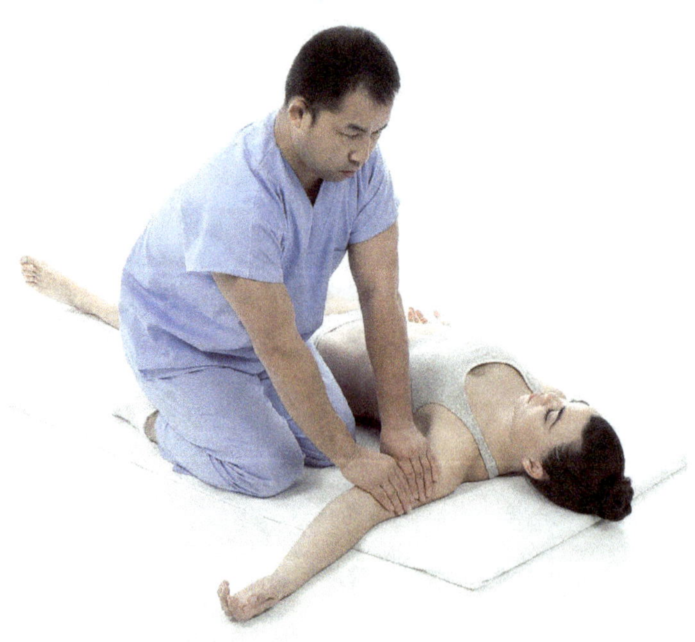

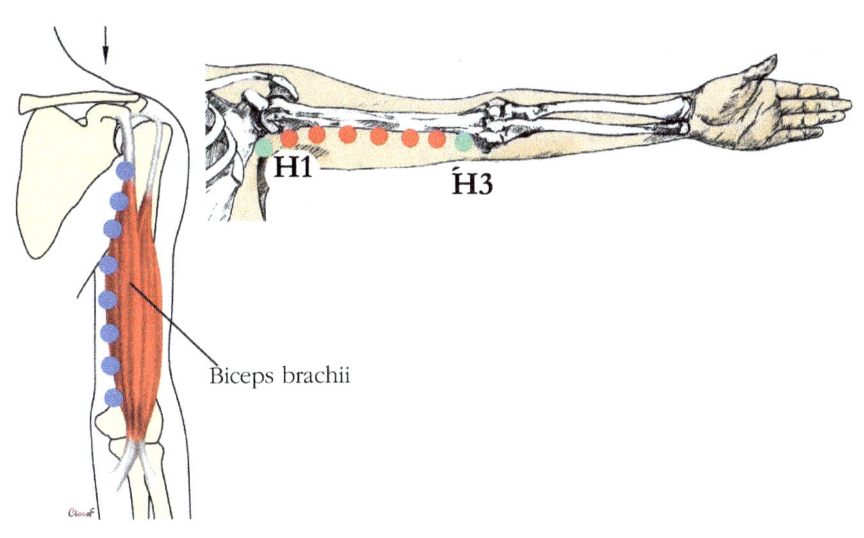

Biceps brachii
H1
H3

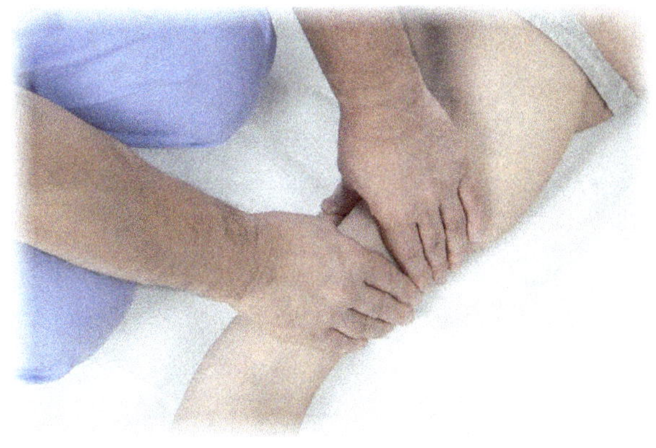

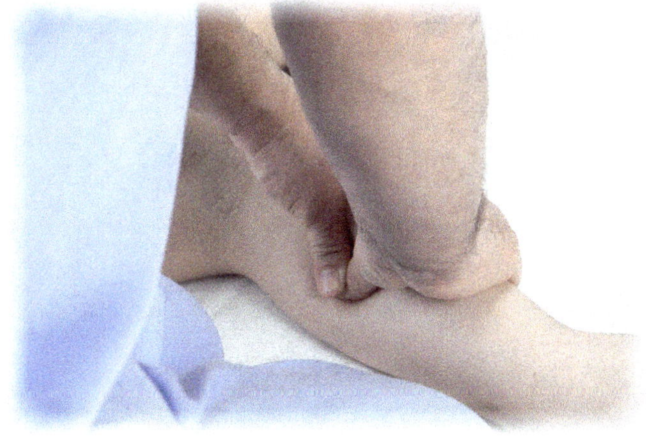

5.3. ULNAR FOSSA REGION

PATIENT'S POSTURE: Supine, arm in 45° abduction and forearm in supine.

THERAPIST'S POSITION: Seiza or kneeling.

TYPE OF PRESSURE: Thumbs in A.

N°. OF POINTS: A five-point line.

DIRECTION OF THE LINE: In the elbow pit joint, from the ulnar to the radial side.

OBSERVATIONS: It is very useful for treating tennis elbow.

The first point coincides with key point H3 (Syoukai); the third with PC3 (Kyokutaku); the fourth with L5 (Syakutaku); fifth with LI11 (Kyokuchi).

Three times for three seconds.

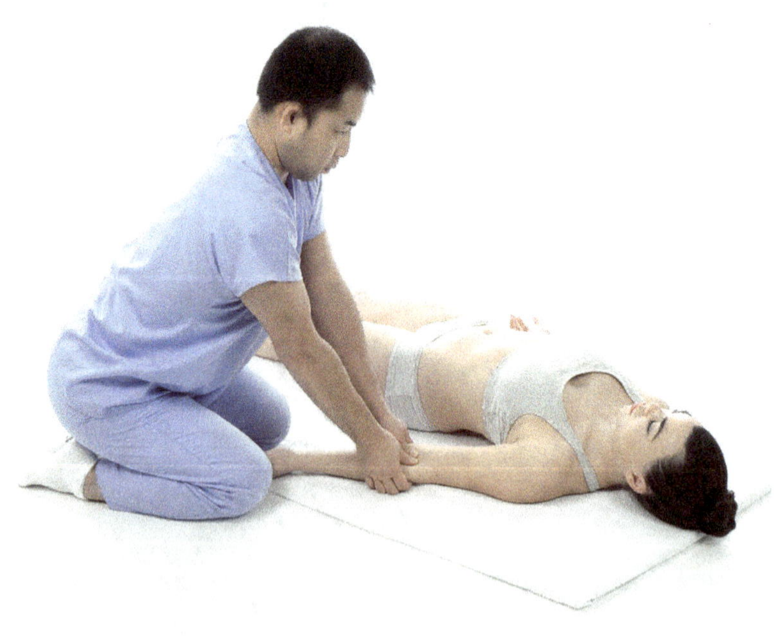

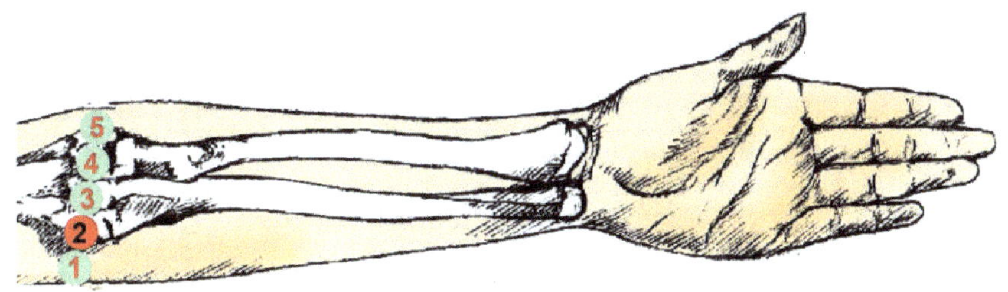

1- H3   4- L5
3- PC3   5- LI11

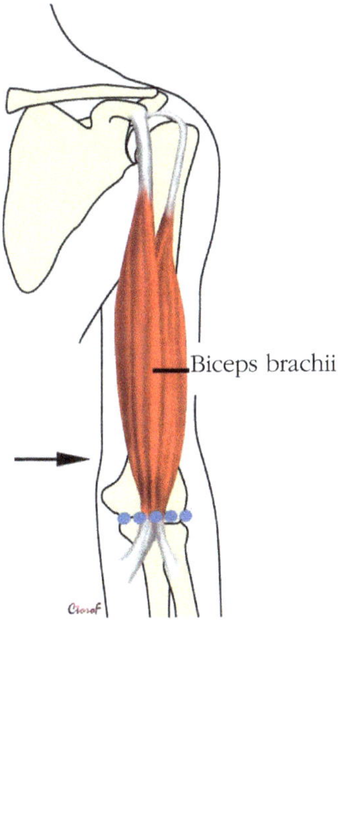

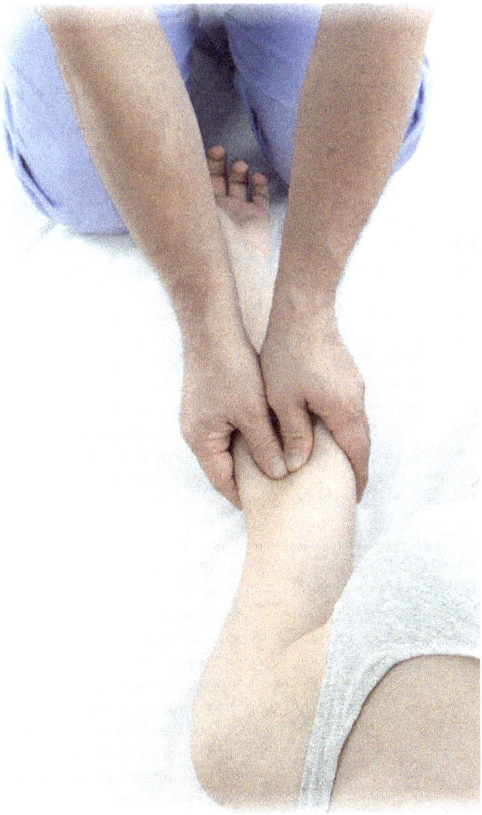

5.4. MEDIAL ANTEBRACHIAL REGION

PATIENT'S POSTURE: Supine, arm in 45° abduction and forearm in supine.

THERAPIST'S POSITION: Seiza or kneeling.

TYPE OF PRESSURE: 1st and 2nd repetitions: Logo.

3rd repetition: Thumb over thumb (right below on the left side).

N°. OF POINTS: Three eight-point line.

Central line: Below the centre point of the ulnar fossa and toward the centre of the medial wrist fold.

Medial line: Below the humeroulnar joint and towards the extreme medial of the wrist fold.

Lateral line: Below the humeroradial joint and towards the extreme lateral of the wrist fold.

DIRECTION OF THE LINE: The first point of each line is located just below the elbow pit. The last point, just above the wrist fold.

Repeat alternately in this order: Central line, medial line (little finger) and lateral line (thumb).

OBSERVATIONS: The fifth point of the central line corresponds to key point PC4 (Gekimon); and the seventh point on the same line with PC6 (Naikan).

Three times for three seconds.

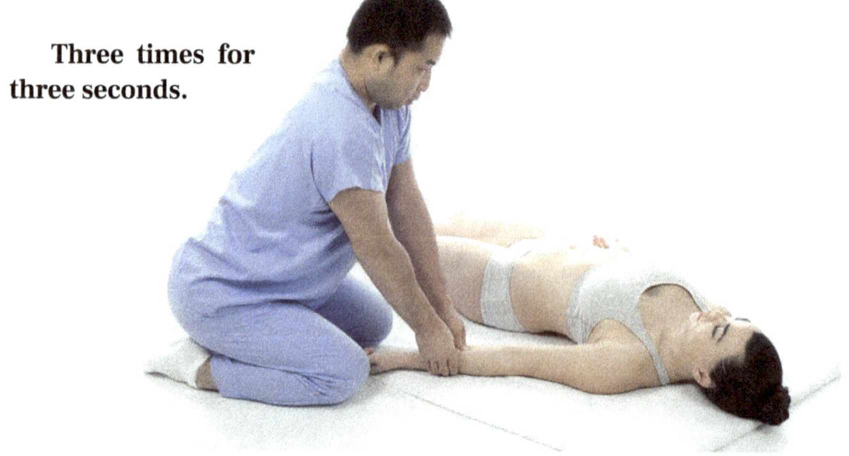

1ª Heart Meridian
2ª Pericardium Meridian
3ª Lung Meridian

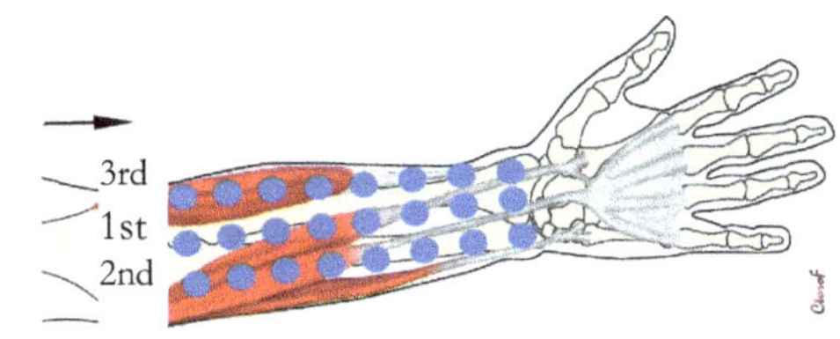

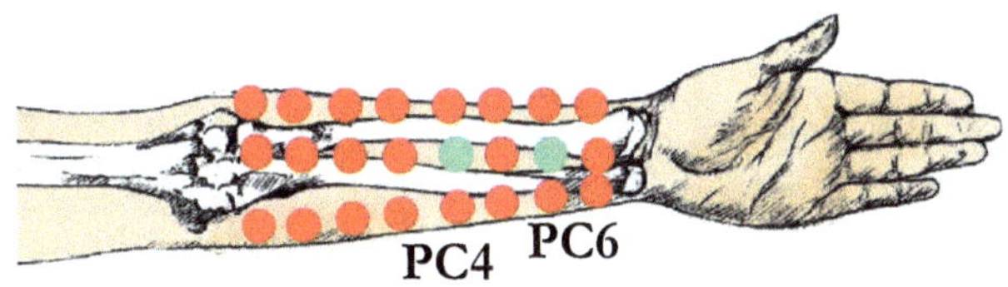

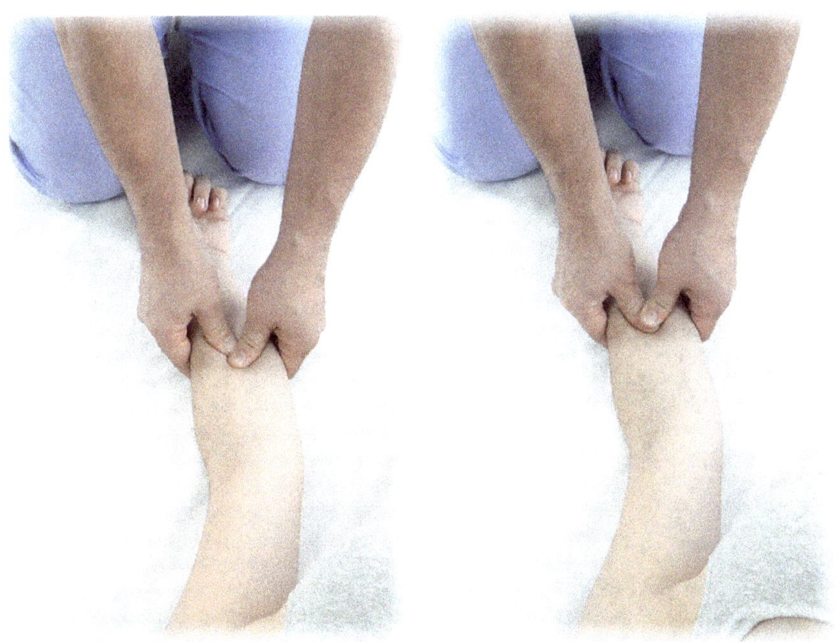

5.5. MEDIAL CARPAL REGION

PATIENT'S POSTURE: Supine, arm in 45° abduction and forearm in supine.

THERAPIST'S POSITION: Seiza or kneeling.

TYPE OF PRESSURE: Thumb over thumb (right below on the left side).

Nº. OF POINTS: A five-point line.

DIRECTION OF THE LINE: On the medial wrist fold, from the ulnar to the radial side.

OBSERVATIONS: The first point corresponds to key point H7 (Shinmon); the third with PC7 (Dairyou); and the fifth with L9 (Taien).

Three times for three seconds.

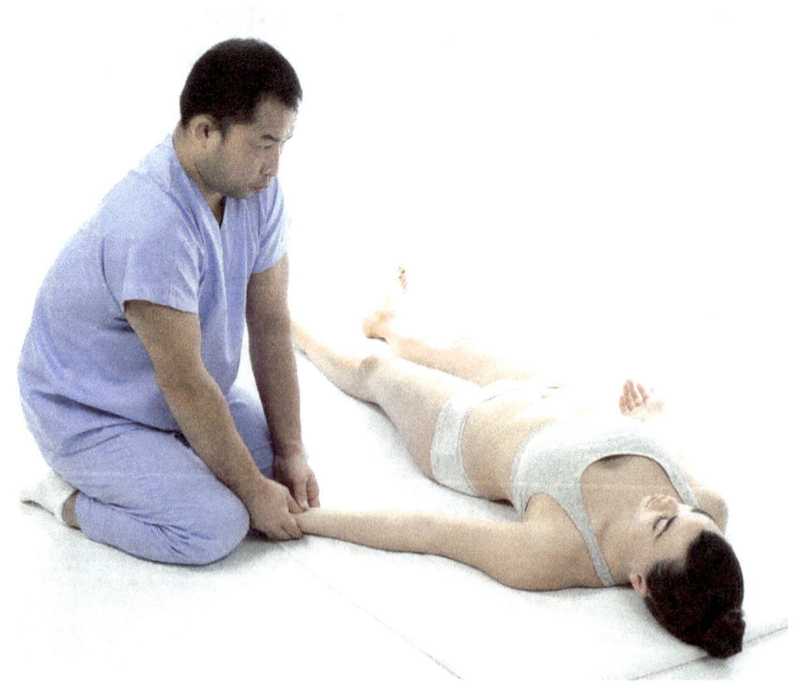

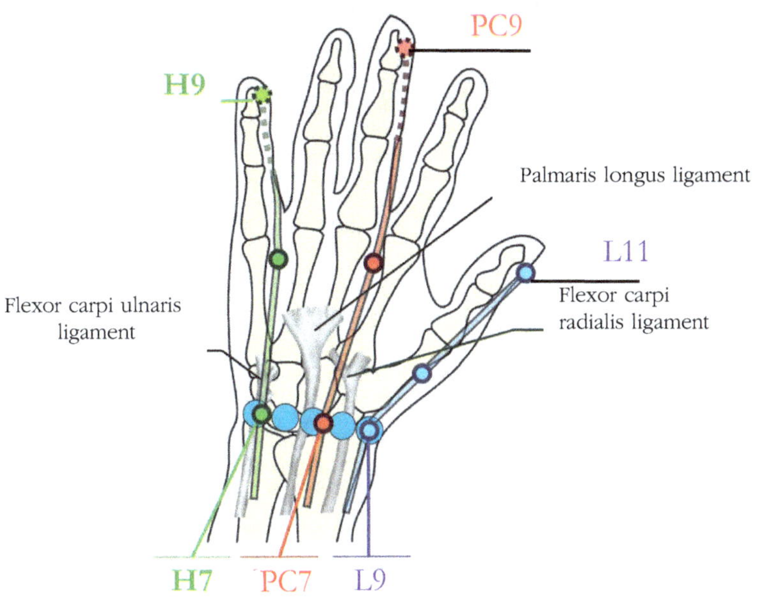

H9
PC9
Palmaris longus ligament
L11
Flexor carpi ulnaris
ligament
Flexor carpi
radialis ligament
H7
PC7
L9

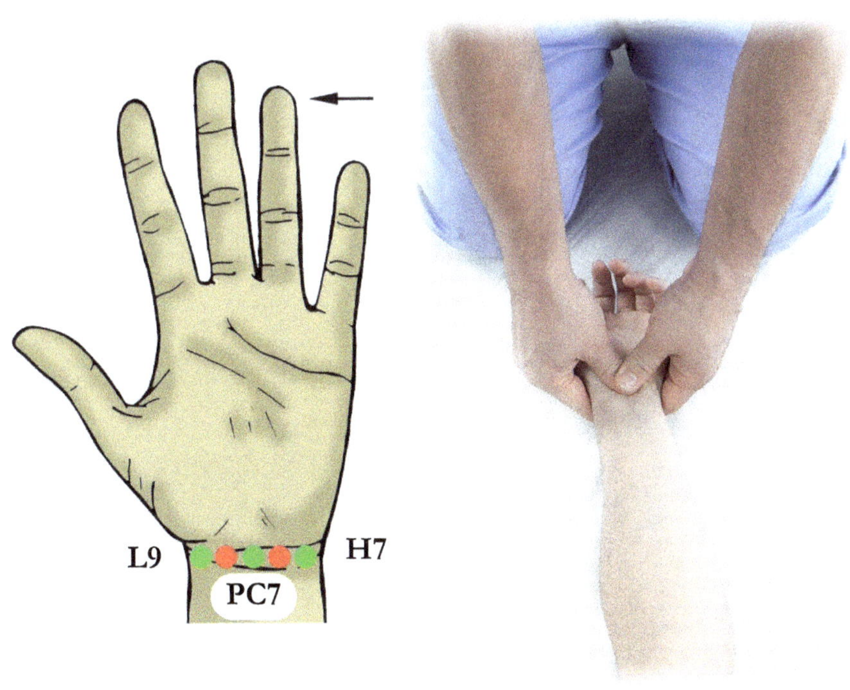

L9
H7
PC7

5.6. PALMAR REGION. CENTRAL LINE

PATIENT'S POSTURE: Supine, arm in 45° abduction and forearm in supine.

THERAPIST'S POSITION: Seiza or kneeling.

TYPE OF PRESSURE: Thumb over thumb (right below on the left side).

N°. OF POINTS: A five-point line.

DIRECTION OF THE LINE: From the wrist to the middle finger.

OBSERVATIONS: Reflective points of different organs are located in the palm of the hand, so work in this region helps to comprehensively regulate the body.

The third point approximates the location of key point 8PC (Roukyuu) (see 5.9. PALMAR REGION. CENTRAL POINT).

Three times for three seconds.

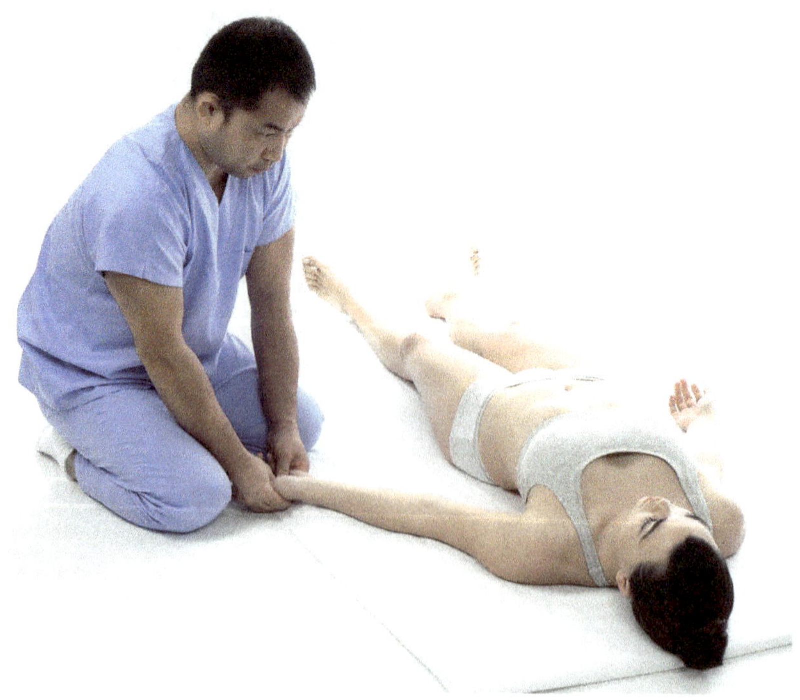

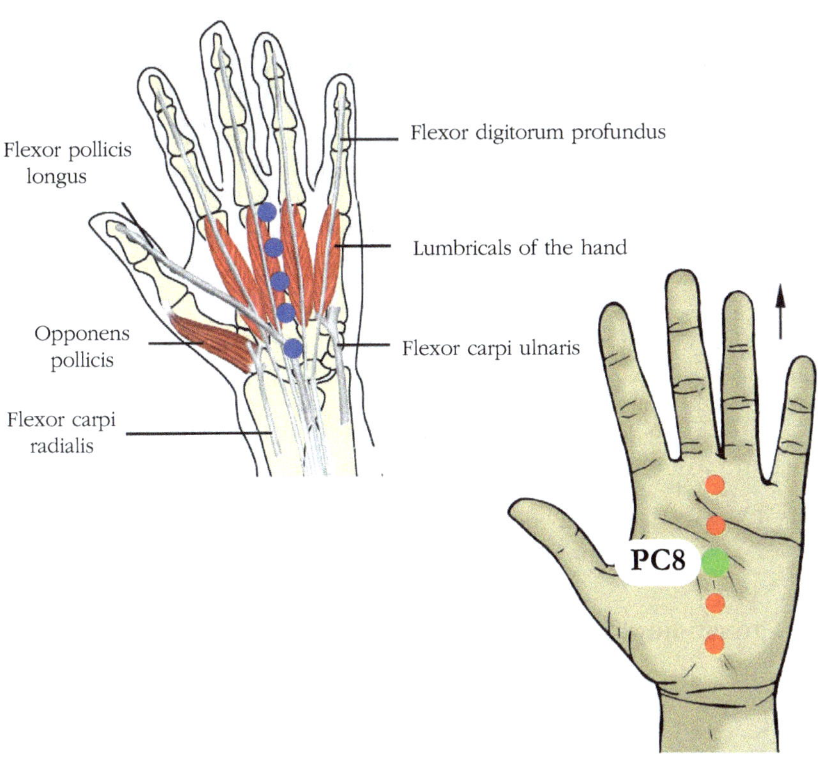

Flexor pollicis longus
Opponens pollicis
Flexor carpi radialis
Flexor digitorum profundus
Lumbricals of the hand
Flexor carpi ulnaris
PC8

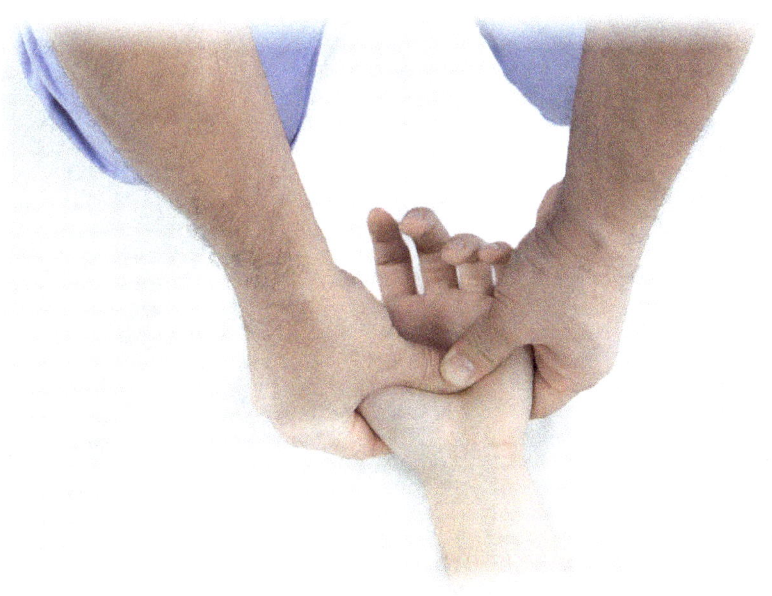

5.7. PALMAR REGION. LATERAL LINES

PATIENT'S POSTURE: Supine, arm in 45° abduction and forearm in supine.

THERAPIST'S POSITION: Seiza or kneeling.

TYPE OF PRESSURE: With both thumbs.

N°. OF POINTS: Five five-point lines on each side; sharing the central point.

DIRECTION OF THE LINE: Starting from the central line to the laterals and from the carpus to the fingers.

OBSERVATIONS: Work on the palm stimulates brain activity.

Three times for three seconds.

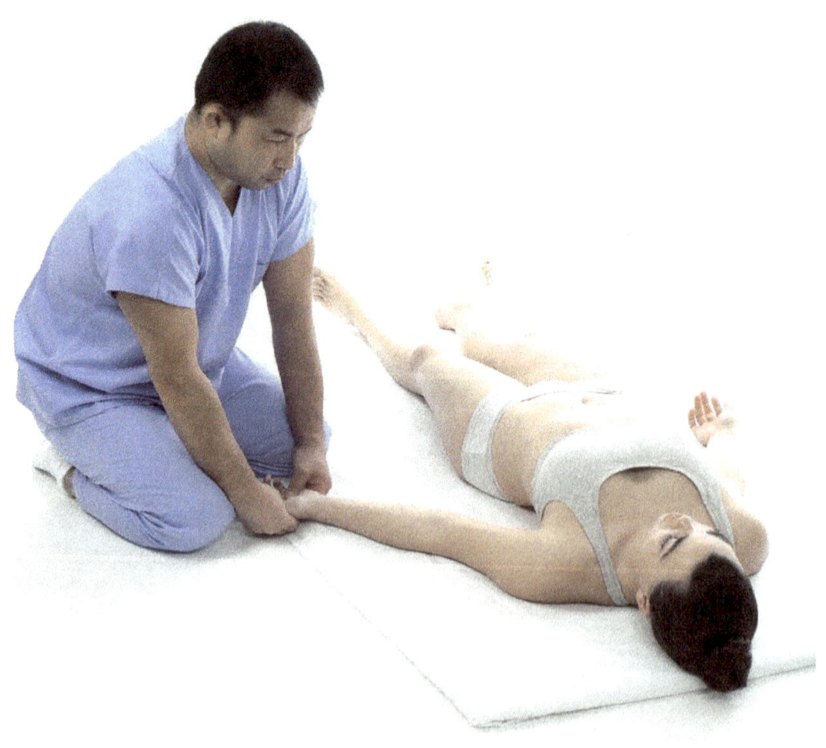

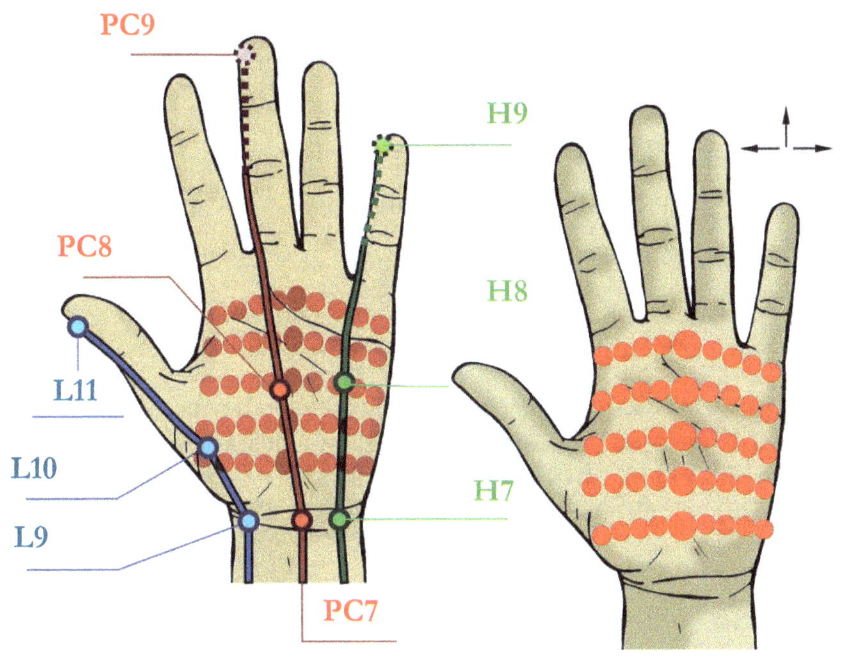

PC9
PC8
L11
L10
L9
PC7
H9
H8
H7

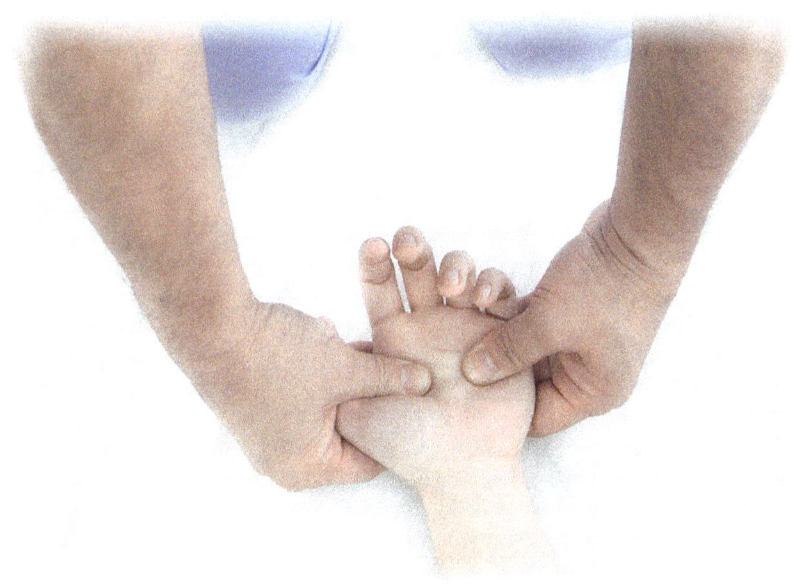

5.8. PALMAR REGION. EMINENCES

PATIENT'S POSTURE: Supine, arm in 45° abduction and forearm in supine.

THERAPIST'S POSITION: Seiza or kneeling.

TYPE OF PRESSURE: With both thumbs.

Nº. OF POINTS: Two five-point lines.

DIRECTION OF THE LINE: From the centre of the carpus to the laterals, on the thenar and hypothenar eminences.

OBSERVATIONS: At the centre of the thenar eminence is located key point L10 (Gyosai). This area is a digestive function reflection. For patients with chronic bad digestion, while applying pincer pressure to point L10, we also work point LI4 (Goukoku).

Three times for three seconds.

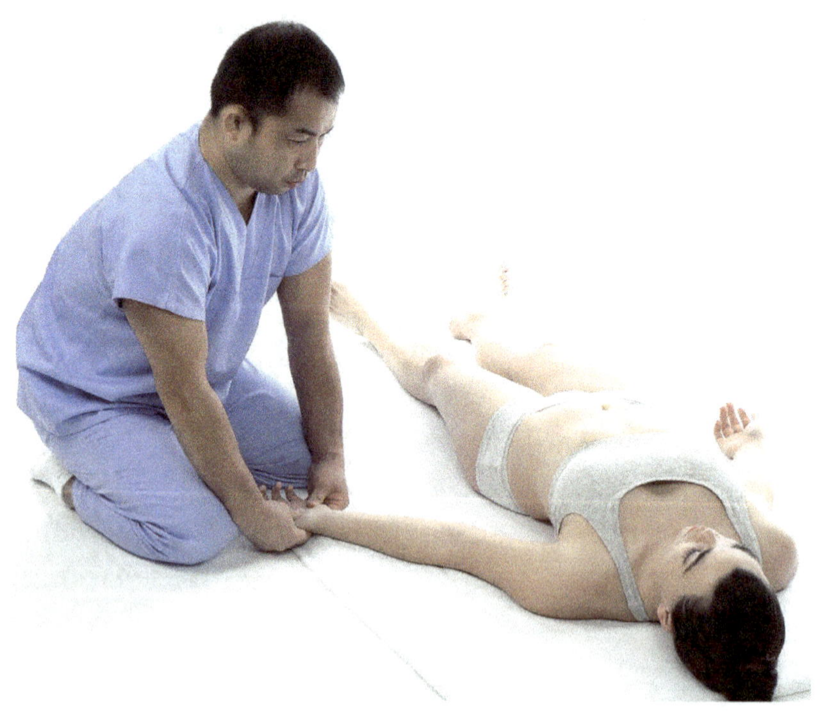

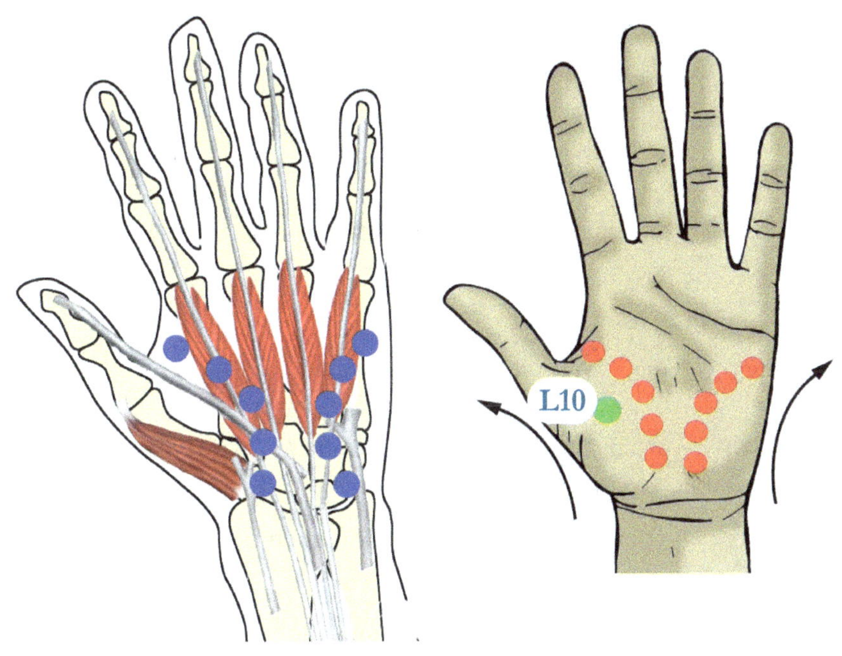

L10

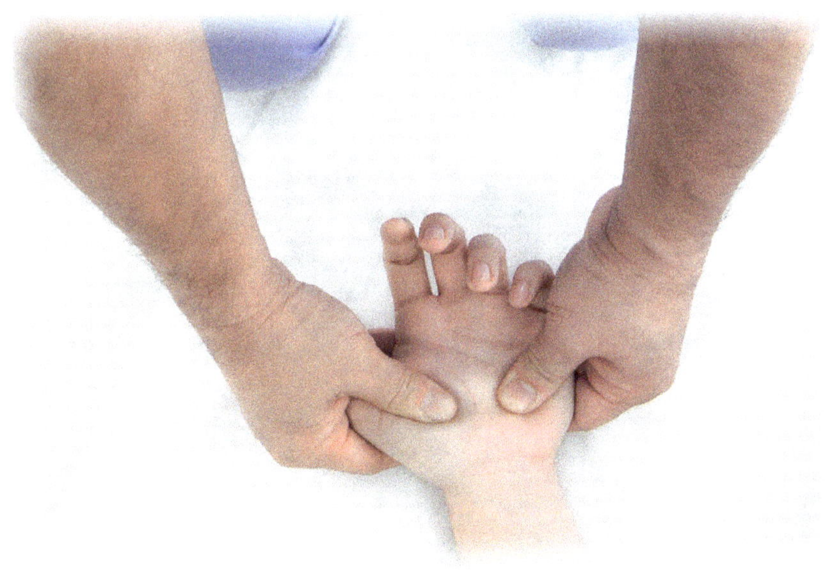

5.9. PALMAR REGION. CENTRAL POINT

PATIENT'S POSTURE: Supine, arm in 45° abduction and forearm in supine.

THERAPIST'S POSITION: Seiza or kneeling.

TYPE OF PRESSURE: Thumb over thumb (right below on the left side).

N°. OF POINTS: One.

OBSERVATIONS: By flexing the fourth finger in the direction of the middle horizontal fold, called the "head line" of the palm, we find PC8 (Roukyuu) according to our theory of Aze Shiatsu, which in Chinese traditional medicine corresponds to the flexing of the third finger.

Very close, we find point H8 (Shoufu), on the superior part of the hypothenar eminence, between the fourth and fifth metacarpal, which the little fingertip rubs when in a closed fist.

Three times for five seconds.

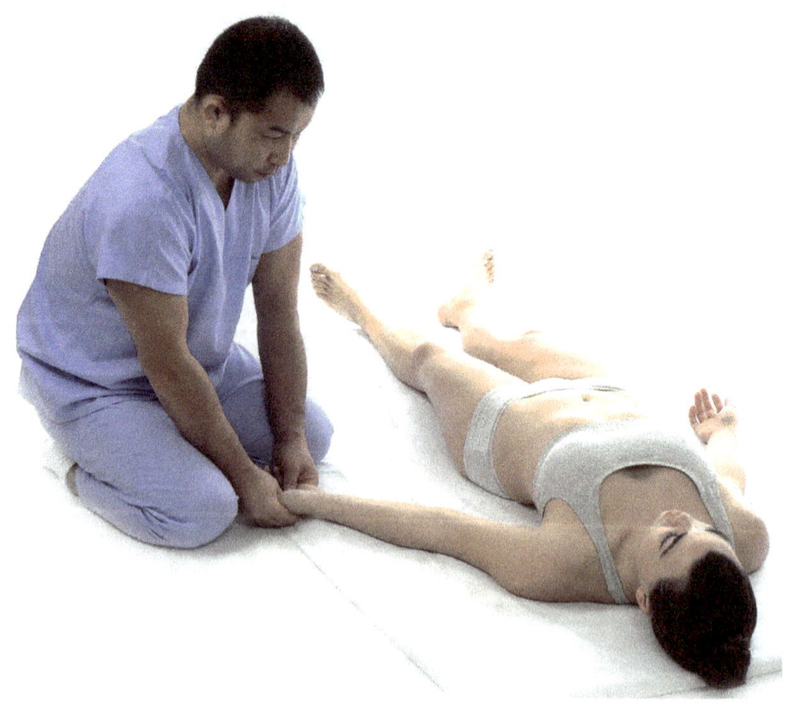

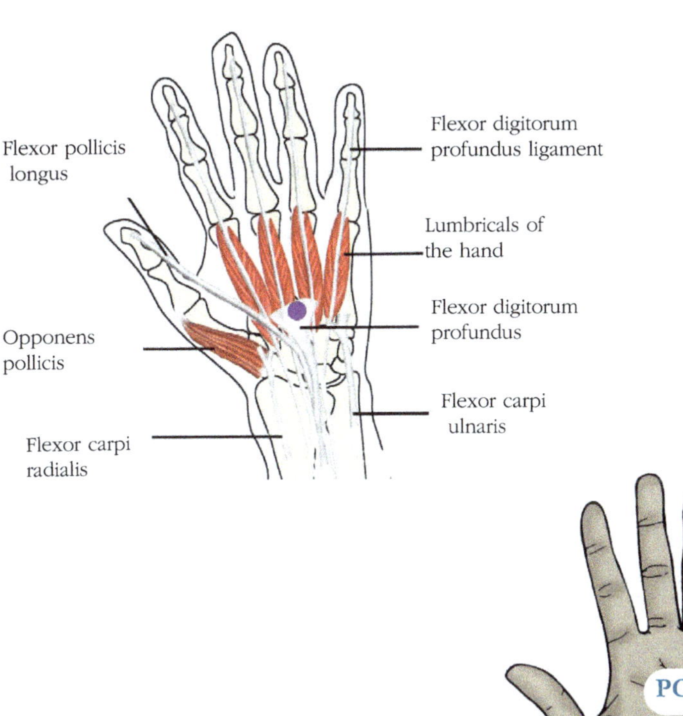

Flexor pollicis
longus
Flexor digitorum
profundus ligament
Lumbricals of
the hand
Flexor digitorum
profundus
Opponens
pollicis
Flexor carpi
ulnaris
Flexor carpi
radialis
PC8
H8
PC7
PC6

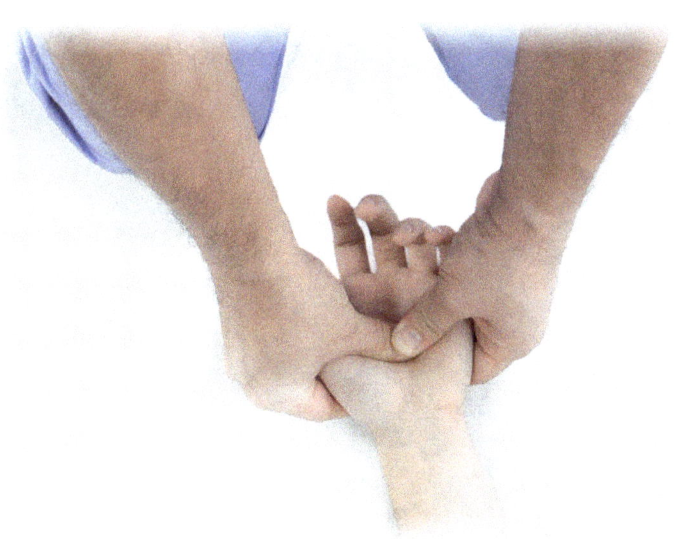

5.10. DELTOPECTORAL REGION

PATIENT'S POSTURE: Supine, arm in 45° abduction and forearm in supine.

THERAPIST'S POSITION: Kneeling.

TYPE OF PRESSURE: Thumb over thumb (left below on the left side). Work with thumbs in A if the area is very sensitive.

N°. OF POINTS: A five-point line.

DIRECTION OF THE LINE: Following the groove that forms between the deltoid muscle and the pectoralis major, from the clavicular to the axillar.

OBSERVATIONS: The first point corresponds to key point L2 (Unmon) and the second to L1 (Chuufu). In general, this region is related to the state of respiratory function.

Three times for three seconds.

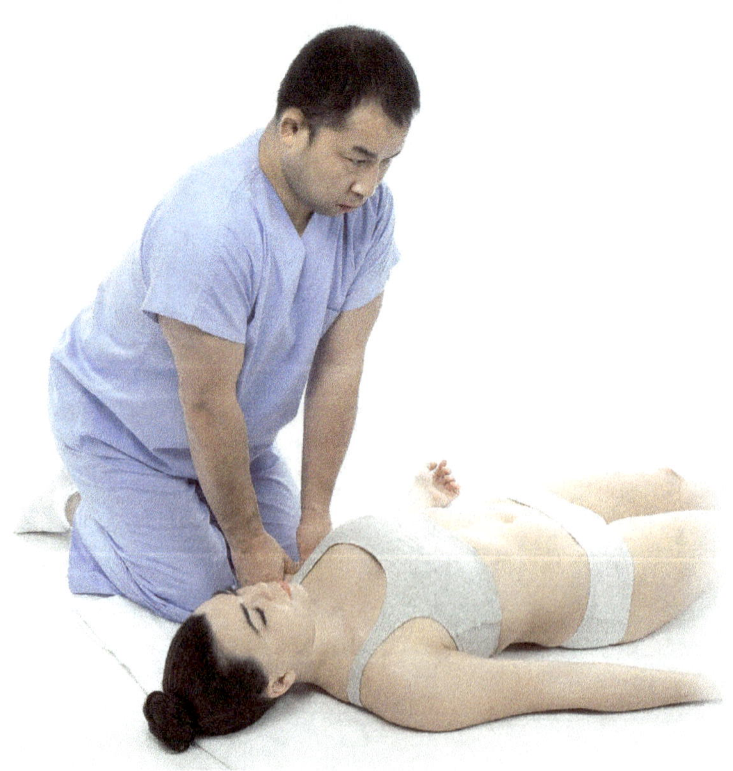

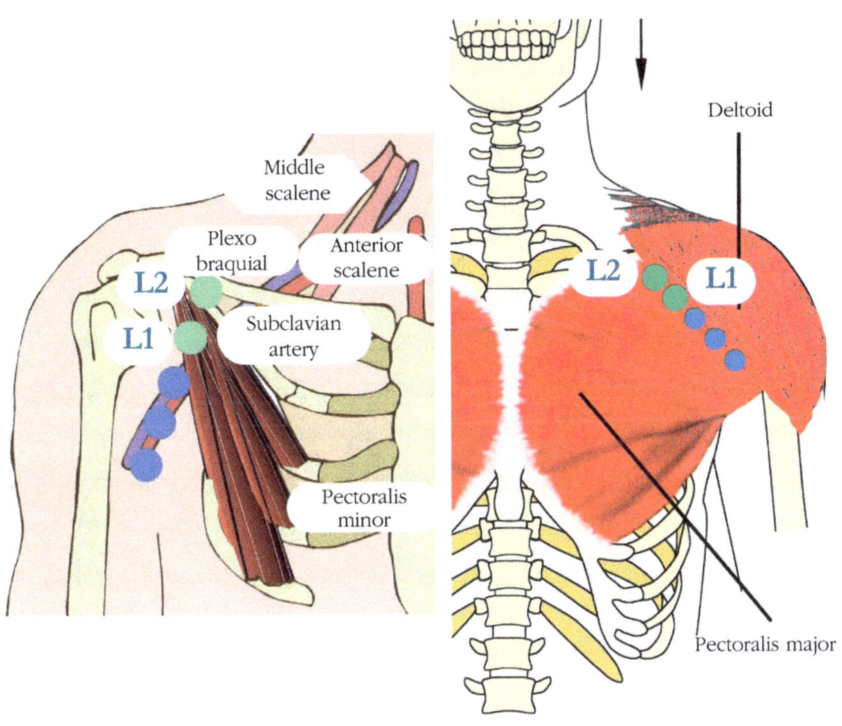

Middle
scalene
Plexo
braquial
L2
L1
Anterior
scalene
Subclavian
artery
Pectoralis
minor
Deltoid
L2
L1
Pectoralis major

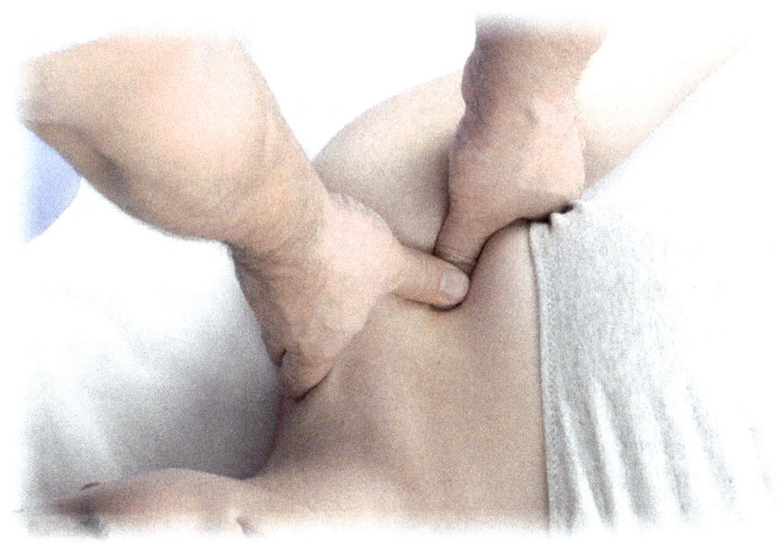

5.11. LATERAL BRACHIAL REGION

PATIENT'S POSTURE: Supine, arm in abduction, elbow bent and forearm in prone.

THERAPIST'S POSITION: Seiza, facing the area to work.

TYPE OF PRESSURE: Thumb over thumb in a V-shape (left below on the left side).

N°. OF POINTS: An eight-point line.

DIRECTION OF THE LINE: From the acromion, on the deltoids, and to the olecranana fossa. The line runs along the brachial triceps.

OBSERVATIONS: Suitable area for treating a frozen shoulder and colds.

The first point, below the acromion, corresponds to key point LI15 (Kenguu).

Three times for three seconds.

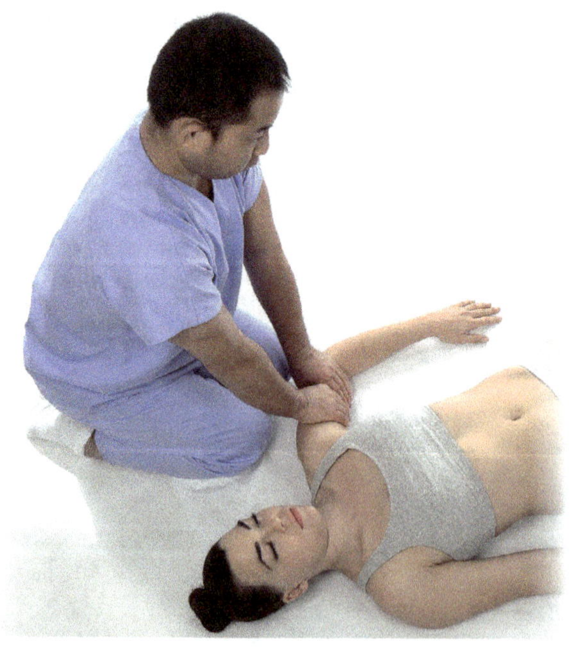

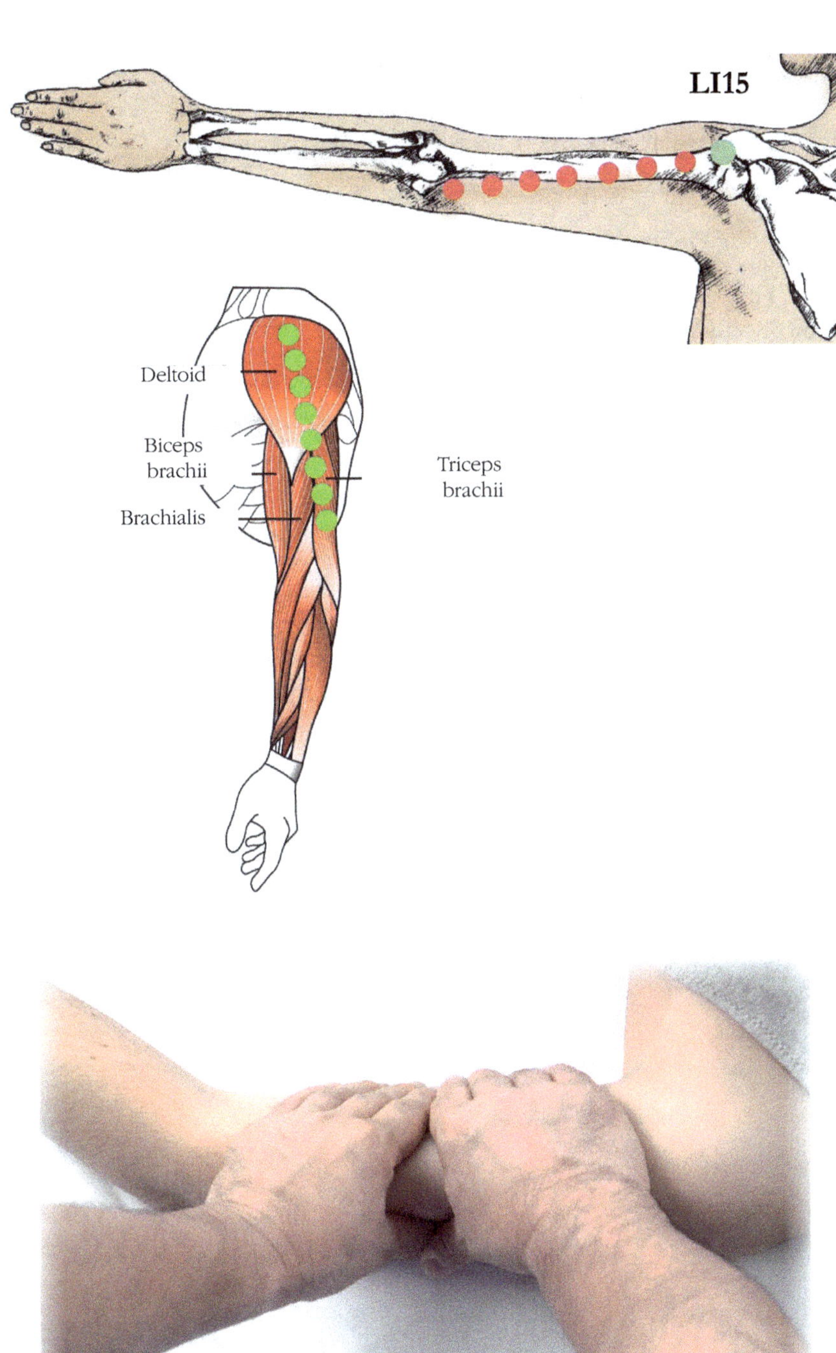

241

5.12. LATERAL ELBOW PIT REGION

PATIENT'S POSTURE: Supine, arm in abduction, elbow bent and forearm in prone.

THERAPIST'S POSITION: Seiza, facing the forearm.

TYPE OF PRESSURE: One thumb (right on the left side). The other hand holds the patient's wrist.

Nº. OF POINTS: A five-point line.

DIRECTION OF THE LINE: From the biceps tendon to the lateral epicondyl of the elbow.

OBSERVATIONS: For treating tennis elbow and sore throats.

The first point coincides with key point L5 (Syakutaku); and the fourth with LI11 (Kyokuchi).

Three times for three seconds.

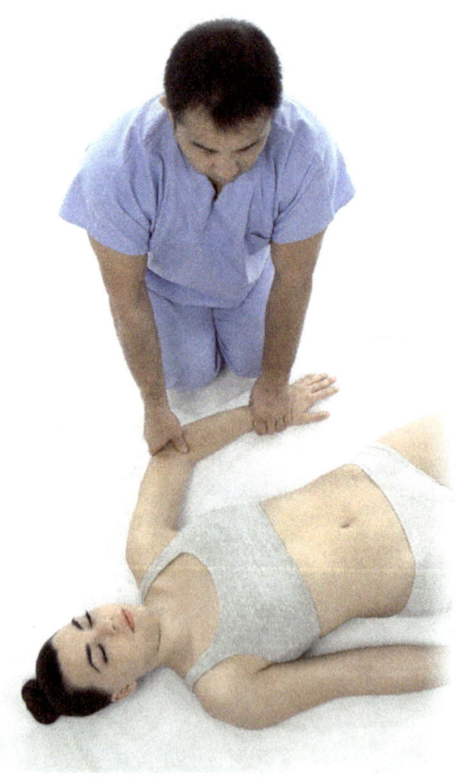

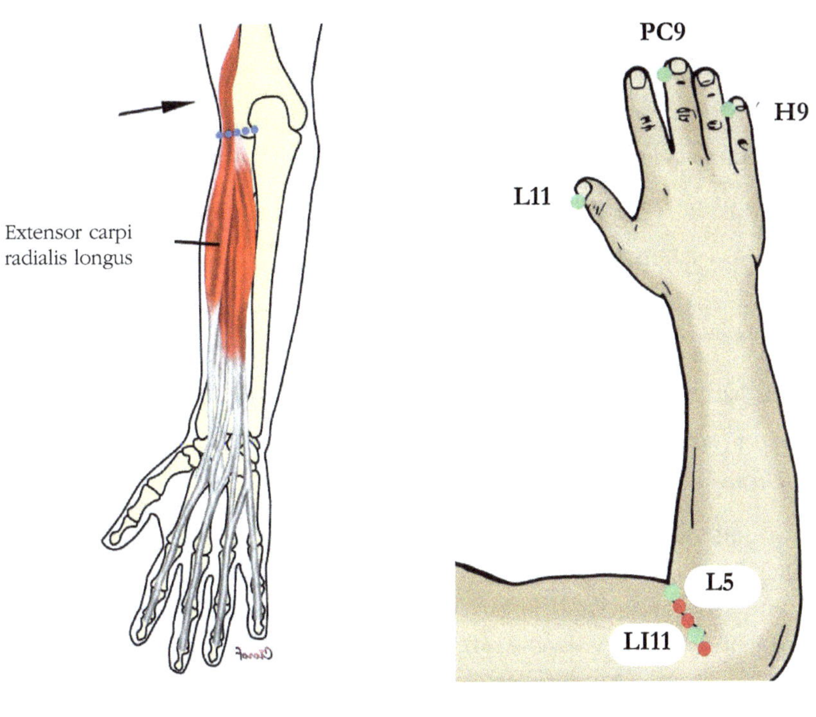

Extensor carpi radialis longus
PC9
H9
L11
L5
LI11

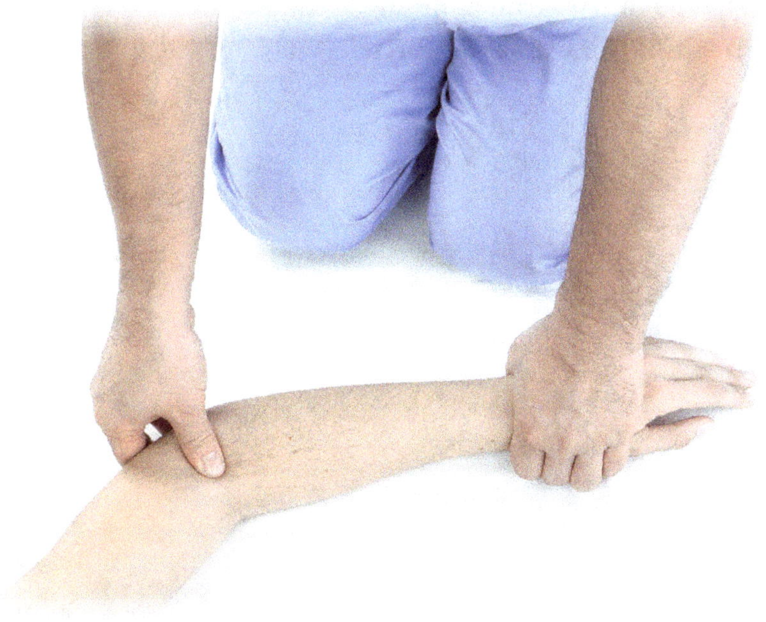

5.13. LATERAL ANTEBRACHIAL REGION

PATIENT'S POSTURE: Supine, forearm in prone. The hand rests on the therapist's leg.

THERAPIST'S POSITION: Seiza, 45° to the patient.

TYPE OF PRESSURE: Thumb over thumb (right below on the left side). When pressure is applied, the therapist performs traction of the patient's arm.

N°. OF POINTS: An eight-point line.

DIRECTION OF THE LINE: From the lateral elbow pit to the lateral wrist fold.

OBSERVATIONS: The first point coincides with key point LI10 (Te no Sanri) and is located three fingers below the lateral elbow pit. For treating arm fatigue and improving hand circulation. The seventh point corresponds to key point TB5 (Gaikan); and the eighth with TB4 (Youchi).

First point: Three times for five seconds.
The rest: Three times for three seconds.

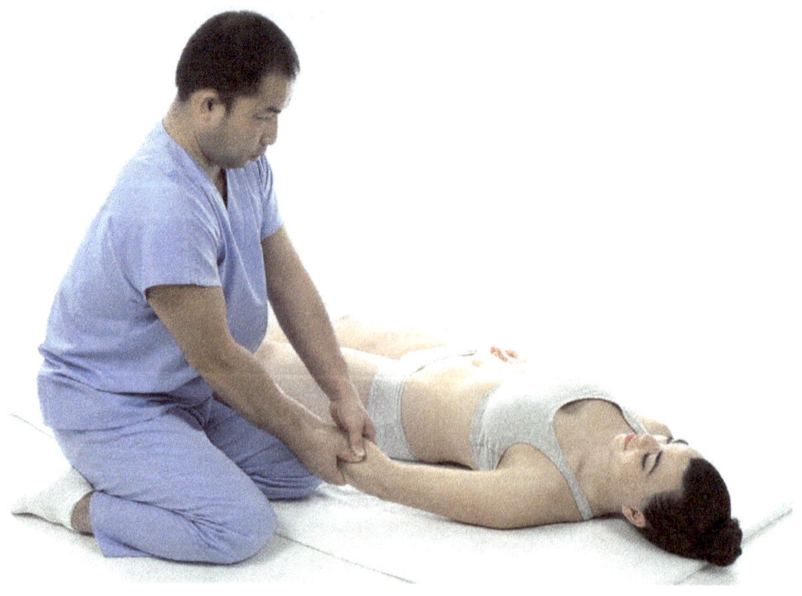

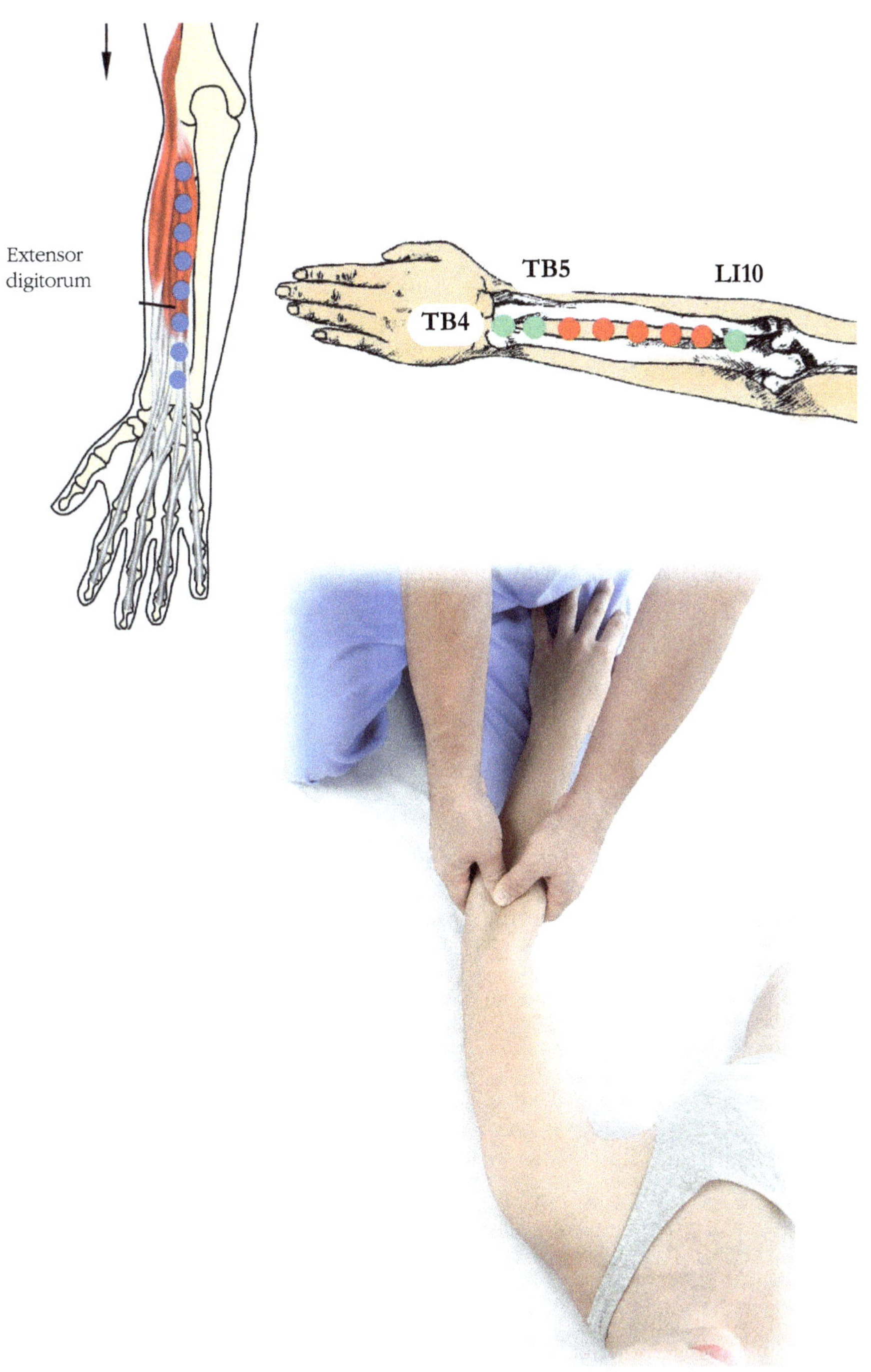

Extensor
digitorum
TB4
TB5
LI10

5.14. LATERAL REGION OF THE WRIST

PATIENT'S POSTURE: Supine, forearm in prone. The hand rests on the therapist's leg.

THERAPIST'S POSITION: Seiza, maintaining the previous position.

TYPE OF PRESSURE: Thumb over thumb (right under left side).

N°. OF POINTS: A five-point line.

DIRECTION OF THE LINE: On the lateral wrist fold, from the extreme radial to the ulnar.

OBSERVATIONS: The first point corresponds to key point LI5 (Youkei); third with TB4 (Youchi); and the fifth with SI5 (Youkoku).

Three times for three seconds.

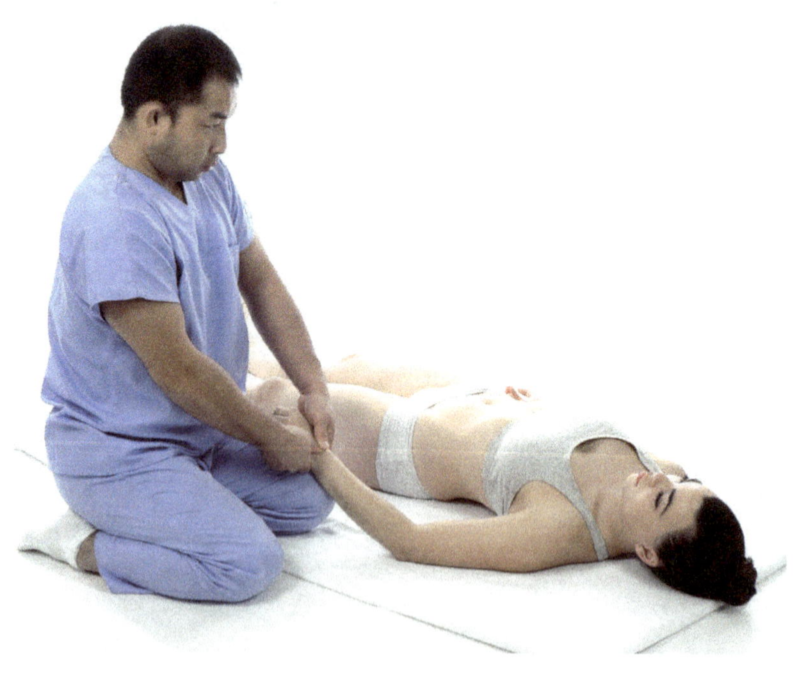

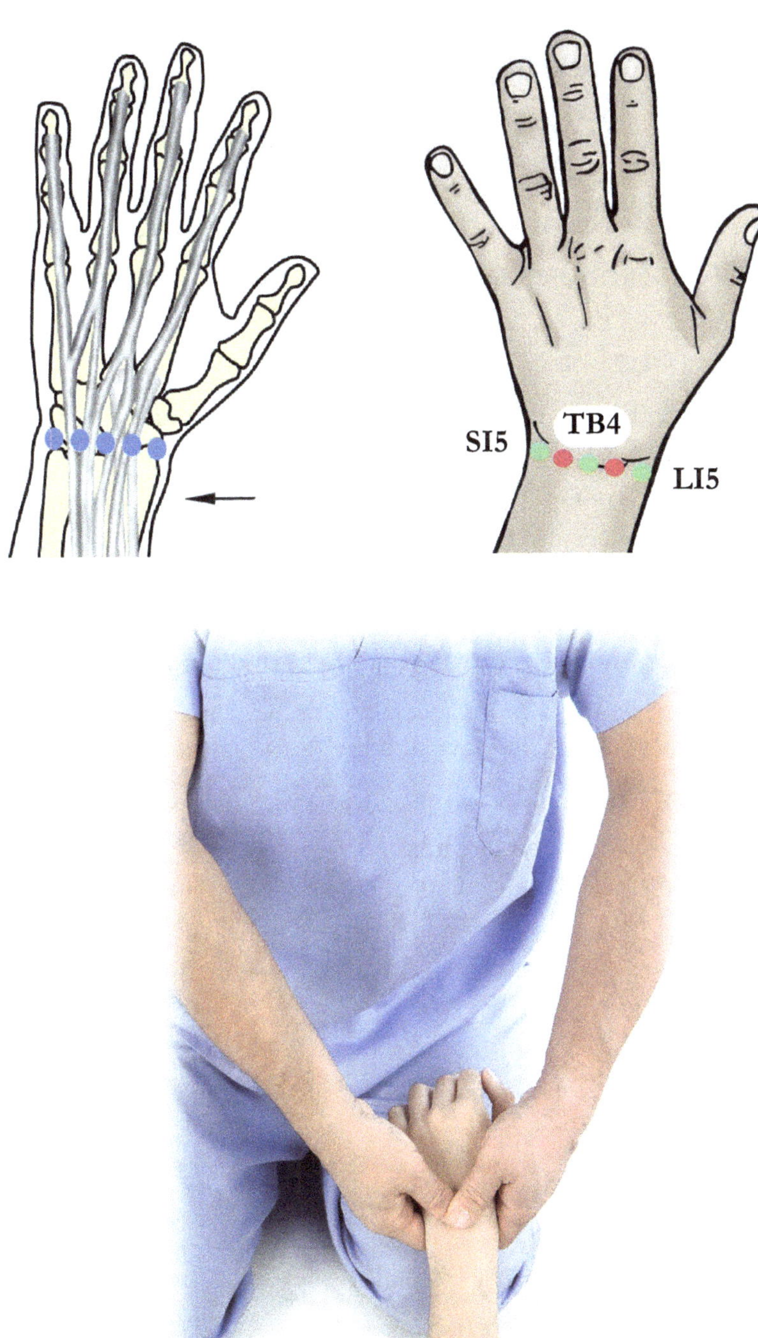

SI5
TB4
LI5

5.15. DORSAL REGION OF THE HAND

PATIENT'S POSTURE: Supine, forearm in prone. The hand rests on the therapist's leg.

THERAPIST'S POSITION: Seiza, maintaining the previous position.

TYPE OF PRESSURE: One thumb. The other hand holds the patient's hand.

N°. OF POINTS: Four five-point lines.

1st and 2nd lines, with left thumb; 3rd and 4th lines, with right thumb (on the left side).

DIRECTION OF THE LINE: In the intermetacarpal grooves. From the carpus to the fingers and from the first groove to the fourth.

OBSERVATIONS: The third point of the first line corresponds to key point LI4 (Goukoku). We call this point the "aspirin point" for its general analgesic effect and specifically for toothache and frontal headaches.

This region has two important points for treating lumbar problems: the first point of the second line, and the first point of the fourth line.

Three times for three seconds.

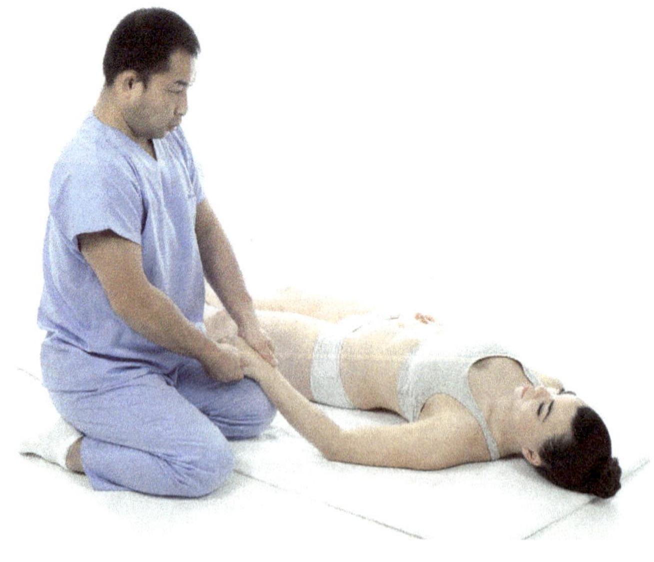

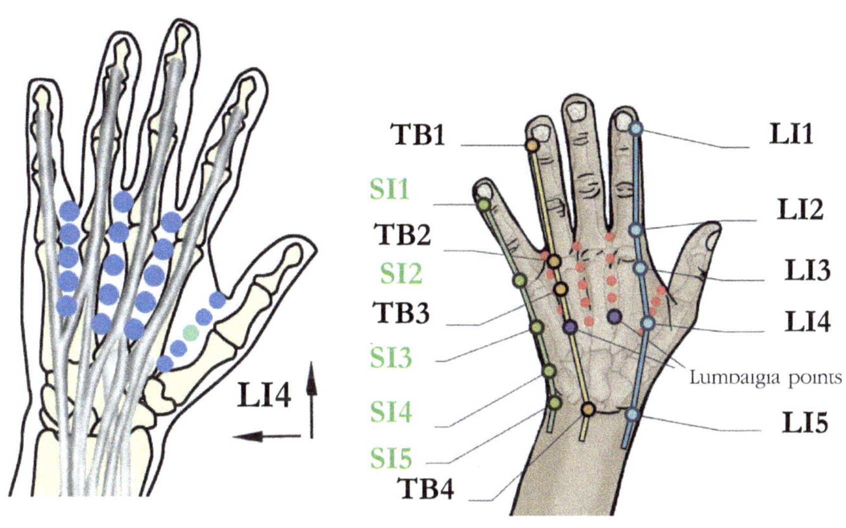

LI4
TB1
SI1
TB2
SI2
TB3
SI3
SI4
SI5
TB4
LI1
LI2
LI3
LI4
Lumbalgia points
LI5

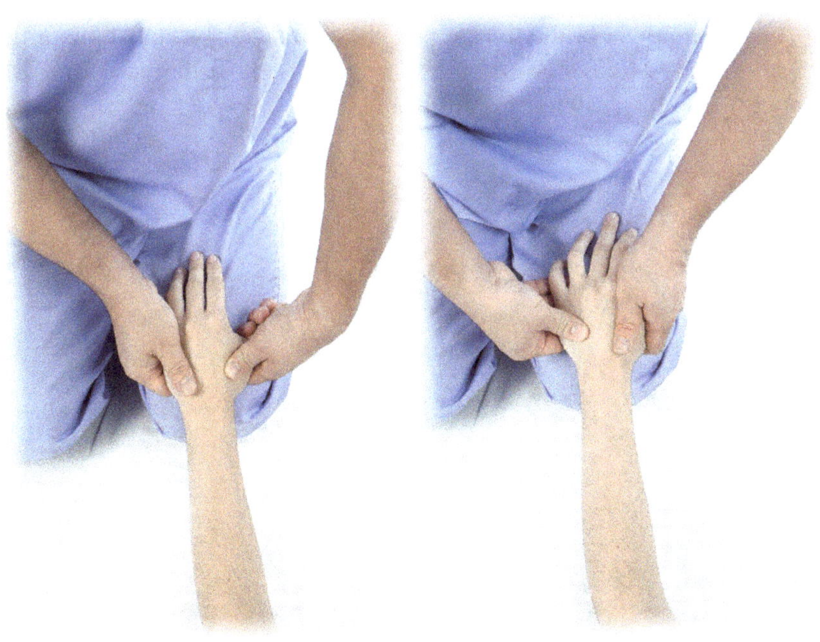

5.16. DORSAL-PALMAR AND LATERAL DIGITAL RE-GION

PATIENT'S POSTURE: Supine, forearm in prone. The hand rests on the therapist's leg.

THERAPIST'S POSITION: Seiza, maintaining the previous position.

TYPE OF PRESSURE: Thumb and index. The first three fingers with the left hand and the other two with the right (on the left side).

N°. OF POINTS: A three-point line (thumb); four four-point lines (rest).

DIRECTION OF THE LINE: From the knuckles to the nails, and from the thumb to the little finger. First on the phalanges and then in the lateral regions.

OBSERVATIONS: Pressure points are located on the joints and on the nail.

This exercise stimulates the key points that are located at the ends of your fingers. They are as follows: L11 (Syousyou, radial angle of the thumbnail); LI1 (Syouyou, radial angle of the second nail); PC9 (Chu-usyou, radial angle of the third nail); TB1 (Kansyou, cubital angle of the fourth nail); H9 (Syousyou, radial angle of the fifth nail); and SI1 (Syoutaku, cubital angle of the fifth nail).

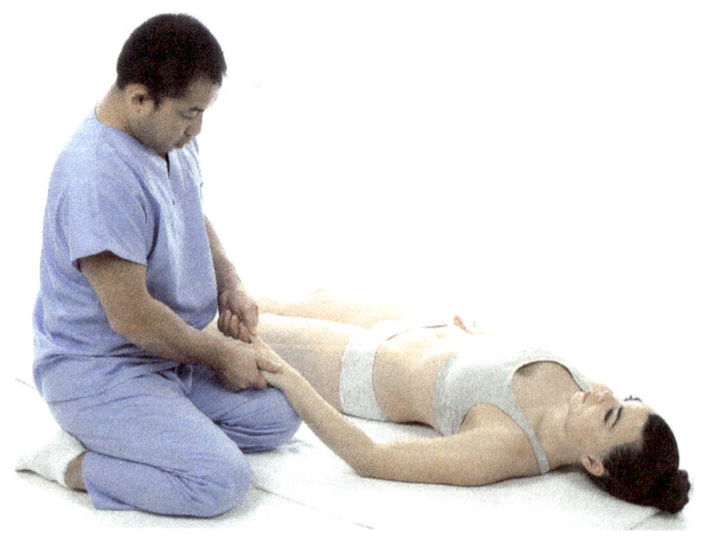

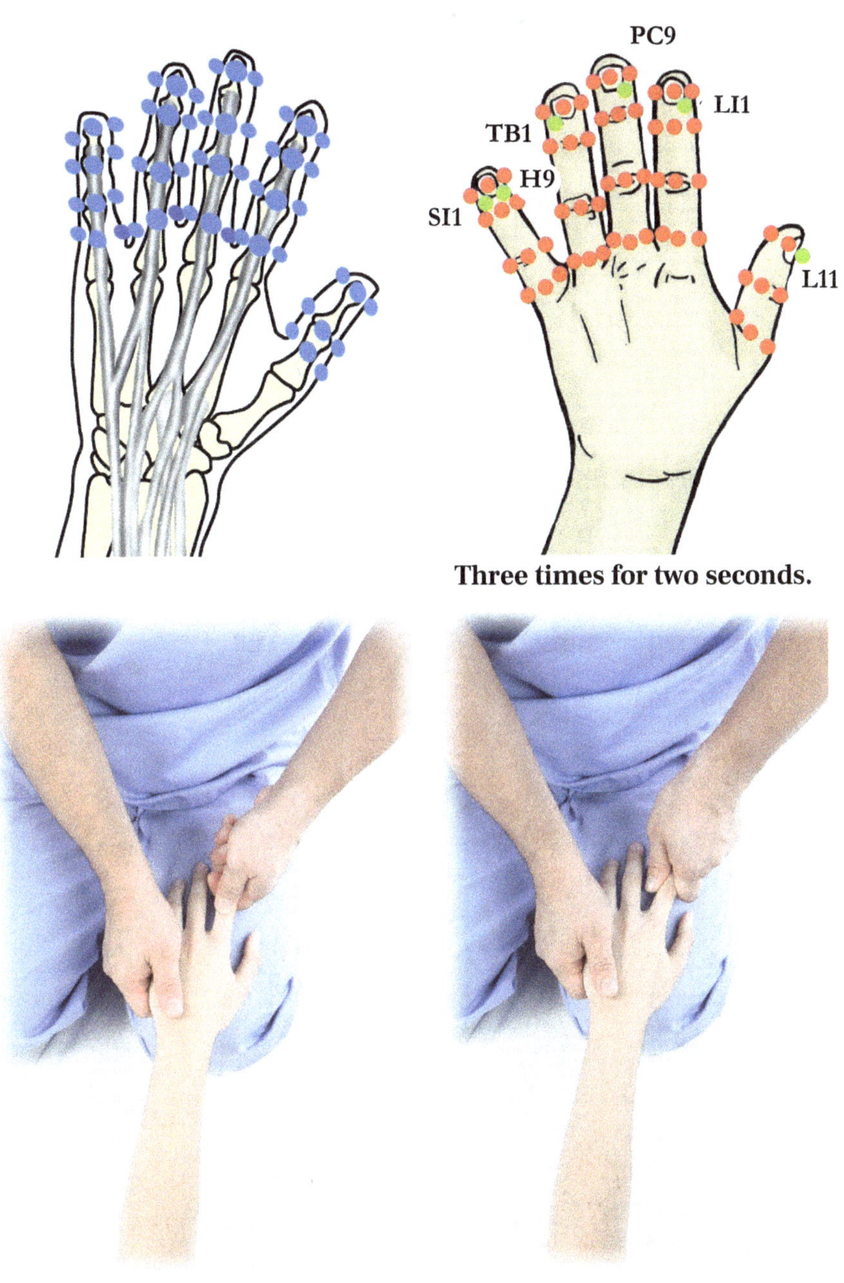

Three times for two seconds.

Repeat the upper limb work on the right arm.

6. Abdomen

6.1. Palm pressure.

6.2. Hand-over-hand pressure.

6.3. Pressure with both thumbs.

6.4. Kidney region.

6.5. Diaphragm region.

6.6. Sigmoid colon region.

6.7. Undulating pressure.

6.8. Circular pressure.

6.9. Vibrational pressure.

6.10. Relaxation.

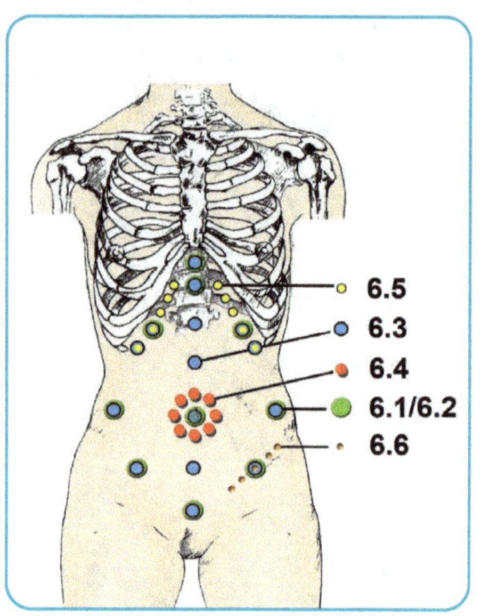

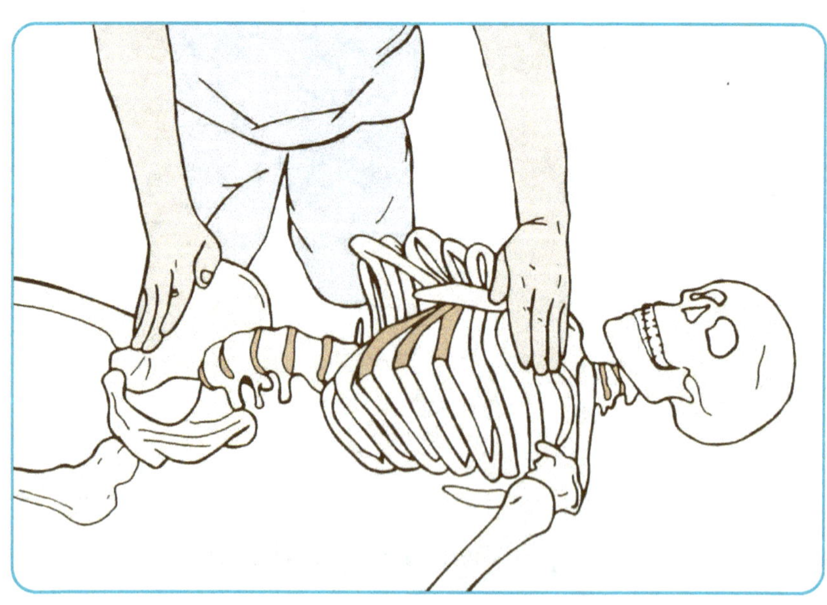

6. TO KEEP IN MIND: ABDOMEN

The abdomen is worked on from the patient's right side.

- It's a very important and fundamental area.
- Working the abdomen for a few minutes rebalances the body.
- Almost the entire abdomen routine is done in a seiza posture.
- The first pressures are applied slower, to see the patient's receptivity.

- Three pressures:

– 1st time: Soft pressure.
– 2nd time: The pressure is deeper.
– 3rd time: You have to find the contracture.

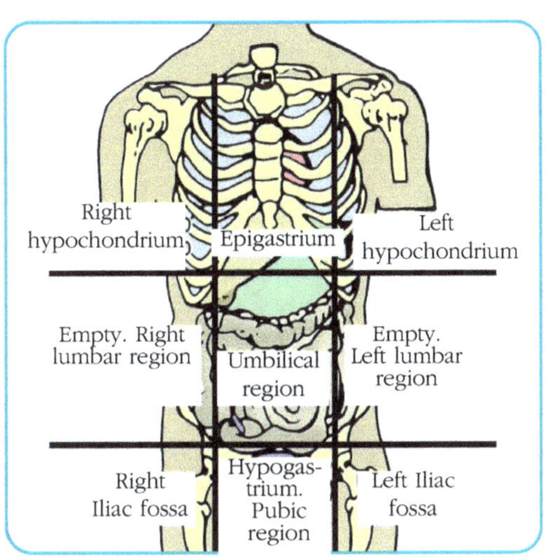

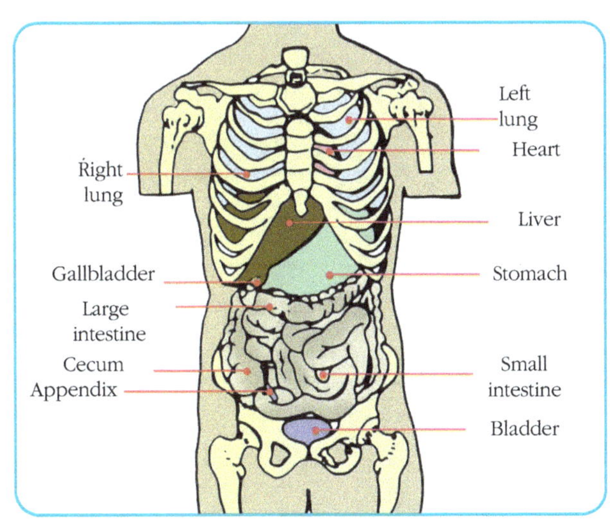

PATIENT-THERAPIST POSITION

PATIENT'S POSTURE: Supine, right arm in 90° abduction.

THERAPIST'S POSITION: Seiza, perpendicular to the patient's right side.

TYPE OF PRESSURE: Palm (pressure is applied with the right hand, left hand rests on the patient's shoulder).

OBSERVATIONS: This posture is maintained for all regions except region 6.3 Thumb pressure (basic posture).

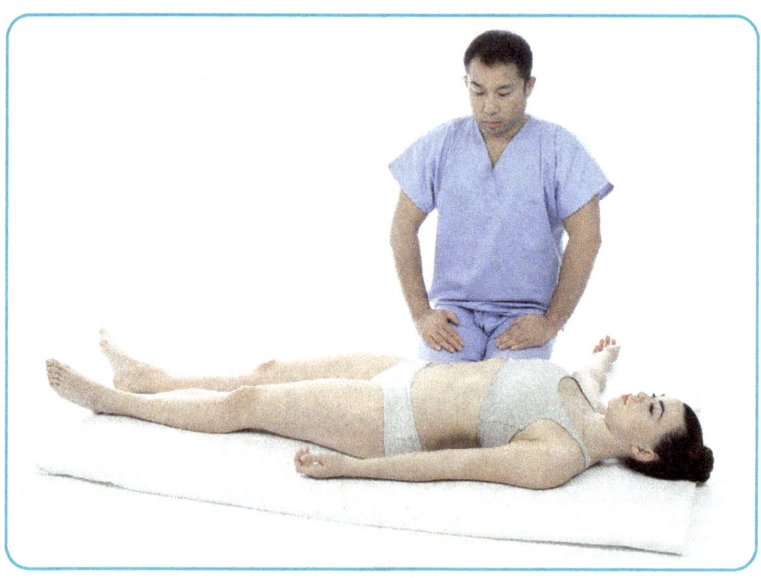

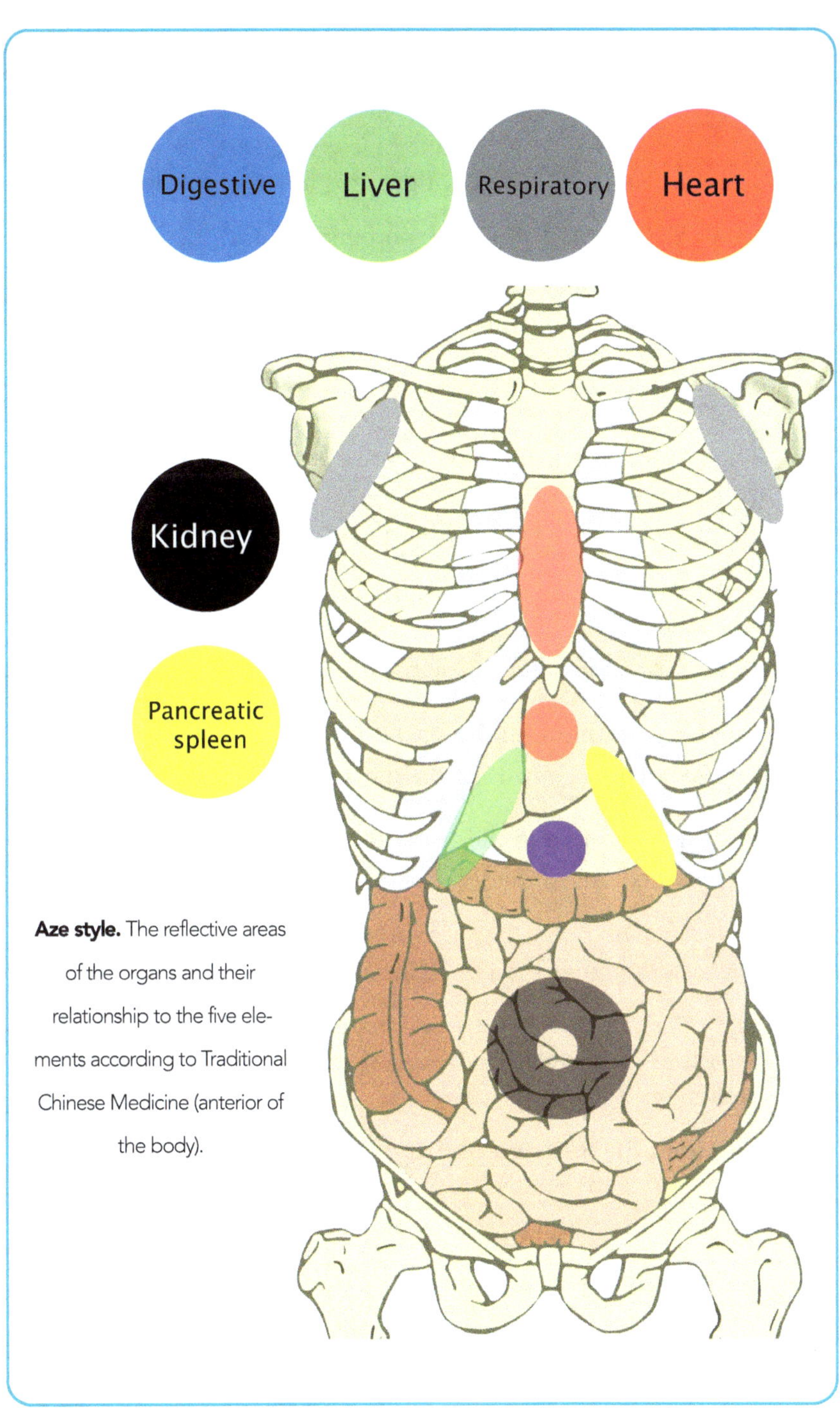

Aze style. The reflective areas of the organs and their relationship to the five elements according to Traditional Chinese Medicine (anterior of the body).

6.1. PALM PRESSURE

PATIENT'S POSTURE: Supine, right arm in 90° abduction.

THERAPIST'S POSITION: Seiza, perpendicular to the patient.

TYPE OF PRESSURE: Palm. The right hand applies pressure while the left hand rests on the patient's shoulder.

N°. OF POINTS: Ten pressures (nine plus repetition of the epigastrium).

1. Epigastrium (Heart/Emotion): In the epigastric fossa.

2. Kidney: On the navel.

3. Bladder: Above the pubic symphysis.

4. Caecum: In the right iliac fossa.

5. Ascending colon: In the right flank.

6. Right Hypochondrium (L and GB): In the centre of the right hypochondrium.

7. Repeat epigastrium: In the epigastric fossa.

8. Left hypochondrium (SP): In the centre of the left hypochondrium.

9. Descending colon: In the left flank.

10. Sigmoid colon: In the left iliac fossa.

DIRECTION OF THE LINE: It works circularly clockwise, between the hypochondrium and the iliac ridges.

OBSERVATIONS: The hand works naturally with the fingers always pointing towards the patient's left flank. Pressure accompanying the patient's breathing.

Three times for three seconds.

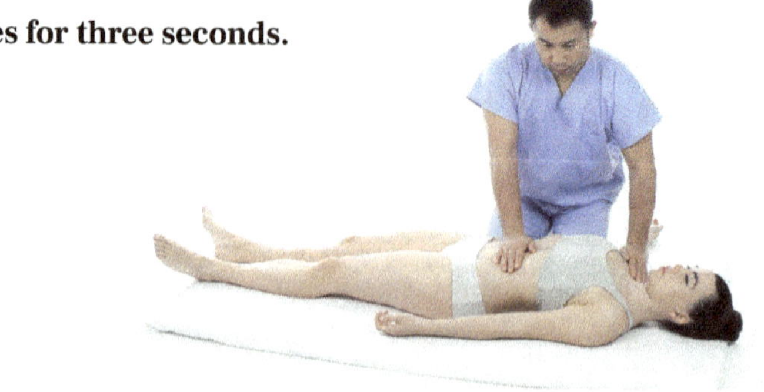

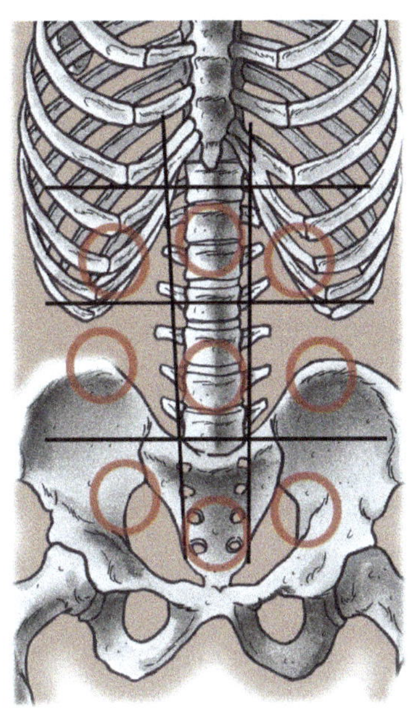

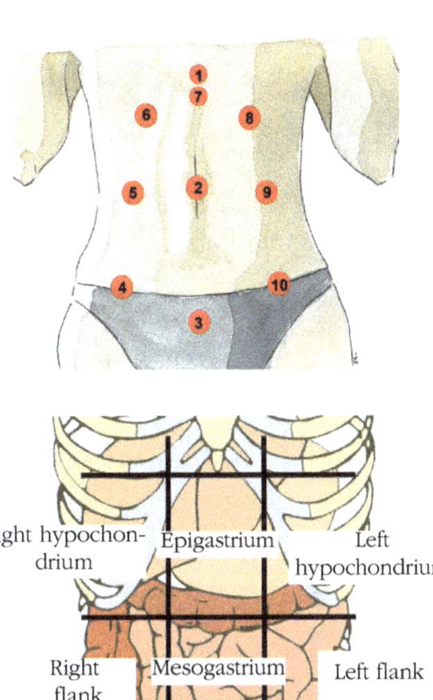

Right hypochon-
drium
Epigastrium
Left
hypochondrium
Right
flank
Mesogastrium
Left flank
Right Iliac
fossa
Hypogastrium
Left Iliac
fossa

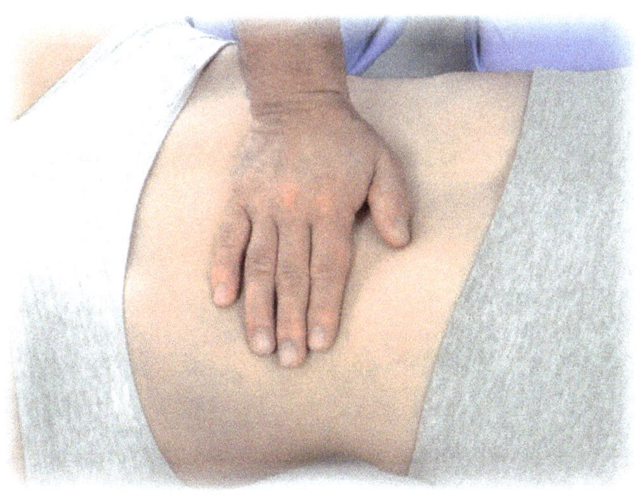

6.2. HAND-OVER-HAND PRESSURE

PATIENT'S POSTURE: Supine, right arm in 90° abduction.

THERAPIST'S POSITION: Seiza, perpendicular to the patient.

TYPE OF PRESSURE: Palm over palm. The whole palm in contact, but concentrated at the end of the fingers.

Nº. OF POINTS: Ten (nine plus repetition of the epigastrium).

1. Epigastrium (Heart/Emotion); 2. Kidney; 3. Bladder; 4. Caecum; 5. Ascending colon; 6. Right hypochondrium (L and GB); 7. Repeat epigastrium; 8. Left hypocondrium (SP); 9. Descending Colon, and 10. Sigmoid colon.

DIRECTION OF THE LINE: Same as in the previous region.

OBSERVATIONS: Fingers always point towards the patient's left flank.

Three times for three seconds.

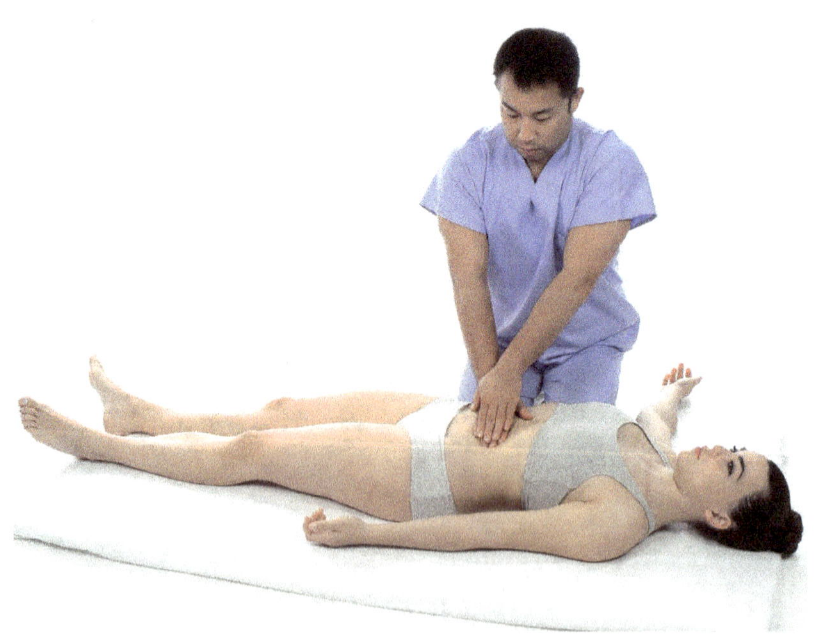

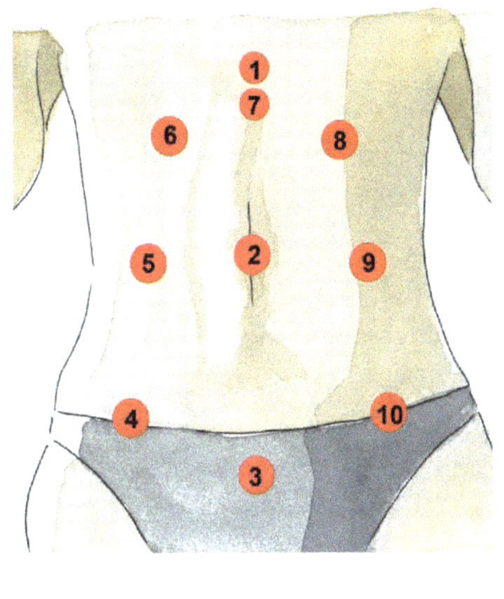

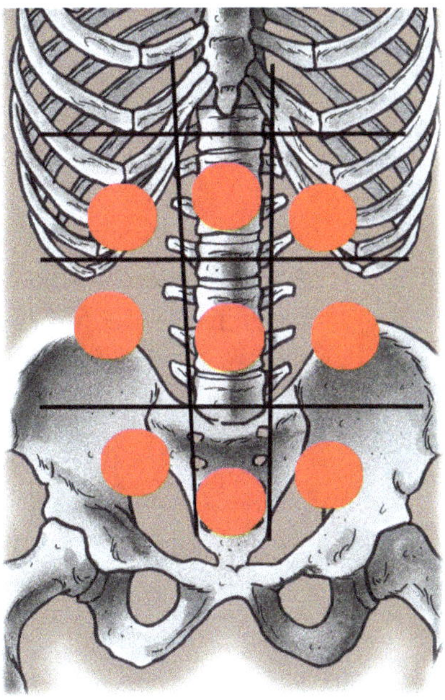

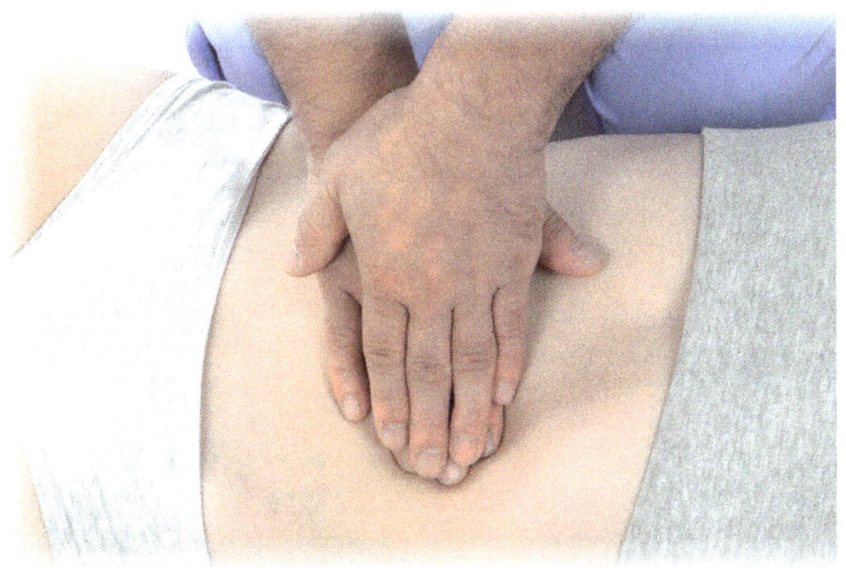

6.3. PRESSURE WITH BOTH THUMBS

PATIENT'S POSTURE: Supine, right arm in 90° abduction.

THERAPIST'S POSITION: Basic.

TYPE OF PRESSURE: Thumbs in A.

N°. OF POINTS: Fifteen (fourteen plus repetition of the epigastrium).

1. Epigastrium (Heart/Emotion): In the epigastric fossa.
2. Stomach: Between the epigastric fossa and the navel.
3. Kidney: Above the navel:
4. Small intestine: Below the navel.
5. Tanden: Between the navel and the pubic symphysis.
6. Bladder (rectum, uterus, prostate): Above pubic symphysis.
7. Caecum: In the right iliac fossa.
8. Ascending colon: In the right flank.
9. Liver 1: In the right hypochondrium.
10. Liver 2: In the right hypochondrium.
11. Epigastrium/Diaphragm (repeat): In the epigastric fossa.
12. Spleen 1: In the left hypochondrium.
13. Spleen 2: In the left hypochondrium.
14. Descending colon: In the left flank.
15. Sigmoid colon: In the left iliac fossa.

DIRECTION OF THE LINE: Same as in the previous region.

OBSERVATIONS: Pressure is applied perpendicularly, but at points 9, 10, 12 and 13 you enter slightly below the rib cage.

Three times for three seconds.

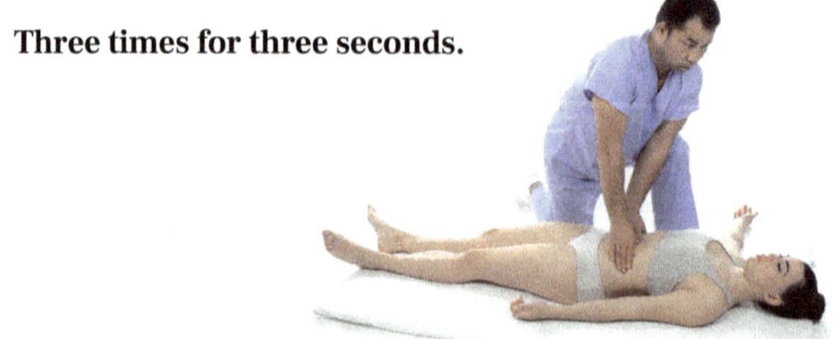

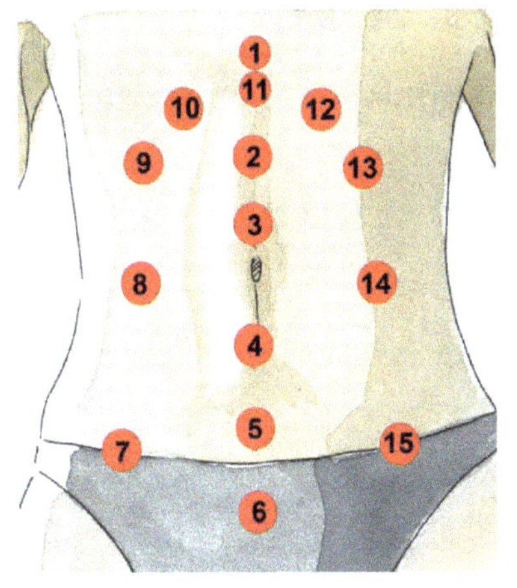

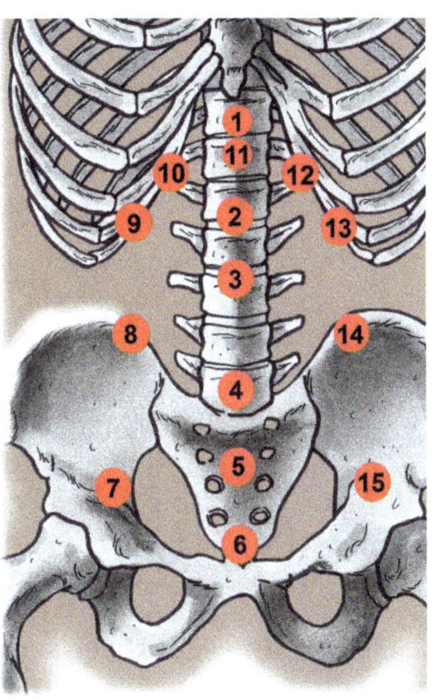

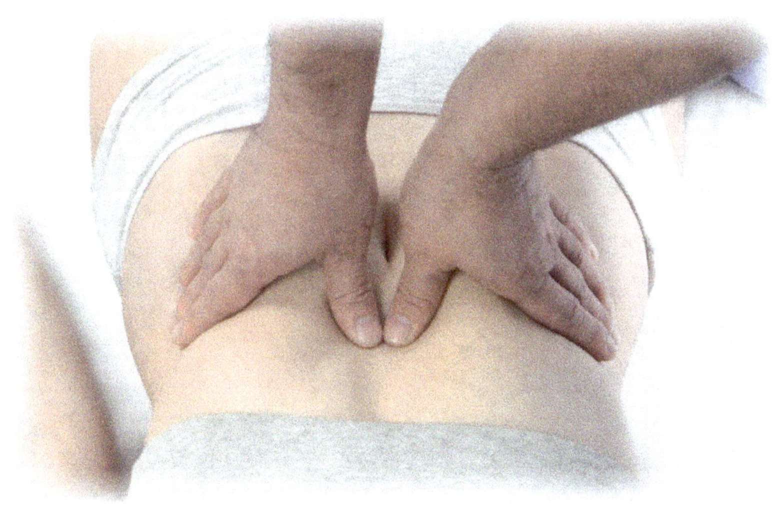

6.4. KIDNEY REGION

PATIENT'S POSTURE: Supine, right arm in 90° abduction.

THERAPIST'S POSITION: Seiza, perpendicular to the patient.

TYPE OF PRESSURE: Palm over palm. The whole palm in contact, but concentrated at the end of the fingers.

N°. OF POINTS: Eight.

DIRECTION OF THE LINE: Around the navel, from the superior mid-line clockwise.

OBSERVATIONS: Stimulates the kidney region.

In the area we can highlight two key points: **CV9 (Suibun)**, which calms abdominal pain and gastroenteritis diarrhea, and **K16 (Kouyu)** indicated to relieve tension and abdominal swelling.

Three times for three seconds.

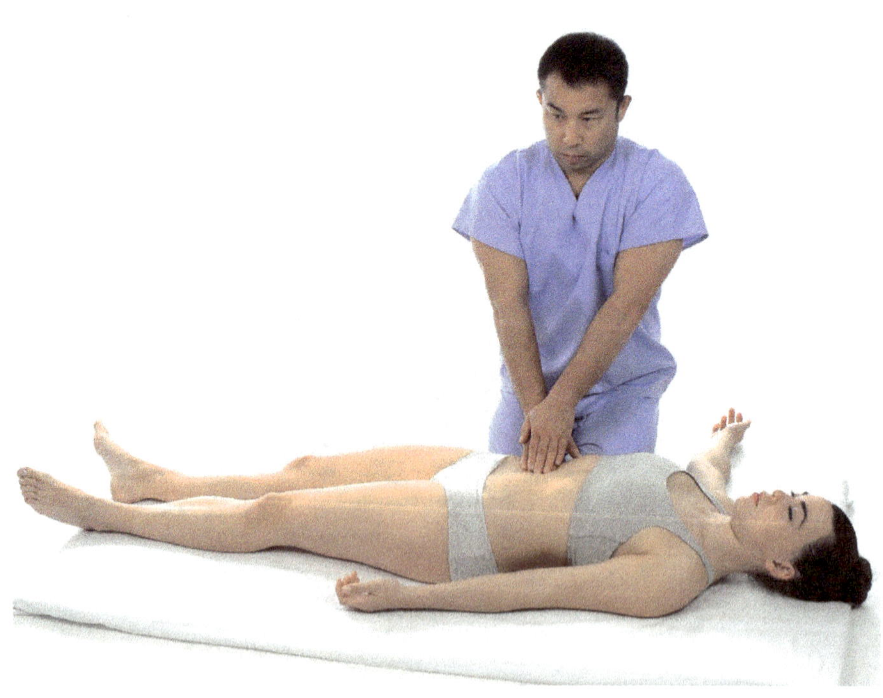

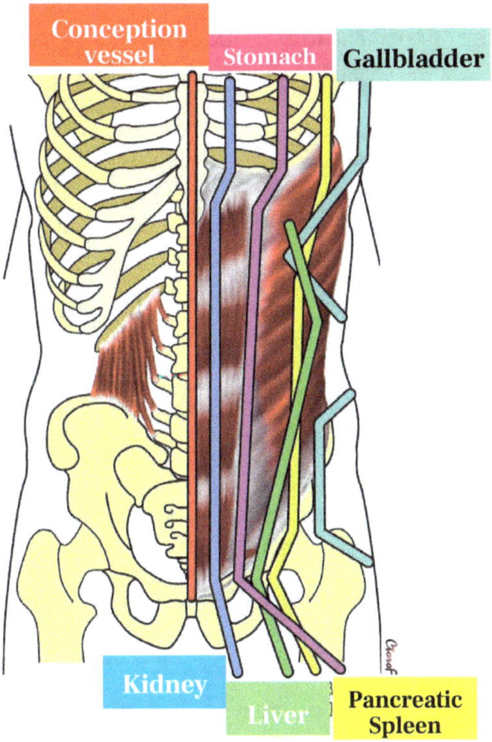

Conception vessel
Stomach
Gallbladder
Kidney
Liver
Pancreatic Spleen

CV9
K16
1
2
3
4
5
6
7
8

1
2
3
4
5
6
7
8

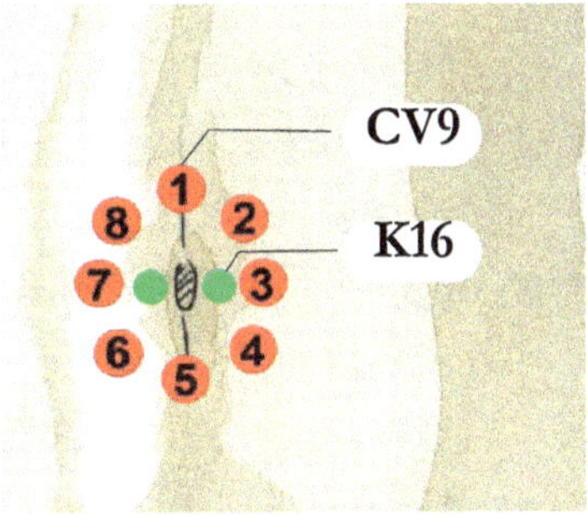

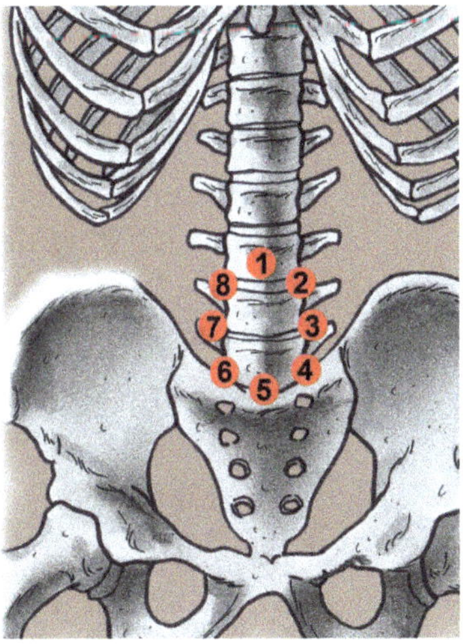

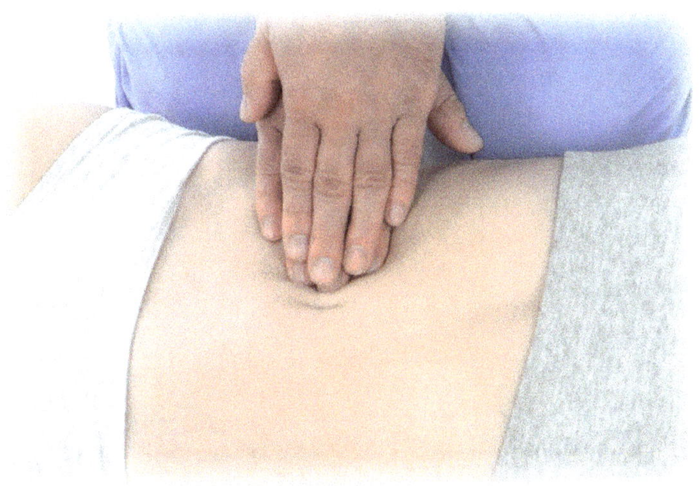

6.5. DIAPHRAGM REGION

PATIENT'S POSTURE: Supine, right arm in 90° abduction.

THERAPIST'S POSITION: Seiza, 45° angle to the patient's left shoulder.

TYPE OF PRESSURE: Palm over palm. The whole palm in contact, but concentrated at the end of the fingers.

N°. OF POINTS: Two five-point lines + solar plexus.

1st Solar Plexus. CV14 (Koketsu)

2nd Right Hypochondrium (Liver Region).

3rd Left Hypochondrium (Spleen-Pancreatic Region).

DIRECTION OF THE LINE: From the solar plexus laterally.

OBSERVATIONS: One slow pressure is applied accompanying the patient's breathing.

In addition to working the Liver and Spleen-Pancreas, it works directly on the diaphragm, applying pressure to the key point **14CV** (Koketsu) indicated for heart pathologies and psychic disorders.

Pressure enters properly when the body is healthy (stress-free) and the diaphragm area is empty (Kyo).

Point **CV6** (**Kikai**, Sea of Energy) is the point where energy, Ki, is generated and stored.

Although the exact position may vary depending on each person, it is located in the middle line of the abdomen, about two to three centimeters below the navel (1.5 cun).

Three times for three

seconds.

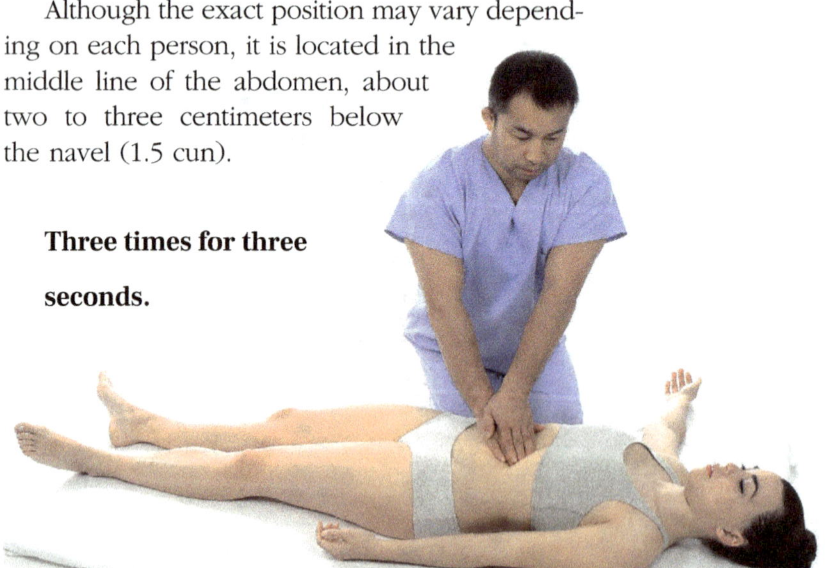

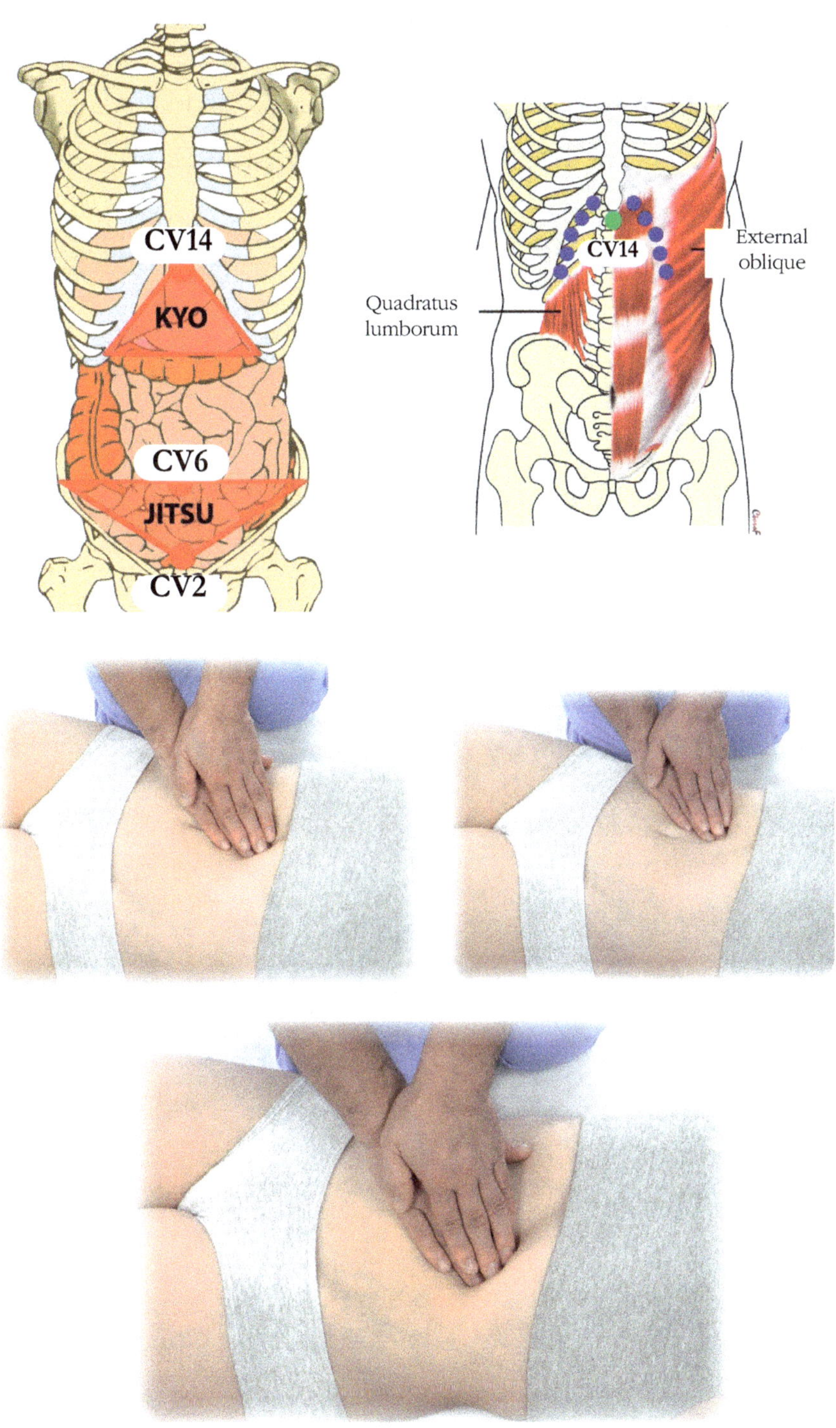

CV14
KYO
CV6
JITSU
CV2
CV14
External oblique
Quadratus lumborum

6.6. SIGMOID COLON REGION

PATIENT'S POSTURE: Supine, right arm in 90° abduction.

THERAPIST'S POSITION: Seiza or kneeling, perpendicular to the patient.

TYPE OF PRESSURE: Both eminences of the right hand. The left hand rests on the patient's shoulder.

Nº. OF POINTS: A five-point line.

DIRECTION OF THE LINE: In the left iliac fossa, from the antero-superior iliac spine to the pubis.

Three times for three seconds.

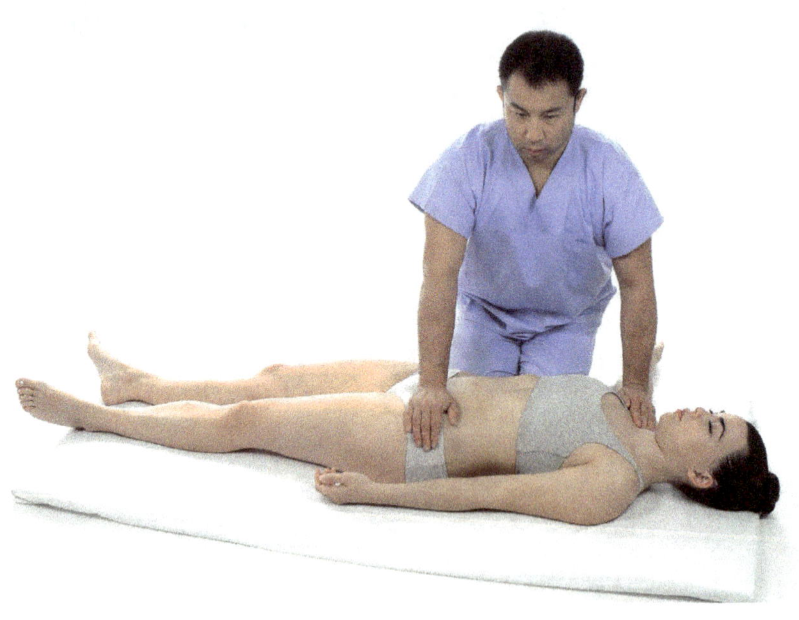

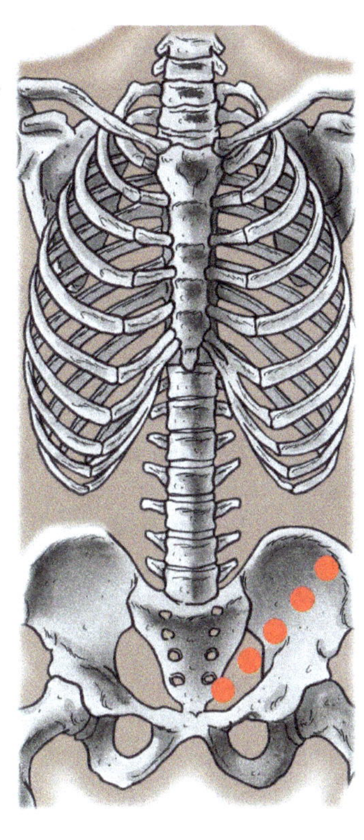

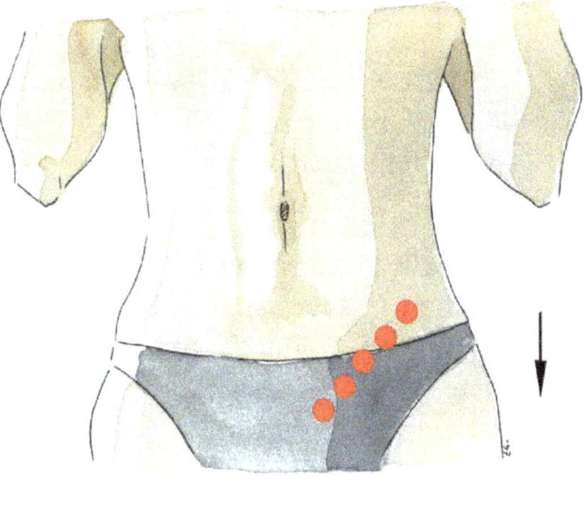

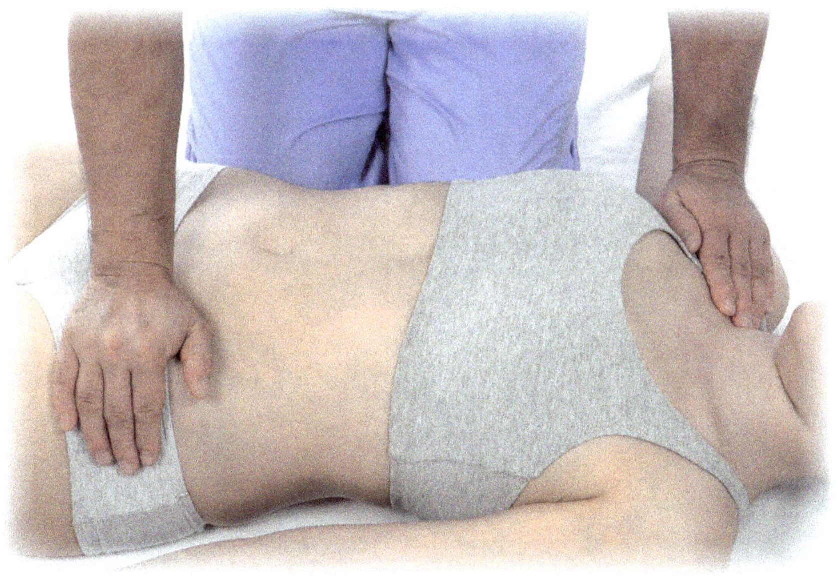

6.7. UNDULATING PRESSURE

PATIENT'S POSTURE: Supine, right arm in 90° abduction.

THERAPIST'S POSITION: Seiza or kneeling, perpendicular to the patient.

TYPE OF PRESSURE: Wave movement with both hands, with the eminences pushing the ascending colon and abdominal pack, while with the fingers pulling towards the descending colon and abdominal pack.

OBSERVATIONS: Do not separate palms from the abdomen. Normally the pressure is applied with both palms at the same time. Palm over palm is performed, only in the case that the patient has a small abdomen.

Ten movements back and forth.

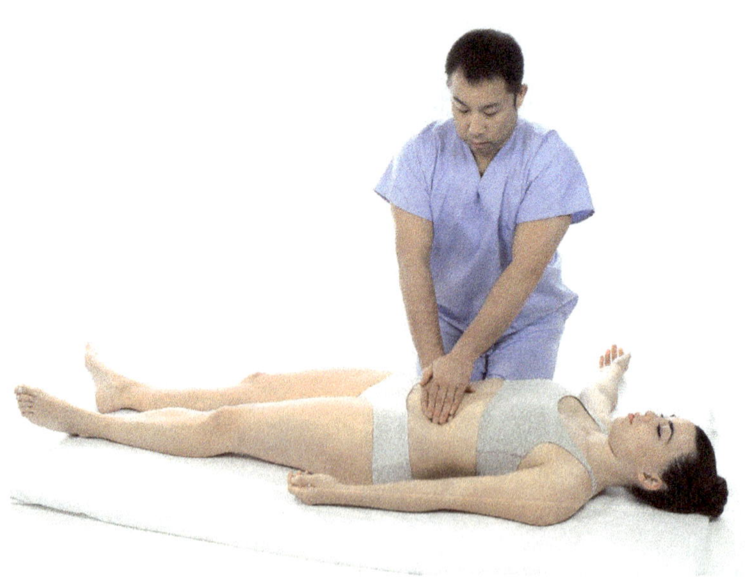

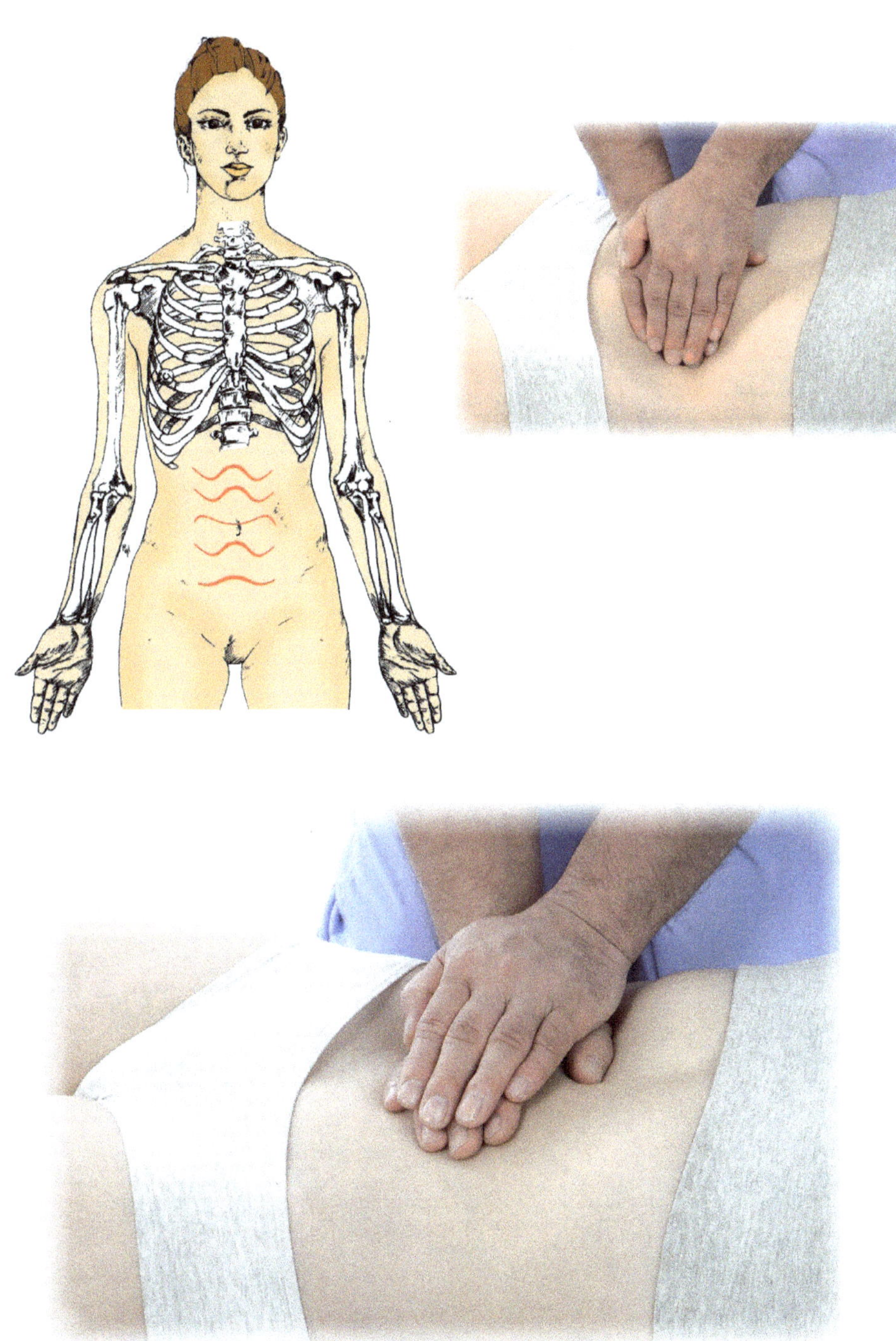

6.8. CIRCULAR PRESSURE

PATIENT'S POSTURE: Supine, right arm in 90° abduction.

THERAPIST'S POSITION: Kneeling, perpendicular to the patient.

TYPE OF PRESSURE: Circular pressure with both hands.

OBSERVATIONS: We perform ten movements in a circular clockwise direction, placing both palms on the patient's navel.

Do not separate palms from the abdomen.

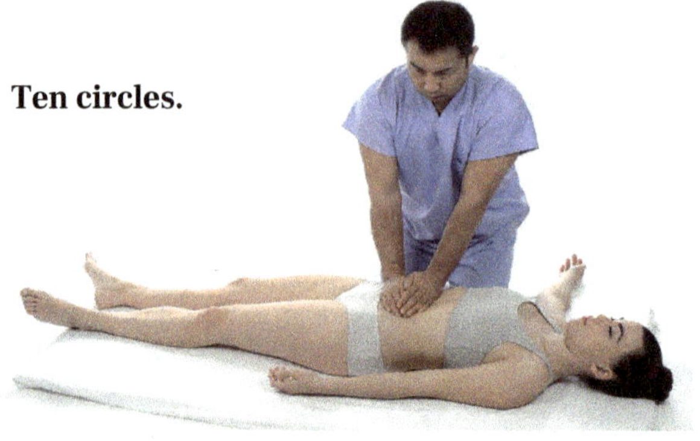

Ten circles.

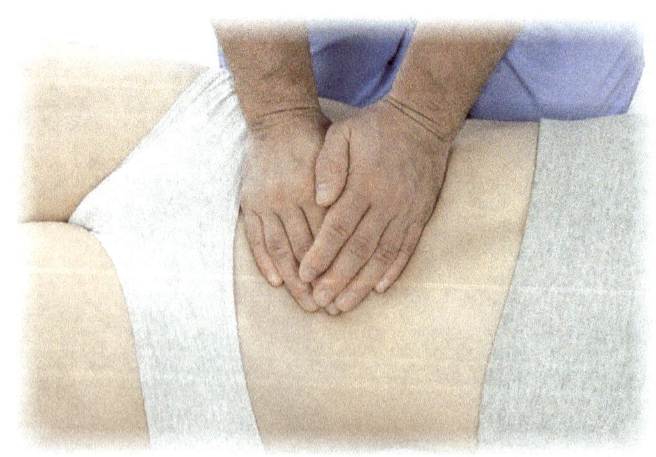

6.9. VIBRATIONAL PRESSURE

PATIENT'S POSTURE: Supine, right arm in 90° abduction.

THERAPIST'S POSITION: Kneeling, perpendicular to the patient.

TYPE OF PRESSURE: Apply a sustained pressure with both hands to the patient's naval and then vibrate both hands.

OBSERVATIONS: To apply vibration, the therapist must tighten the muscles in his arms and maintain position while expeling air.

Ten seconds.

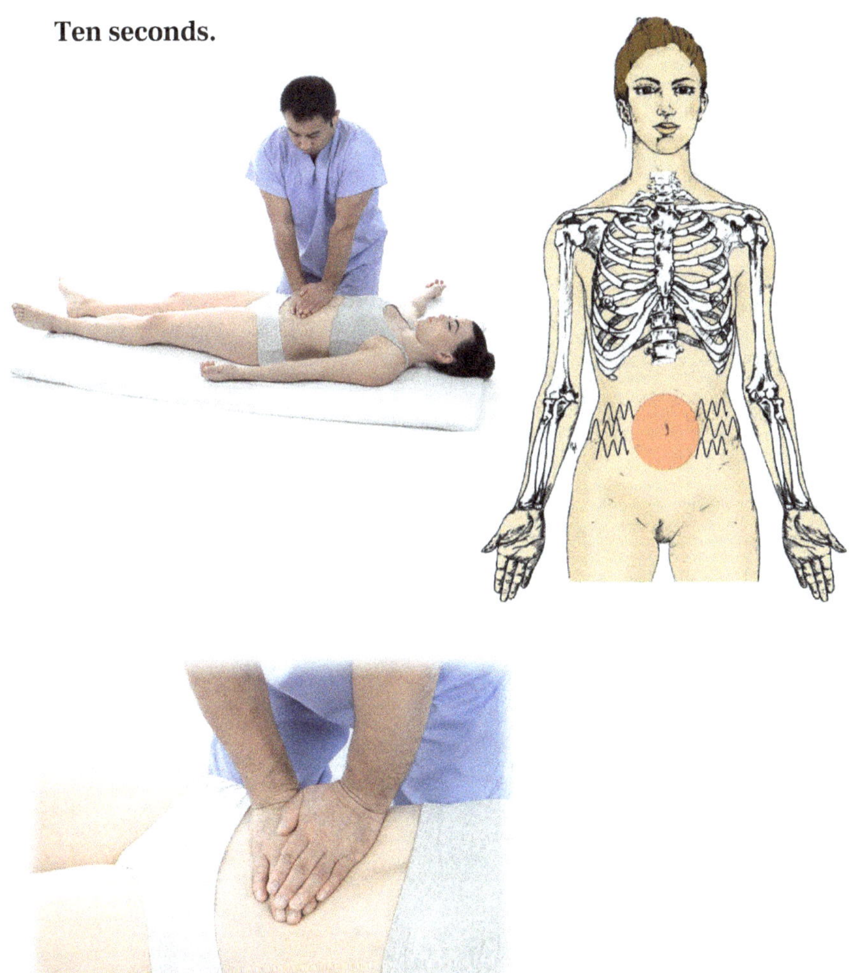

6.10. RELAXATION

PATIENT'S POSTURE: Supine, right arm in 90° abduction.

THERAPIST'S POSITION: Seiza perpendicular to the patient.

TYPE OF PRESSURE: The righthand rests on the abdomen at tanden level (CV4, Kangen; CV5, Sekimon; CV6, Kikai). The left hand rests in the centre of the sternum (CV17, Danchuu).

OBSERVATIONS: Stay for a few minutes breathing deeply and try to connect with the patient's breathing. There is no pressure. This exercise serves to inform the patient that the session has come to an end.

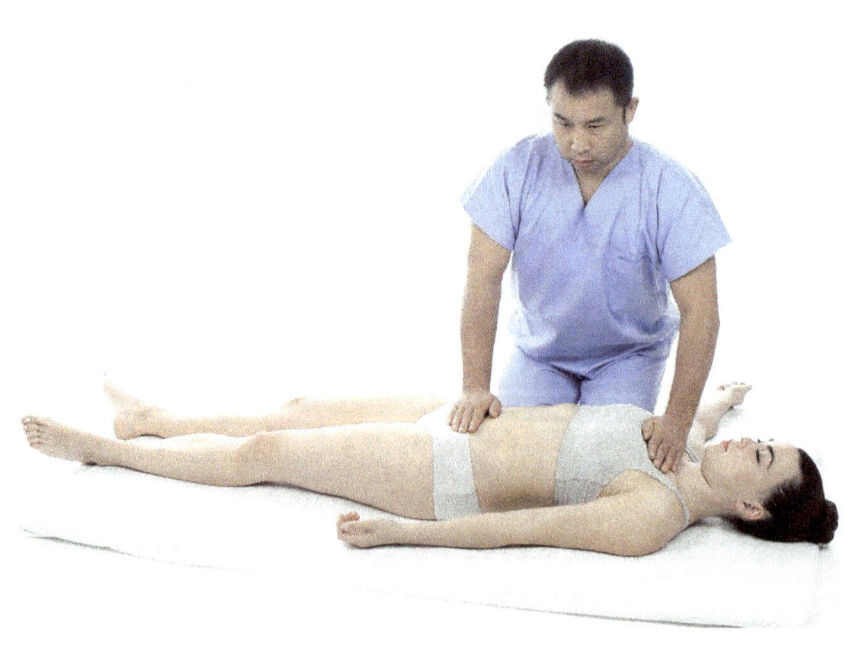

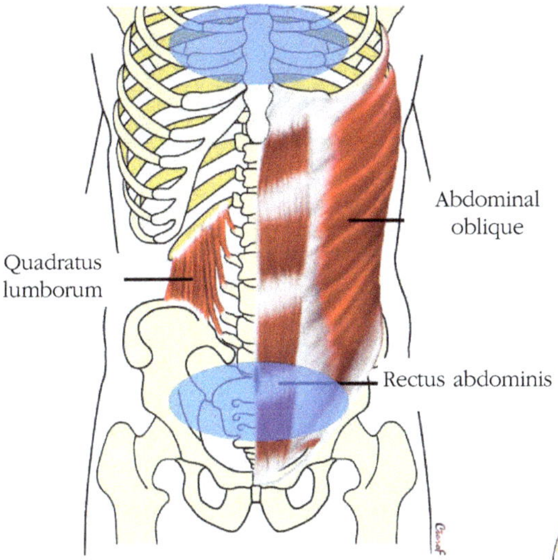

Quadratus
lumborum
Abdominal
oblique
Rectus abdominis

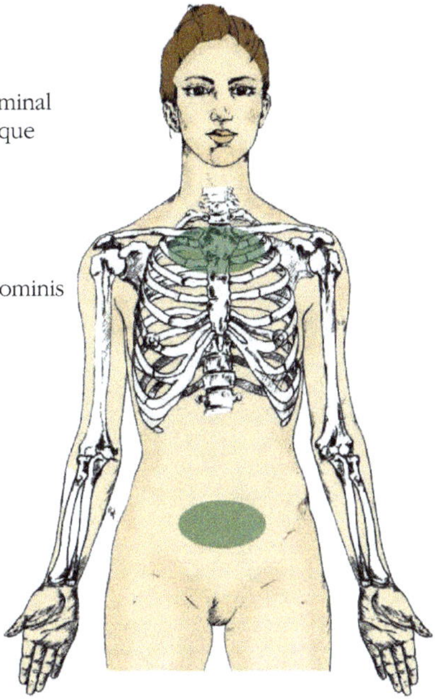

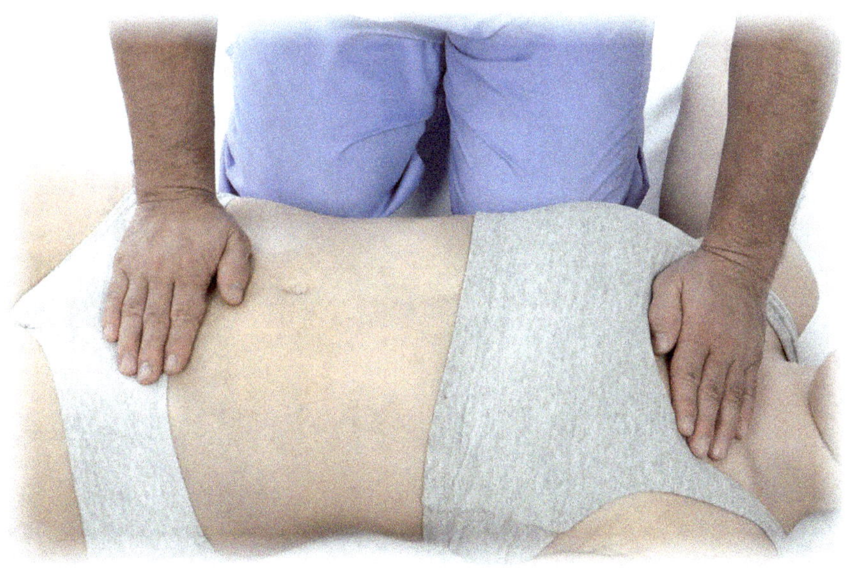

WHAT IS MENKEN?

瞑眩

In Shiatsu the body's reaction after receiving a session is called Menken. This reaction can appear as pain, stiffness, tiredness or even slight discomfort. Despite what it may seem to Western eyes, this reaction is not only productive, but is considered part of the recovery process. It doesn't always happen and, if it does, it isn't always with the same intensity. It usually occurs, especially in the case of a patient receiving a Shiatsu session for the first time or if they are in a process of significant imbalance.

Over time, the body accumulates tiredness and tension. The body learns to live with them in such a way that they remain secret, hidden and inactive. The therapist needs to apply treatment with the intention of stimulating the body and correcting the mismatches. As they correct, old stresses emerge to the surface and reveal themselves in the patient's general condition. The patient's feeling changes; he feels heavy, but at the same time he notices more and better energy.

Shiatsu, compared to other types of massages, stimulates not only the surface, but also at deeper levels. That's why tsubos or surface contractures disappear and, little by little, the deeper stresses begin to move to the surface.

Really the Menken effect refers to the detoxification of the body, revealing itself in various ways depending on the person's problem. It is important to know this and make the patient understand that the treatment is progressive; for full effect you have to rebalance.

MENKEN EFFECTS

The effects or sensations that the Menken effect produces in patients are very different. Some patients feel a little tired or even feel worse the day after receiving a session. Other times, they notice that they go to the bathroom more often, eczema can appear or some women start menstruating.

In the case of people of a certain age, with hormonal problems, after a shiatsu session their body begins to react. If the patient is a woman, their menstrual flow may be darker and denser. If in menopause, menstrual flow may even reappear.

There are people who, although they sweat, do not give off any smell, but after being treated by Shiatsu some odour may appear produced by this reaction. The same can happen with urine. There are even reactions such as the onset of facial acne. These are all symptoms of detoxification. The body needs to expel accumulated remains and thereby remove toxins. There may, of course, also appear feelings of relief, of the pain area changing, becoming more localized, and so on. Even if the patient does not feel perfectly well and still has discomfort, he will feel more energetic, more flexible and released.

These effects should not last longer than two days. After this period, the discomfort should go away. If this does not happen, it is not about the Menken effect. When a person with a lot of stagnant energy (Jitsu state) comes for Shiatsu and treatment is applied too quickly, the reaction can be very strong due to overstimulation. The effects may be quite unpleasant (increased pain, inflammation, etc.) and will likely last several days. You have to know how to differentiate between an abnormal reaction and the Menken effect. Not all after-treatment sensations should be attributed to Menken. An ineperienced therapist or overstimulation after a Shiatsu session may cause discomfort that is unnecessary or unbeneficial for the treatment. These effects do not mean a worsening of the patient's pathology, but they do delay the recovery.

AREA FOR MITIGATING THE MENKEN EFFECTS

Although the Menken state is considered part of the improvement process, Shiatsu therapists always try to mitigate its effects. There are various basic Shiatsu routine regions that are used for this purpose.

They are as follows:

— Occipital region: The accumulated body tension from negative stimuli is alleviated and increases flexibility of the muscle insertion area of the neck.
— Abdomen Region: Work on the hara eliminates internal organ tension, preventing toxins and negative energy from accumulating.
— Lateral Sural Region and, above all, work on point **S36**, as it is a very energetic and endorphin-releasing point.

SWEEPING PRESSURE: NAGARE OSHI

流れ圧し

DEFINITION

What is known at our School as Sweeping Pressure is called Nagare Oshi in Japan.

Nagare: It means getting carried away, getting carried away by the facts, just as the water flows in a river.

Oshi: It means force with pressure or pushing.

Therefore, the metaphorical concept contained in the Japanese words leads us to the definition of sweeping pressure. Contractures are a cluster of toxins in muscle fibers, like boulders accumulating on the riverbed. The Nagare Oshi-type pressure would be like the river, which fluidly sweeps the stones into its current. The therapist's fingers never separate from the patient's body; as they come out of pressure, the thumbs sweep to the next point. During this movement we perceive/diagnose the state of the area at the general level (macro work).This enables us to locate the contractures for further work (micro work).

WAY OF WORKING

When we apply sweeping pressure, we work along the whole line, not just on the points of the basic routine. The same sweeping pressure will be applied to all points on the line so that we can define a diagnosis and treatment at the same time. In this way we can more easily find the contractures between points of the treated area.

After applying pressure to a point and when we notice that the body signals that we have reached the penetration "limit", we will slowly move back up and, without completely removing the pressure from the thumbs, we will sweep them slowly to the next point of the line. So, we will continue to sweep the surface, without losing contact with the patient's body, to the next point and apply pressure again. It is important to note that if ever contractures appear, we work them with a little inclination while applying pressure. A common mistake is to understand the sweep as sliding the thumbs along the patient's body while maintaining pressure.

For this type of pressure, we use thumbs in Logo or thumbs in A. Sometimes, we can also use thumb over thumb, although this type of pressure is considered too strong to use throughout the treatment. For this reason we will use it only occasionally after locating some contracture by sweeping pressure; then we will maintain the thumb over thumb pressure until the contracture changes, decreases or disappears. Bearing Kyo Jitsu theory in mind, you cannot work the area with contractures with sweeping pressure when it is Jitsu type on the surface or in the case of recent pain.

If it is Kyo type on the surface, and it is an old injury (internally Jitsu), we can work on the deep contracture that we find with sweeping pressure; the pressure here should be stronger.

THUMB OVER THUMB.

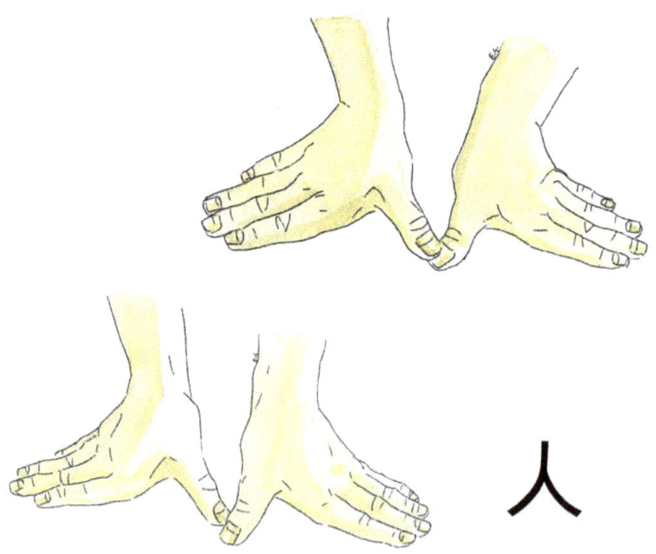

THUMB IN THE SHAPE OF «HITO».

CHARACTERISTICS

Sweeping pressure has the following characteristics:

• It's a really professional pressure

This type of pressure is considered suitable only for professionals. It requires greater concentration and practice to make it fluid and effective. It is harder for the therapist to correctly apply pressure on the tsubo, so a person without enough hours of practice will not be able to use the technique properly, turning it into a kind of superficial, ineffective kneading.

It should not be forgotten that the recommended position of the hands to perform this technique is that of "logo". This posture requires greater dexterity on the part of the therapist.

• It's a pressure performed without extra force

The stronger pressure is applied when entering the tsubo, and corresponds to the first part of the undulating sweeping pressure. The sweep itself begins when coming out of that pressure. Thumbs sweep over the muscles, without separating from the skin.

In my classes, I always point out to my students not to confuse the sweeping technique with grabbing the skin and trying to drag it. This is a common mistake among Shiatsu novices.

• It's an untiring pressure

One of the advantages for the therapist is that this technique does not make them excessively tired. The therapist follows our Shiatsu's basic routine smoothly, quickly and effortlessly. This way of working is very different from the slow and deep pressure to be used later with therapeutic purpose.

In any case, this pressure must be applied without forgetting the work comes from the therapist's hara, and his proper centre of gravity in each applied pressure. Pressure should enter each tsubo properly. I always repeat that the speed of this technique should not be detrimental to the quality of the pressure, which should never be light and without any effect.

• It enables a quick search

Sweeping pressure aims to quickly find the patient's deepest contractures. By having a comprehensive view of the state of the contractures in a given area, a more appropriate treatment can be established.

I often insist that by using slow pressure the therapist receives too much information, so the location of deep contractures can escape. A quick search locates all contractures with a "bird's eye view". The use of the hand palm is also recommended for generally searching for contractures.

• It brings the contracture to the surface

In Japanese, the action of "bringing the contracture" to the surface of the body is called Ukabu ("sprouting"). The interesting thing about this rapid, fluid pressure technique is that enough stimulus is created to sprout the deep contractures towards the surface of the body. Therefore, you can later work on them with slow thumb over thumb pressure.

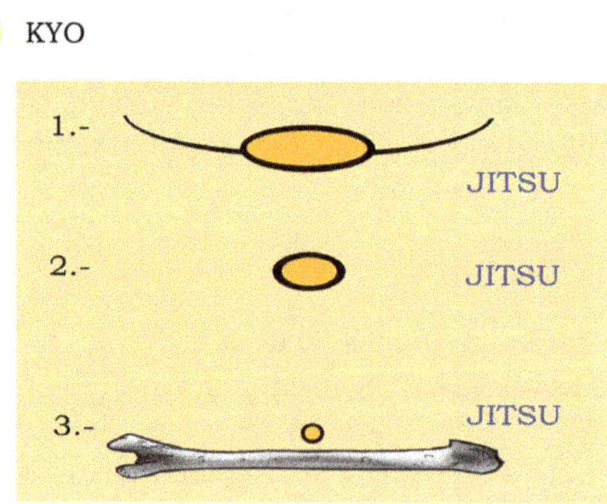

• It reduces treatment time

Another star characteristic of this type of pressure is that by creating greater stimulus in the patient, the patient has the feeling of having received a longer session. For this reason, a twenty-five or thirty minute sweeping-pressure session is comparable to a fifty-minute or one-hour session with normal Shiatsu pressure.

MENKEN. BY BREAKING CAPILLAR VESSELS

It should be borne in mind that, when many pressures are applied in a short period of time, the treated area can become overstimulated, especially if this area has accumulated a lot of tension. A type of Menken is then produced as capillary vessels rupture, which causes small blood congestions and skin redness. The therapist should warn the patient of this possibility before performing pressure.

OLDER OR KYO-TYPE PEOPLE

I always recommend my students to be very careful with this type of pressure when treating older people. Because their biorhythms are slower, sweeping pressure overstimulation is not adequate for the treated area. Physically and mentally, older people are accustomed to a more leisurely pace of life. That's why they prefer slower pressure; Shiatsu's usual pressure. However, young people are accustomed to a more frantic pace of life, so slow pressure can cause them the same distress as the fast to the elderly.

Kyo-type people (empty typology) are also hypersensitive to sweeping pressure. The therapist should take this into account during treatment.

ADVANTAGES AND DISADVANTAGES OF SWEEPING PRESSURE

Advantages:

— Helps diagnosis.
— Helps find contractures.
— Enables treatment and diagnosis at the same time.
— Takes care of the therapist's thumbs.
— Follows the energy flows we can work on along the meridian path, in the same way as acupuncture.

Disadvantages:

— It is a greater stimulus for the body, so the reaction the next day can be strong.

— We shouldn't work on recent inflammations or acute problems
for the above reason.

— We should not work in areas that are Jitsu on the surface (Kyo-
Jitsu theory).
— You should not work on older and general Kyo-type people.

Sweeping pressure should not be used on the whole body. The
usual treatment areas using the sweeping pressure are:

— Infrascapular and lumbar, intending to separate.
— B52 region.
— Popliteal fossa.
— Tarsus.
— Brachial.
— Medial femoral.
— Lateral sural, three lines, separating.
— Scapular edge.

THERAPEUTIC PRESSURE

After locating the most contractured points with the sweeping pressure, they are worked on longer and deeper. In this case the usual
thumb over thumb pressure is used. The pressure will now be slow and
maintained until the contracture changes or even disappears.

Cold	Head	Hot	Feet

頭寒足熱

Zu   **Kan**   **Soku**   **Netsu**

The human body constantly evolves to adapt to the environment in which it lives and grows. This is a natural and inexorable principle. Until the beginning of the last Century, in the Western world, people had styles of life in which movement was implicit, both because of the type of activity they did and because the means of moving from one place to another was scarce. A large section of the population lived in the countryside, involved in more physical tasks. And many of those who worked in the cities, in the midst of the expanding industrial sector, were doing manual labour. It was a lifestyle where body movement and physical exercise were daily actions for most people.

We are currently in the information age. A period characterized by a technological revolution focused on digital information and communication technologies, which affect all areas of human activity. The need for immediate information and the computerization of social and work-sphere processes have changed our style of life. With computers, we access a global market from our armchair at home or at work. The accelerated development processes have increased exponentially, making time a very valuable element. At times, this makes us live our lives at a frenetic pace.

This change in our lifestyle has been faster than our ability to adapt to it, which has caused and continues to cause diseases that did not exist before. Many of these diseases are related to the changing habits of modern society: buildings with hardly any windows to the outside, the abusive use of mobile telephones, the lack of movement in front of computer screens, stressful negotiations, the use of air conditioning, driving and public transport, continued air travel, labour disputes, the tightness of shoes and modern family conflicts.

With regard to the lack of physical movement, it is important to remember that the human body is designed for movement and, in turn, feeds on it to stay in balance. This lack of physical activity and the demand for almost permanent mental activity leads to a imbalance in how heat is distributed in the body, since blood stays longer where it is most needed. This, for physiological purposes, causes the legs to cool and excess heat in the upper body.

When this imbalance is maintained over time, it begins to affect organ functions in general, and may cause diseases such as fibromyalgia, chronic fatigue syndrome, allergy, hypertension, genitourinary disorders, migraines, edema, leg swelling and stress; it also affects our character, making us more irascible and sensitive to everything around us and making it easier to have depression, fears and anxiety crises.

That concentration of blood in the upper body overworks the heart. In the East, the legs are called the second heart, because their movement assists blood circulation, and not having good blood supply in the lower limbs is as if the upper half is floating in the air due to the lack of connection with the ground. Cool feet also makes it difficult to sleep and an overstimulated head makes it difficult to concentrate on any type of activity.

The ideal state of the body would be that the lower half (below the navel) was feeling a tense strength, with a lot of energy, as if it were glued to the ground, providing balance and stability, and that the upper half (above the navel) was loose and light.

Zu kan soku netsu is an ancient Japanese expression meaning "cold head and hot feet". With this simple phrase our ancestors taught us how to take care of our health, as that is the healthiest state. Staying true to that expression helps us stay relaxed, focused, and stress-free, as well as keeping our muscles and joints flexible. Oriental Medicine considers that the body in Zu kan soku netsu has awakened its own natural healing and high self-defenses.

According to Traditional Chinese Medicine, six meridians pass through the legs; three of them through the inner part, which in women is related to the genital tract. A lack of mobility results in insufficient circulation which makes it easier to have hormonal and genitourinary system imbalances.

These days, people do not take the state of their health into account and always think about the latest fashion without worrying about the consequences that this lack of care will bring in the future. Young girls dress in very short clothes that expose the stomach area (navel) and, at the back, the sacrum and lumbar area. This part of the body, in addition to the inner legs, is also related to the genital organs, so it should be kept at a certain temperature (always warm).

Of course, we must take into account that the lumbar region corresponds to the centre of the body and, if an imbalance appears in this region, it will affect the whole body, especially the abdominal area. In Japan, children in the past tucked their pyjama top into the trousers to protect areas sensitive to the cold. At night, everyone should protect the lower back, abdomen and genital area from the cold. When the abdominal part cools it disrupts viscera movements (diarrhoea), so we must always protect this area from the wind. Women in Japan said that the habit of wearing socks was very healthy, as it prevents the cold from rising up from the soles of the feet and protects the sacrolumbar and abdominal area from getting cold.

The treatment that we should apply to this type of body heat decompensation should be aimed at providing better blood flow from the navel downwards. To do this, we must massage well the soles of the feet, fingers and especially the inner legs.

Bad postures, inappropriate footwear and lack of exercise cause the ankles to become excessively stiff, so we must keep in mind how important it is to work on them, making wide rotations in both directions to improve elasticity in that narrow region, taking the importance of the joint into account as it bears the full weight of the body structure.

It would be obvious to say that walking every day is the ideal exercise to alleviate these kinds of problems, but often we walk incorrectly which has the opposite effect. Many people do not support the big toe when walking, and that hinders concentration and work on the inner legs, whose importance has already been mentioned. When walking, initial support should be done with the heel, but lifting up the foot should be done by putting weight on the big toe and concentrating the movement and tension on the inner part of both legs. This will increase heat in this area, improving overall blood flow.

Generally, in the same way that this type of imbalance reveals itself throughout the body (macro), it also does so in a reflective way in the abdomen (micro). That is why we must pay special attention to this area. In the general body treatment, when the back is tight, we work on the abdomen. In it we will find that, in many cases, the epigastrium or stomach pit is tense (jitsu) in an sphere-like area about four centimeters in diameter. This is caused by the tensions the body is subjected to, since, when it is not balanced, there is also an imbalance of the autonomic nervous system, affecting organs and bowels, but especially the stomach. Likewise we will find that the area below the navel, known as the tanden or hara, appears empty and soft (kyo), making it difficult for blood to flow to the legs. The ideal state of the abdomen, therefore, is that the pit of the stomach is empty and relaxed, and the hara is the contrary, with a certain muscle tone to store the body's energy.

To locally correct this imbalance in the abdomen, we must do two things: one, take slow and deep diaphragmatic breaths, invest more time in breathing out than in, and two, especially before sleeping, massage the stomach pit deeply, applying pressure on it while breathing out and relaxing the pressure while breathing in.

The Japanese expression naga iki describes the relationship between breathing correctly and health: naga means "deep", iki means "breathing", but also naga means "long" and iki "to live"; this means that if the breathing is slow and deep, our life will be long. Conversely, if breathing is fast and light, the bowels contract and stress builds up.

Another recommendation for maintaining good balance between the upper and lower body, is to split the day in eight hours for work, eight for free time and eight for rest. During sleep, the body activates the parasympathetic system, which helps the organs to function well, but for this, it is not advisable to eat in the three or four hours before rest, and for the over forties and fifities to avoid animal protein.

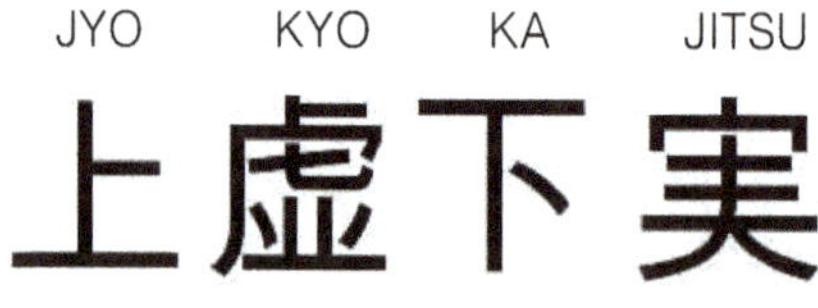

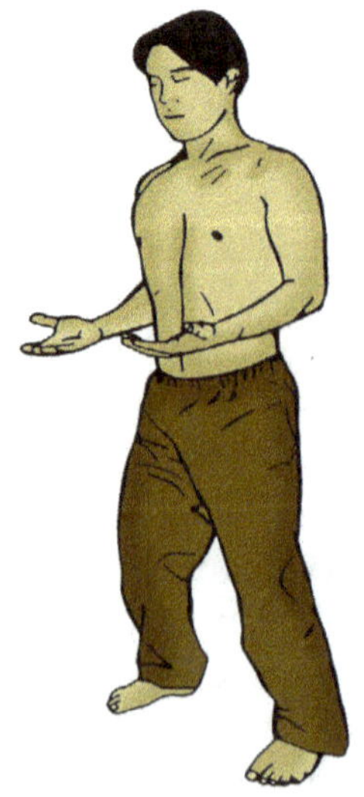

THE UPPER BODY IS RELAXED.

THE LOWER HALF IS CONCENTRATED ON THE BIG TOE AND STORING THE BODY'S ENERGY.

BREATHING, CONCENTRATED THREE FINGERS BELOW THE NAVEL (TANDEN).

BASIC KYO-JITSU CONCEPT APPLIED TO SHIATSU IN AZE STYLE

The Kyo-Jitsu theory refers to the body's energy duality, which is recognized in Eastern traditional medicine. Energy (Qi, Ki, Prana, etc.) manifests itself in different ways in the body; it can qualitatively be found in Kyo state (empty) or Jitsu state (excess). Both states are not, in themselves, either bad or good; both are characteristic of energy and its imbalance; the origin of all pathology. Aze Shiatsu picks up this concept and translates it to how it appears at the muscle and structural level.

Kyo means empty, lacking energy. Applied to Shiatsu, it refers to soft, loose, flaccid, sunken, cold, chronic, and so on. This does not mean that the quality of the energy is poor, but that the amount of energy is poor. So we must think that Kyo needs Jitsu, its opposing state; Kyo needs to receive some energy. Kyo also refers to a chronic problem. When an injury is not treated properly, it remains over time and slowly becomes more internalized. The body learns to live with it and forgets it. Aze Shiatsu says the contracture hides, sticks to the bone, the problem becomes chronic and moves into Kyo state.

Treatment with Shiatsu: A structural Kyo state will likely manifest as a soft and weak area. The pressure will have to be slow and deep. This is how you tone it and help it recover energy. In Japan moxibustion is used to achieve this effect.

Jitsu is defined as excessive or stagnant energy. That doesn't mean the patient has a lot of energy. Stagnant or excessive energy becomes malignant; the accumulated toxins that are difficult to expel from the body. At the muscle level a full, hard, dense, fresh and hot (even inflamed) area is perceived. All pathology, originally, begins as Jitsu and is located at the surface level.

Treatment with Shiatsu: Pressure is applied to a hard and rigid Jitsu zone quickly and shallowy. It's about removing or sedating the accumulated energy. In Japan, acupuncture needles are used in the case of Jitsu pathologies.

THE EVOLUTION OF IMBALANCE

The body's state of equilibrium means having Kyo and Jitsu combined at 50%. A balanced body is able to self-correct these inequalities. So, Shiatsu is about helping the body carry out this task. Therefore, the therapist should look for the deficit areas and tone them, and at the same time eliminate excessive energy from others. The purpose of treatment is to restore the lost balance to the body. The primary goal of Aze Shiatsu: It is very important to look for the source of pain. It's about regaining body balance, and stimulating the self-healing system.

The evolution of structural tension in the human body happens in the following way. Originally, the affected area has a Jitsu character. The contracture is recent, shallow and usually takes up a large space. As we said, Shiatsu seeks to eliminate excess energy by applying the right pressure. If the problem is not resolved, it gradually changes its status. The tension is concentrated into a smaller area and goes deeper and deeper. Finally, it becomes chronic and passes to a Kyo state.

From this point of view you can categorize people as Kyo or Jitsu, or as a mixture of both. This categorization helps the Shiatsu therapist make a first assessment of the pattern of imbalances and the corresponding symptoms that the person will present. But this Kyo-Jitsu duality also manifests itself by applying pressure to every point, in every region of the patient's body. The therapist's thumbs should feel the qualitative state of each part of the patient when performing treatment. With this perception, and making use of one of Shiatsu's characteristics - performing diagnosis and treatment at the same time, the therapist will apply the right type of pressure at all times. Depending on the age of the person, the goal of Shiatsu treatment will be different. Every stage of life brings people closer to the Kyo or Jitsu side. The elderly have accumulated imbalances that bring down the balance on the Kyo side. You have to be careful when working with them. There is no need to stimulate Kyo areas, as hidden alterations that surface can drastically decrease the quality of life. In children, on the contrary, all imbalances are Jitsu. There are no old contractures. Treatment is much simpler and their body's response faster and more effective.

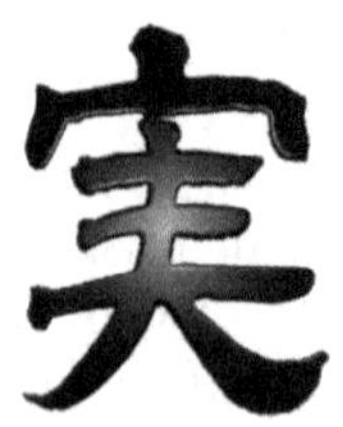

We already know the importance of observing the patient's movement and attitude, as well as touching to diagnose in Shiatsu. The Aze style also combines Kyo-Jitsu theory with these methods to make a more accurate diagnosis and set out a more effective treatment. It is about making a diagnosis by comparing the body's balance from different angles, depending on the Kyo-Jitsu state of the parts.

When the diagnosis is made, treatment is determined and completed. We already know that one of Shiatsu's characteristics is that diagnosis and treatment happen simultaneously.

These are the fundamental diagnostic/treatment methods used by Aze Shiatsu based on the Kyo-Jitsu theory:

1. TOP-BOTTOM
Kyo-Jitsu of the top and bottom

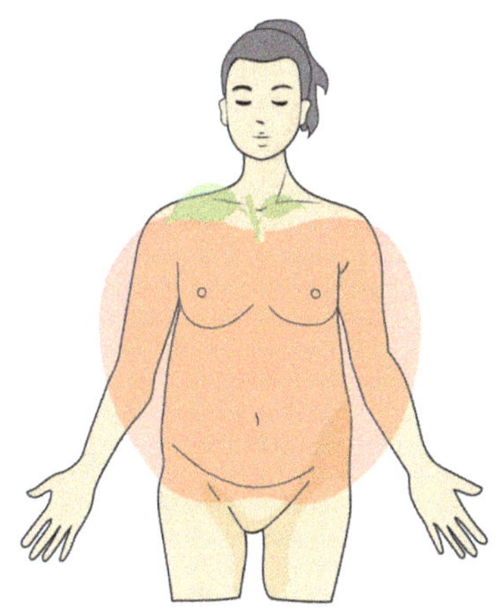

APPLE TYPE

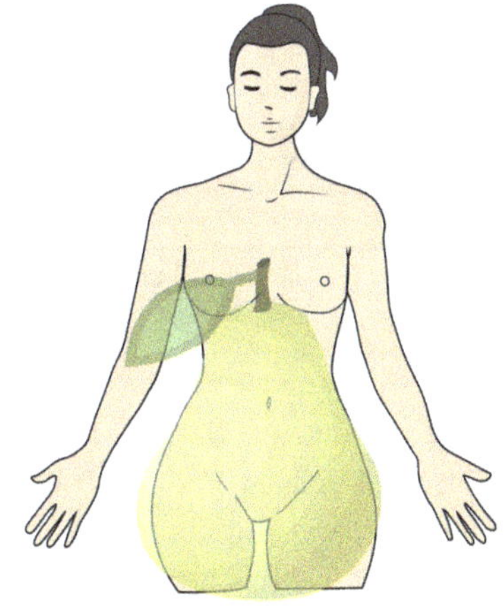

PEAR TYPE

The first diagnostic method divides the body in two from the navel. Comparing both halves can establish two pathological types:

A. **Apple type:** Very thin legs and thick trunk. Top, Jitsu; bottom, Kyo.

Circulatory problems.

B. **Pear type:** Top, normal or prone to Kyo; bottom, Jitsu. Hormonal imbalances (typical of women), poor circulation, fluid retention, genital tract problems.

2. RIGHT-LEFT

a) Kyo-Jitsu of the right and left

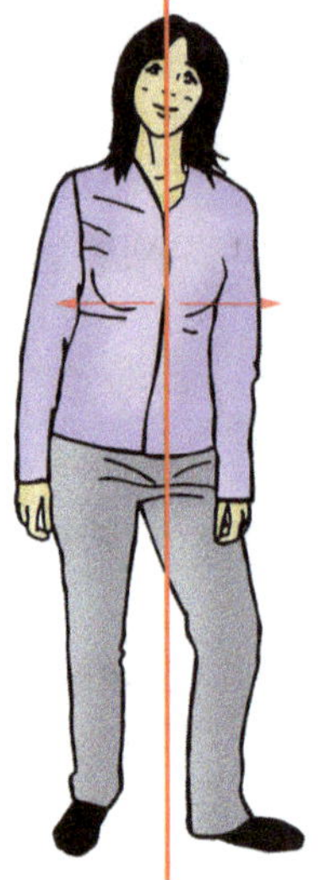

DAILY POSTURE

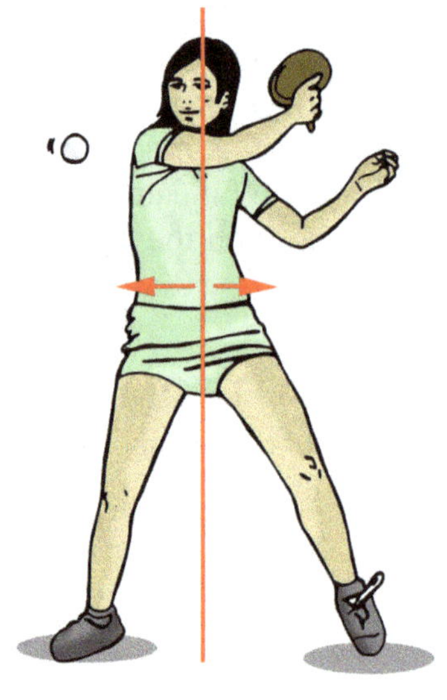

REPETITIVE MOVEMENT

This method divides the body into two halves from its central axis. Compare the overall state of the right and left side to look for where the structural imbalance is.

Everyone has a tendency to carry or distribute their body weight on one side or the other. There are two causes that generate these imbalances. First, everyone's everyday postural habit.

Each person has a tendency to always use the same side; some of us are right-handed and some left-handed, and this conditions our daily actions.

Second, accumulated repetitive movements also generate this type of right-left imbalance. Athletes (tennis, golf, etc.), musicians (violin, guitar, etc.) and other professionals use one side more than the other with the consequential problems that this generates.

b) Kyo-Jitsu in the five warning points

Another variant of the right-left comparison is taking into account the warning points on both sides. By applying pressure on these points the therapist determines their Kyo-Jitsu state and the type of pressure suitable for their treatment.

c) Kyo-Jitsu of each meridian point/key points

As in the previous case, but now applying pressure to the meridians and their key points, the therapist perceives the meridian's qualitative state and determines what type of pressure is necessary in each case.

3. ANTERIOR-POSTERIOR

Kyo-Jitsu of the back and hara

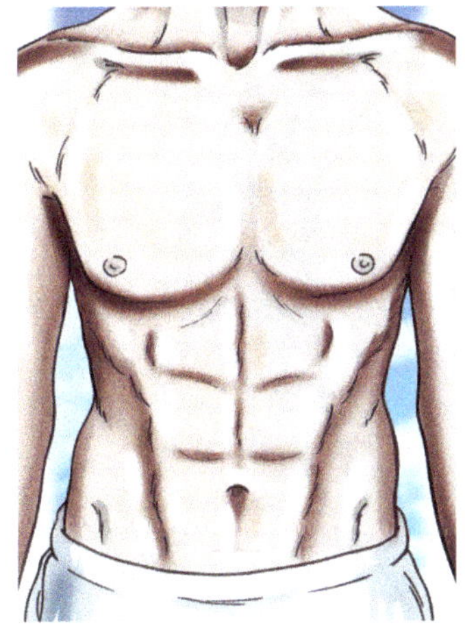
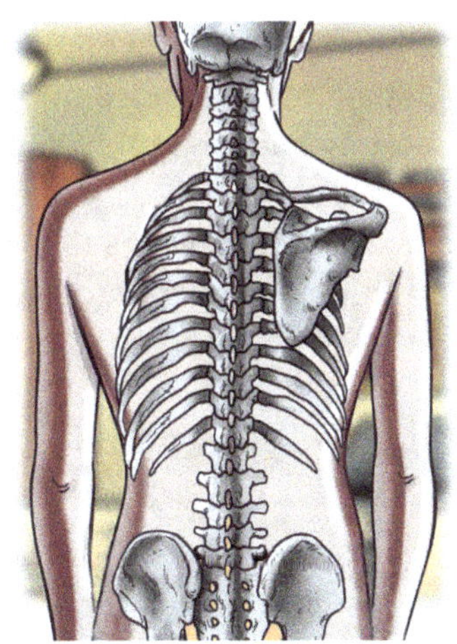

Now it is about comparing the anterior part, represented by the abdomen/hara, with the posterior, especially along the spinal column.

A balanced body must be Jitsu behind and Kyo in front. When one of the sides tends towards the opposite type, the other side does so in reverse, since both coexist in opposite and in complement.

4. PIT OF THE STOMACH AND TANDEN

A balanced body has Kyo state in the stomach pit and Jitsu state in the tanden (three fingers under the navel).

The frenetic pace of life reverses this polarity. Physical and mental stress builds up tension in the stomach pit making it Jitsu. In contrast, the tanden moves to a weak Kyo energy state. It is essential in Aze Shiatsu treatment to restore natural balance to these regions.

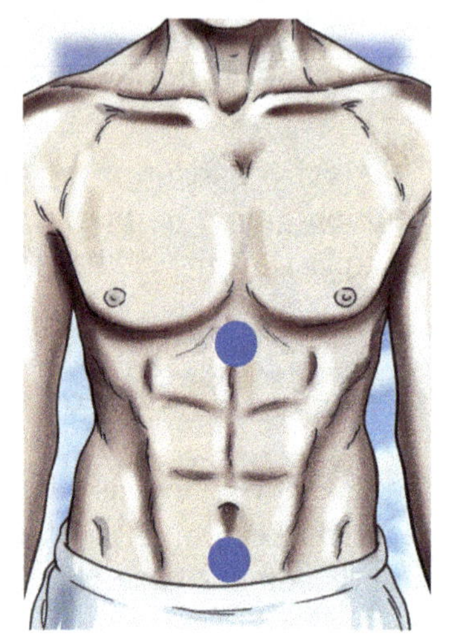

5. KYO-JITSU IN THE ASPA CONCEPT

Combining Kyo-Jitsu theory and Aze Shiatsu's Aspa theory can establish another method of diagnosis and treatment.

Aze Shiatsu uses all these diagnostic methods together and combines them to determine the treatment to follow. It's not about choosing one or more of them. To perform a true holistic treatment, all the parts and relationships they have between them must be taken into account.

THE FIVE WARNING POINTS PLUS TWO COMPLEMENTARY ONES

Getting rid of pain or making the symptom go away is the primary goal of many therapies. It is also the main reason why a person goes to a therapy consultation.

For Aze Shiatsu the function of pain is clear. It is a signal that the body makes when there is some kind of imbalance. In short, it is a warning of the altered state of the homeostatic balance. Therefore, therapy aims to rebalance the body to increase its self-healing capacity. Removing the symptom is important, but the essential thing is to look for the source of the imbalance and get rid of it.

Many years ago, Oriental Medicine established the reflective points of the internal organs located in the back. Through them it is possible to make a diagnosis of their condition and help restore their proper function. Aze Shiatsu takes this principle and, along with over twenty-five years' experience, has created its own diagnostic and treatment system. After many years of working with patients who come to our centres with the most diverse ailments, we have found that back pain is concentrated in recurrent areas. Aze Shiatsu sets out five fundamental points where pain shows as a form of warning that the patient's body is reaching its equilibrium limit; beyond which disease can suddenly arise.

The difference between Shiatsu (area) and Acupuncture (point)

Although almost all of Aze Shiatsu's warning points match acupuncture points, and are located using the same references, the work of both therapies is very different. Acupuncture has to be more accurate when inserting the needle; the location of the point must be as accurate as possible according to the anatomical references. In addition, by remaining inserted under the skin for more than twenty minutes, its effect is greater.

When working with Shiatsu, it is not necessary to be so accurate in the theoretical location of the point. According to Aze Shiatsu, we must look for the most sensitive point (Aze point) around the standard location area. Aze means "to look for where there is tension, discomfort or altered sensitivity, regardless of the meridian's standard points". Thumbs don't penetrate under the skin, nor do they stay with continuous pressure for long. In Shiatsu we think not of a specific point, but of a certain region. That is why you have to work the area and not the point, using different directions, varying the direction of pressure as well as the patient's position. In many cases, the contracture area covers more than one point.

FIVE WARNING POINTS

1. First warning point   B43 Kou Kou   膏肓

Location

It is located in the central portion of the internal edge of the scapula, roughly coinciding with the third point of the scapula region: medial edge. Relating this point to Traditional Chinese Medicine, it is located in the area of points B43 and B44.

"Kou Kou" refers to a disease that is difficult to cure, which has been left until late to intervene.

"Shin Dou" wants to express the place where the spirituality of being resides. When this point is painful, many patients point out that they suffer from a lot of physical and mental stress. It is a pain not directly related to structural or joint problems of the neighbouring vertebrae.

We can establish a relationship between the right side, with digestive problems, and the left side, with circulatory system problems.

Indications

This point is very useful for heart-

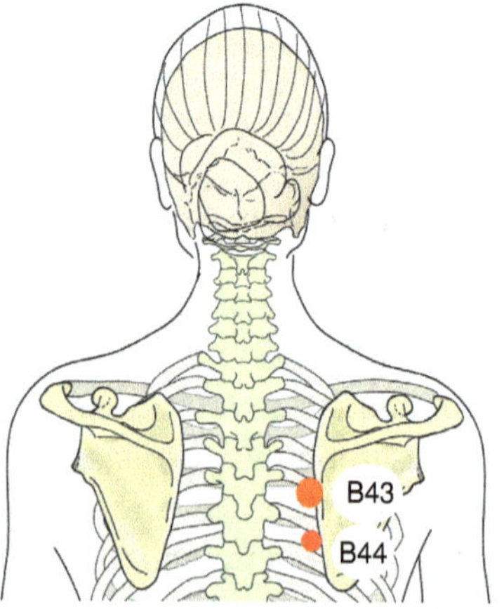

B44 Shin Dou

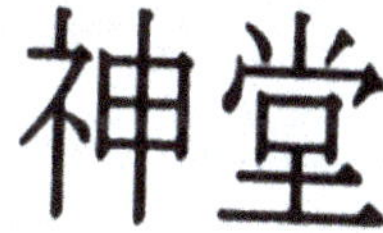

related problems and diseases, both functional (blood circulation, tachycardia, etc.) and emotional.

If there is also chest pain, it will be related to breathing problems: acute and chronic bronchitis, bronchial asthma.

It is also used for digestive problems and localised shoulder snd back problems.

It is related to the state of the suprascapular point on the same side and lateral cervical on the opposite side. For a complete treatment we will work on all these areas.

2. Second warning point

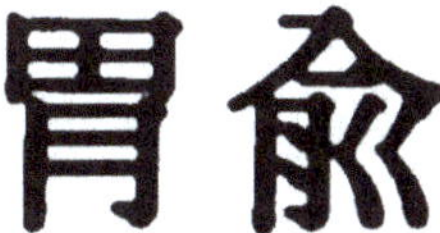

B21 I Yu

B21 I Yu

Location

It is located around the fifth point of the first line of the infrascapular and lumbar region, next to the inferior depression of the twelfth dorsal vertebra spinous process; 1.5 cun laterally. This point roughly corresponds to the acupuncture point 21 of the bladder.

"I Yu" refers to where the disease enters the stomach.

Indications

We usually use it when there are digestive problems, gases, hiatus hernia.

The D12 vertebra tends to move when it is located in an area strained

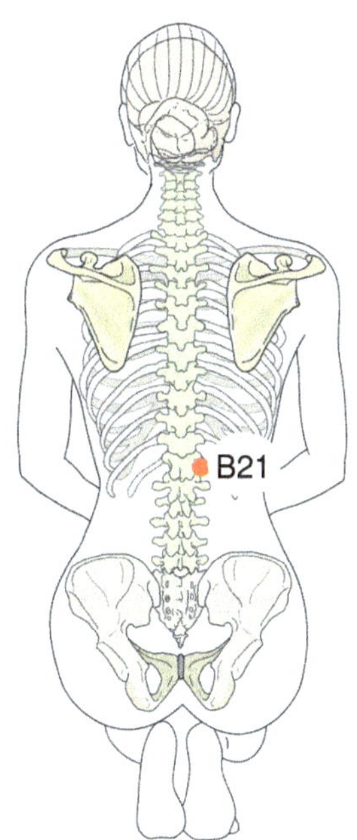

by all movements in the spinal column. It's very difficult for it to reposition itself. That is why mobilization work is fundamental for it to recover: pressure is applied alternately from each side of the spinous process.

B52 SHI SHITSU

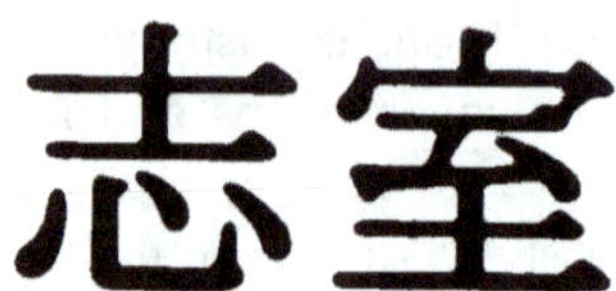

3. Third warning point

Location

It is the third point of the lumbar region. It is located between the end of the tenth rib and the iliac crest, two fingers laterally from the second line of the infrascapular and lumbar region. It corresponds approximately to the acupuncture point 52 of the Bladder.

"SHISHITSU" means a place where the will and vitality for the kidney resides. Physical strength builds up at this point.

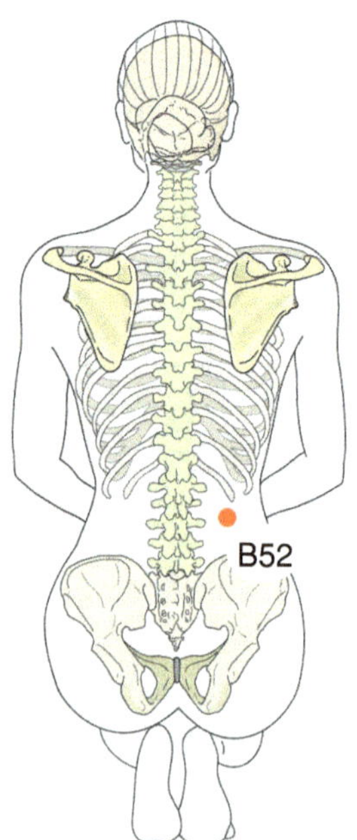

Indications

Lower back pain, sciatica, widespread body tiredness, difficulty urinating, kidney problems, impotence.

Working on the kidneys means helping remove toxins from the body.

4. Fourth warning point

Location

It is the tenth point of the first line of the infrascapular and lumbar region. It is located at 1.5 cun from the central line, at the level of the inferior depression of the fifth lumbar vertebra spinous process, and corresponds approximately to the acupuncture point 26 of the Bladder.

"Kan Gen Yu" means where mood occurs

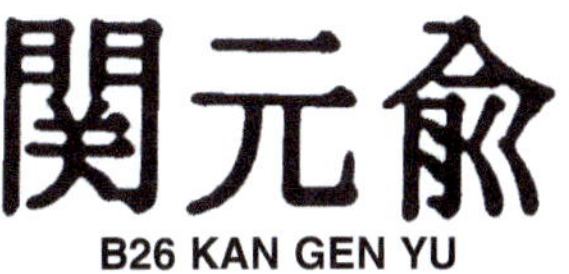

B26 KAN GEN YU

Indications

Being located next to the centre of the body, it is suitable for treating most symptoms or diseases. Although it is more effective for lower back problems, as well as for gynecological, menstrual pains and cold conditions (cystitis).

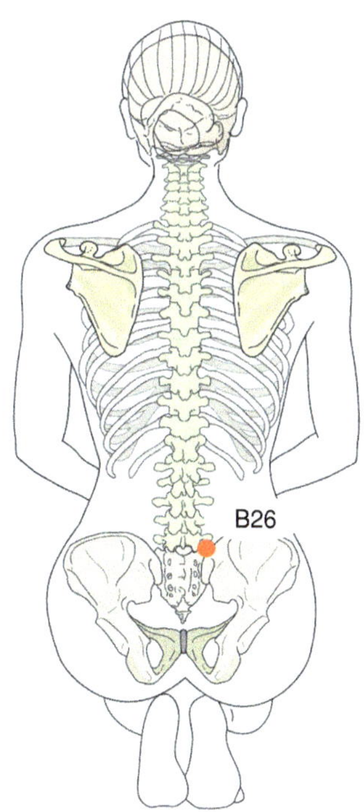

5. Fifth warning point

We call it the iliac ridges, ovaries or lumbalgia point.

Location

It is the highest point of the iliac crest. It roughly coincides with the third point of the second line in the iliac crest region.

Indications

Generally used for problems with the genital tract and lower back. Helps remove accumulated blood and toxins in the pelvic region (oketsu).

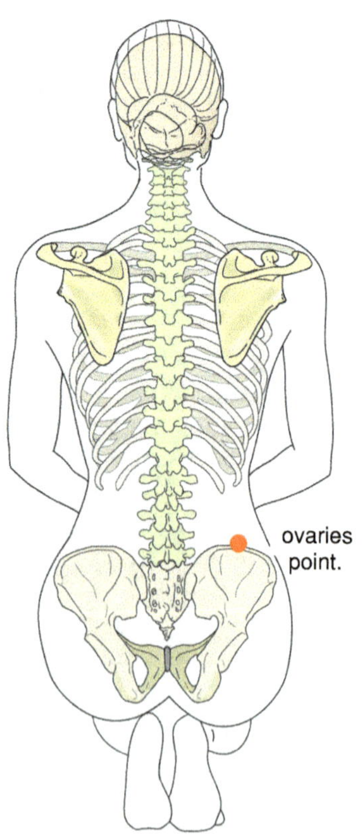

COMPLEMENTARY
WARNING POINTS

These points were added after the previous ones. They are as important and are used to diagnose and treat with Aze Shiatsu.

They are generally used on right-handed patients. For left-handed patients and a percentage of right-handed people, other completely different contractures may come out.

These points are affected by using the body in the wrong way. For example, when writing, right-handed people place the body so that tension builds up in the right cervical area. In addition, by not moving well in the Aspa form to carry out daily activities, contractures come up in the popliteal fossa; if the big toe is not used correctly, the weight of the body moves towards the little toe causing tension in the popliteal fossa.

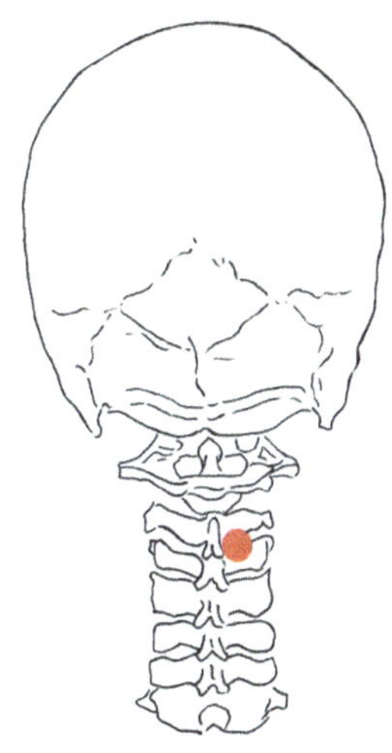

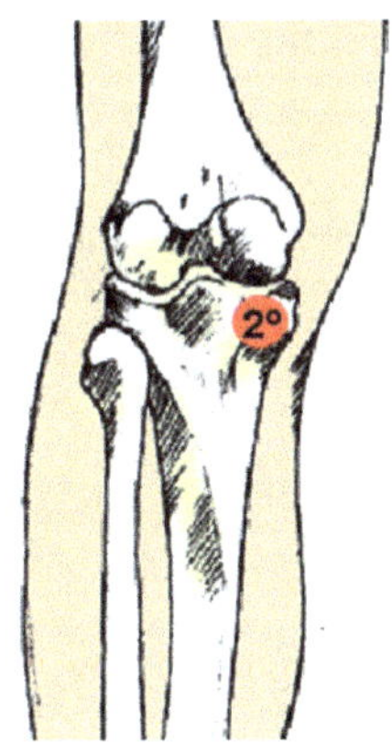

6. First complementary warning point

Location

It is located between the second and third cervical vertebrae, around the second point of the posterior cervical region (right-handed people on the right side, left-handed on the left side).

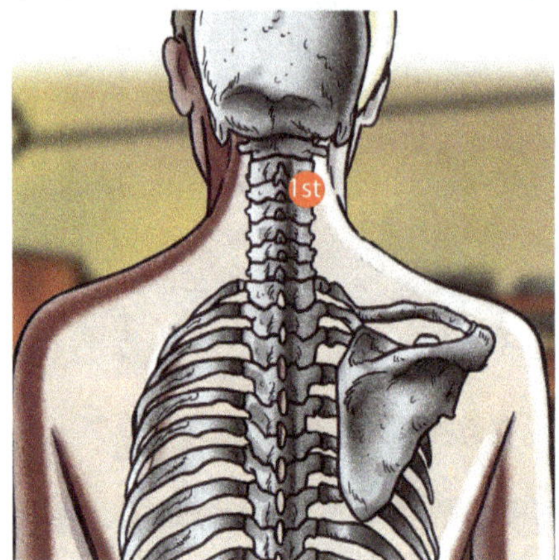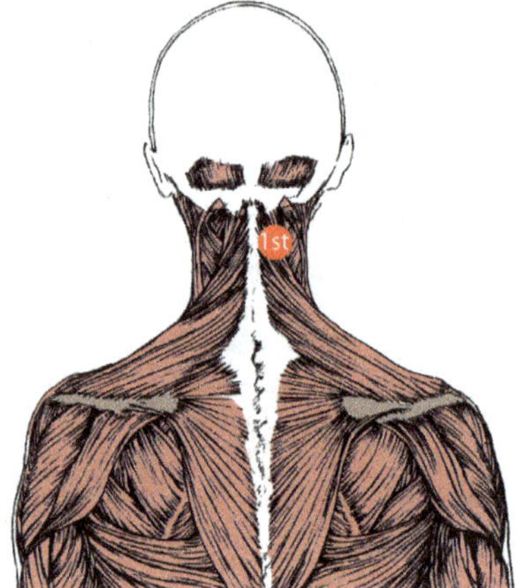

Indications

Bad posture habits and the tendency of each person to use one side of the body more than the other causes neck tensions to appear especially in this area. In addition, mental stress can aggravate symptoms.

7. Second complementary warning point

Location

It is located at the back of the left knee, below the popliteal fossa. Coiciding with the fifth point of the inferior line of the popliteal fossa region.

Depending on the patient's posture habits, this point may show itself on the other leg.

Indications

It is the appearance of structural problems in the lumbar area, especially on the L5-S1 joint. It is very important for work on lumbar problems.

There are many forms of treatment in Aze Shiatsu. One of them is to use the five warning points as standard treatment. Such treatment would consist of the following:

— Ankle rotation.
— Five warning points plus two complementary ones.
— Hara: Especially tanden and stomach pit.
— Foot and occipital sanri: to mitigate the Menken effects.

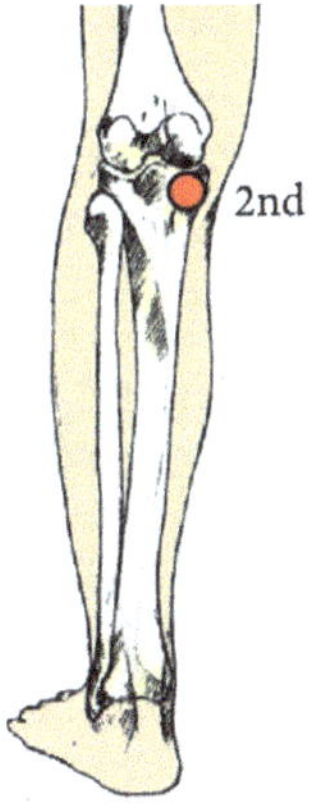

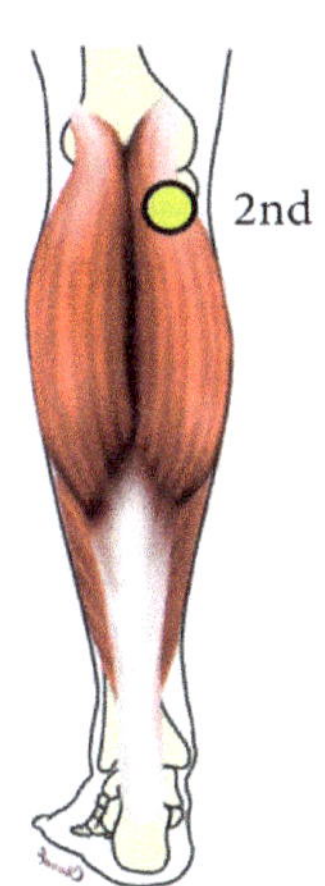

ELIMINATING SLACK

Beneath this concept lies one of the keys to Aze Shiatsu treatment's effectiveness: both pressure as well as stretches must take this concept into account to be effective.

Our body is composed of more than 70% liquid, with different densities depending on the organs and tissues: skin, subcutaneous tissue, fatty tissue, muscle tissue, etc. This characteristic of the tissues makes our joints sufficiently elastic to properly function. Aze Shiatsu's basic technique is based on reducing slack before applying pressure or stretching.

For Shiatsu pressure to be effective, it must reach the deeper layers of the body structure. To achieve this it is necessary to eliminate the slack between the surface and the contracture or deep layers. Applying pressure at this level activates the area's blood and lymphatic circulation and removes the accumulated lactic acid; this action flexes the muscles and keeps the area clean of waste products.

It is easy to apply a force to inanimate objects and transmit it without losing or dispersing it. The result is that it moves or is destroyed. The human body, however, is a living organism that reacts to force applied to the surface. The reaction can be pain, a sense of pleasure, resistance, a rise in temperature, and so on, and the therapist can perceive it in infinite ways. For that bodily reaction to appear more accurately and quickly, the therapist needs to know how to apply force correctly (without losing it or dispersing it); by eliminating surface slack.

Aze Shiatsu employs several techniques to reduce slack:

1. Stretching the area

Perform a stretch in the region to locate the maximum stress point. When the surface layers are tightened, they move closer to the deep layers, eliminating the slack.

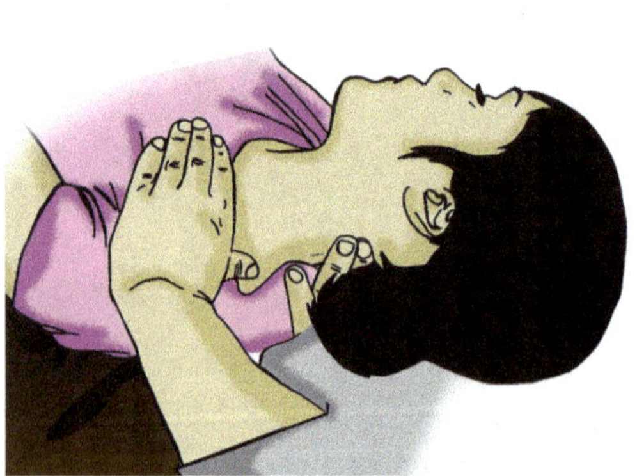

When working the Suprascapular Region, a stretch can be performed on the area with the other hand. This tightens the trapezium muscle and the maximum tension point reveals itself so that pressure is applied to it better.

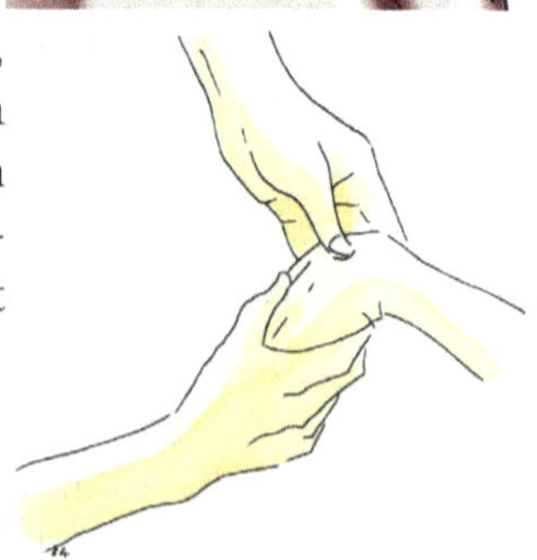

2. Maintaining perpendicular pressure

Two of the fundamental charac-teristics of Shiatsu pressure are to be perpendicular and to be maintained. Using his body weight, the therapist should gradually increase perpendicular pressure and maintain it until reaching the patient's pain threshold when he or she starts to feel pain. This work removes approximately 80% of the slack. To eliminate the remaining slack, the patient's limit must be exceeded.

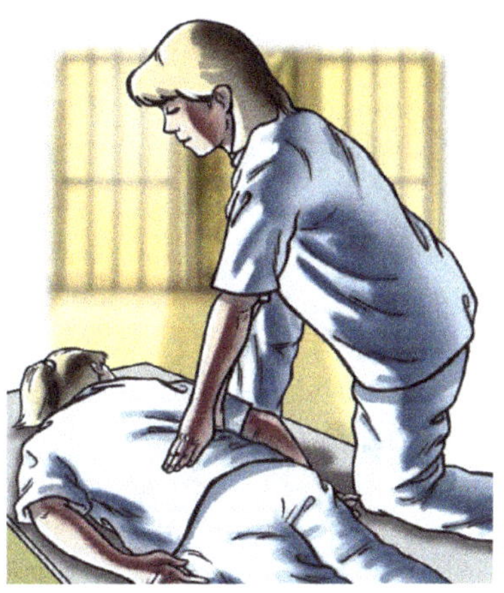

3. Tightening the skin with one hand and applying pressure with the other

Sometimes it is enough to tighten the skin around the point where pressure will be applied, using the other hand. This technique is used in areas where there is an accumulation of tissue between the skin and bone or joint. This is the case with the back of the hand, the elbow joint, the back of the foot and the sacral area.

In the lateral region of the wrist the slack is removed by performing a dorsal joint extension. So, the area's key points are more accessible for pressure to be applied.

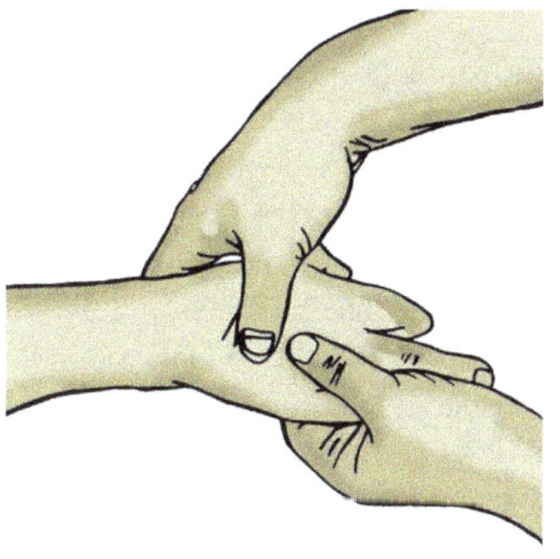
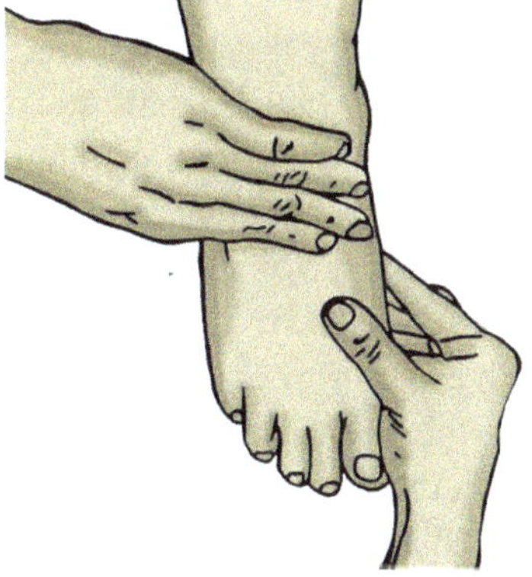

4. Sliding pressure

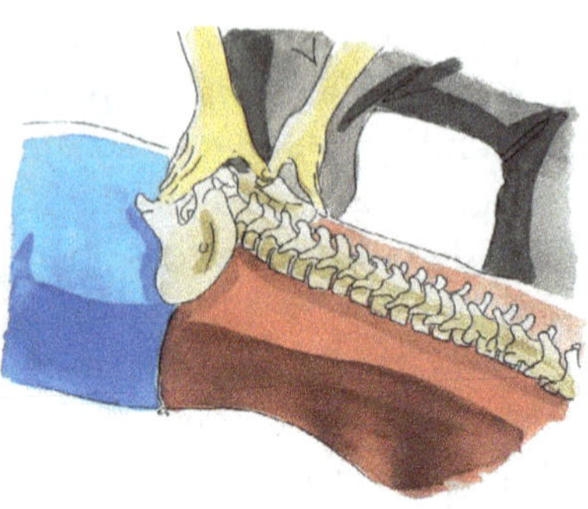

Another way to eliminate slack is by using a sliding thumb over thumb pressure or with thumbs together. This pressure consists of applying pressure that's not perpendicular, but a little upwards, and when reaching the patient's threshold change the direction downwards, while always maintaining pressure. This slides the pressure as if the area is being scraped. This technique can be used in areas such as occipital or lumbo-sacral joint.

These techniques can be used individually or combined for better performance. Shiatsu should be applied gradually, eliminating surface slack, testing once, twice and three times cautiously and prudently while observing the body's reaction.

Aze Shiatsu uses stretches in its therapy to try to release, above all, the patient's joints. To perform these, it is also essential to eliminate slack. We are, therefore, talking about a first phase of preparation to try to eliminate slack and a second of executing movement.

In the preparation phase, the therapist elongates the joints as much as possible, performing a traction from a distal point.

In the execution phase, stretching or manipulation starts from the previous position.

We consider the lumbar traction movement, one of the eight spinal column movements. In the preparation phase, the therapist performs a slight traction of the entire spinal column from the patient's knees. A movement of the patient's trunk is considered to the point from which the patient's body would be pulled. From that point, the therapist performs the stretch itself by dropping his weight back onto his heels.

These movements are only for milliseconds and are only possible when the joint's mobility has been pushed to its limit, otherwise the slack between the joint's components does not allow it to reach its objective. Eliminating slack is not an easy technique. It requires a lot of training to combine pressure with the removal of slack. But we are confident that its use increases the effectiveness of Aze Shiatsu treatment.

THE EIGHT SPINAL COLUMN MOVEMENTS

Both Eastern medicine and the different traditional Japanese arts consider the hara to be the centre of the body's balance. It is located in the lower belly area and in the pelvic waist. From this point arise all the possible body movements; interlocked joints and muscles that enable us to perform daily activities such as walking, running, jumping, turning, standing, etc. Dance, theatre, painting, floral art, martial arts and Japanese meditation emphasize using the hara as a balance point of physical and energetic movement.

This area is so important that it is considered that when some imbalance occurs, it ends up affecting the rest of our body. When the body is unbalanced, the hara is not in its place. This imbalance affects the bone and muscle system as well as the body as a whole. When there are tensions in some part of the body, they can be transmitted to the internal organs via the autonomic nervous system and viscerocutaneous reflections.

When there is an imbalance, movements are not performed properly. The job of a Shiatsu therapist is to balance the body in order to return the hara to its centre.

ANTERIOR PART OF THE BODY

Hara (Tanden) (literally "sea of energy") is an energy centre that plays an important role in various disciplines of Eastern tradition.

The hara is complemented by the movement of koshi (hip/lumbar area). Koshi literally means the most important area of the body.

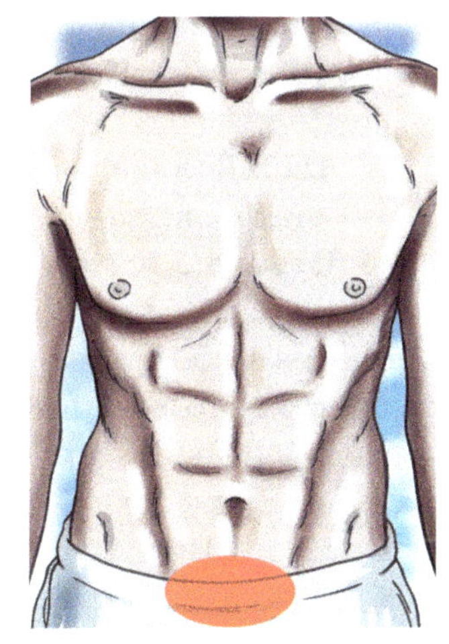

Koshi means "the lower back". This character is divided into two: "body" and "most important", so we can say that it indicates the most important area of the body.

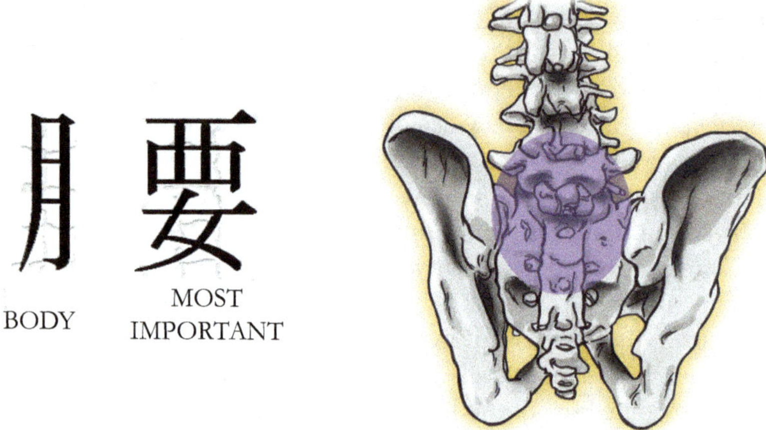

The eight movements in the spinal column represent all movements made from the hara. The Shiatsu therapist must know them in depth. They serve as diagnosis and treatment. Looking at the the range of each one's mobility can establish which parts of the patient's body have tension, or where imbalance appears.

For treatment, the therapist can use them in two ways:

1. **Auto:** Recommending the patient to do these exercises daily on their own.
2. **With a therapist:** Using these exercises in the Shiatsu session.

Aze Shiatsu uses these movements following Sotai Ho technique guidelines. Choosing the easiest movement that the patient can do, between two opposite movements (flexion / extension, left rotation / right rotation, etc.) and is worked repeatedly. Therefore, both the choice of most appropriate exercise and the way of executing it is made according to Sotai Ho therapy's principles: choose the exercise that effects the affected area, compare its mobility in the two directions of the movement and choose the one that is easiest to perform. Oriental medicine understands that, as the human body is a whole, stretching a joint in a given direction directly affects its opposite. Likewise, Shiatsu thinks and works in the same way: we do not apply pressure on areas where there is pain and are full, but in areas that have a sense of emptiness.

FLEXION

Muscles involved: The muscles of the dorsal and lumbar area (paravertebral muscles: spinalis, longissimus, iliocostal, multifids, etc.) are stretched and the abdomen and belly flexor muscles contract. If your knees can extend fully, the muscles in the back of your leg (hamstrings) are also stretched.

Auto: Movement starts in the hara, (1) the person moves the hip backwards by shifting the body weight to the back of the feet, (2) this movement causes the trunk to bend from the hip so that (3) it propels the arms downwards (no need to touch the ground)

With a therapist: The patient lies in supine position with their legs bent. The therapist, kneeling, takes the patient's legs below the patella and bends them back towards the chest. This movement causes retropulsion of the hip, relieving tension in the lower back. It is particularly beneficial in those with lumbar hyperlordosis.

The therapist can perform this exercise on each leg independently.

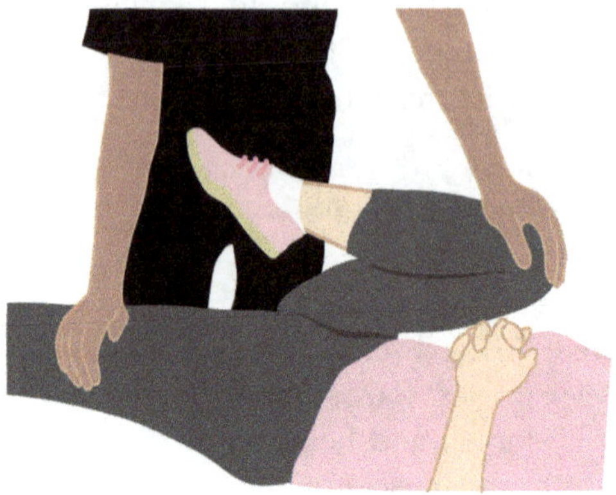

EXTENSION

Muscles involved: The abdomen flexor muscles (rectus abdominis, external and internal oblique and psoas, which is the hip flexor) are stretched while the dorsal and lumbar muscles area contract.

Auto: With semi-flexed knees and the movement starting from the hara, (1) the hip moves forward bringing the weight to the front of the foot. This movement (2) causes the spine to extend to the neck and head. There's no need to force your position.

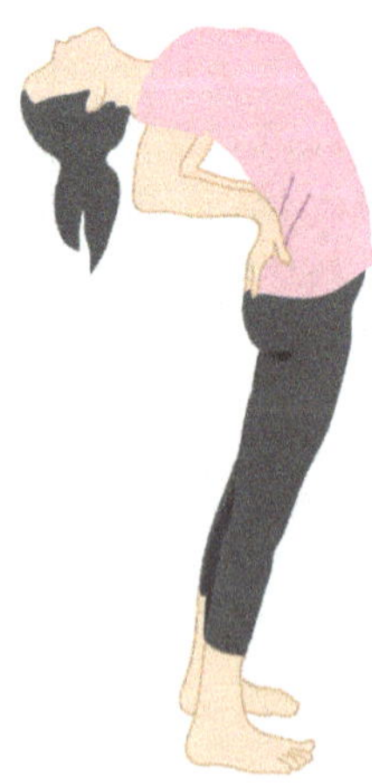

With a therapist: The patient lies in prone position with legs stretched out. The therapist bends the patient's knees from his feet, towards the gluteus. This movement causes an anteversion of the hip, so special care must be taken when the person has lumbar problems.

You can do this exercise on each leg independently.

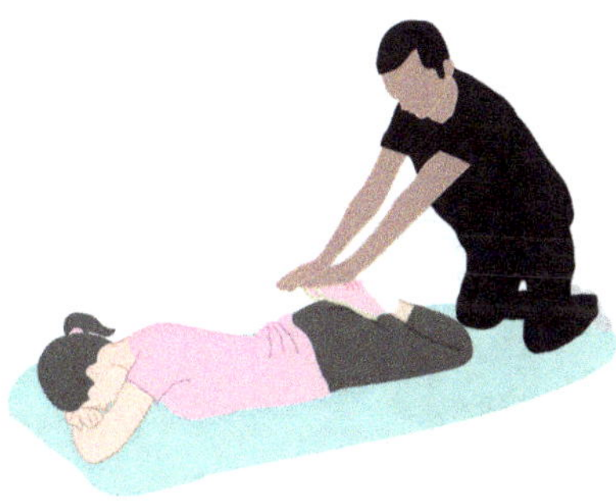

RIGHT AND LEFT LATERAL INCLINATIONS

Muscles involved: Stretching unilaterally from the side which moves the weight of the quadratus lumborum body, spinalis, longissimus, iliocostal, external oblique, internal oblique, intertransverse and latissimus dorsi. With the same leg the gluteus medius, maximus, minimus, fascia lata tensor and sartorio are stretched. The other leg stretches adductors, internal rectum, psoas major, iliac and inferior fibers of the gluteus maximus.

Auto: Moving the hara (1) displaces the hip onto the leg and the body's weight onto that foot. (2) This movement moves the trunk to the other side causing the stretch; (3) stretching the arm sharpens the movement.

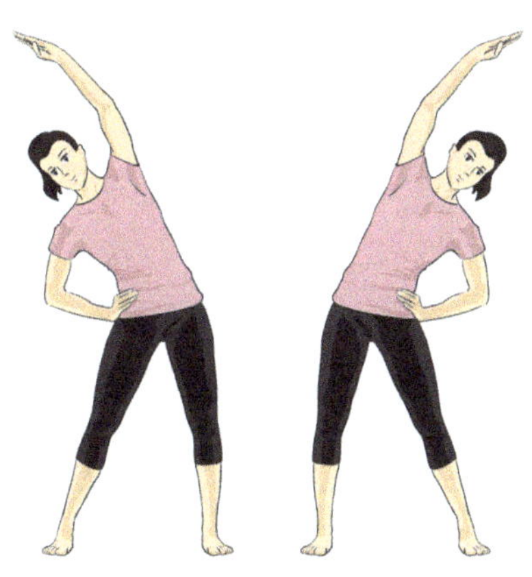

With a therapist: The person lies in supine position. The therapist is facing the patient in Shiatsu's basic position and places the patient's legs on their raised leg. The patient's hips and knees should be bent at ninety degrees. From this position the therapist turns his body causing the patient's legs to move so that the person's hip moves causing the lateral inclination of the spinal column. Normally you work in the direction of most range of movement.

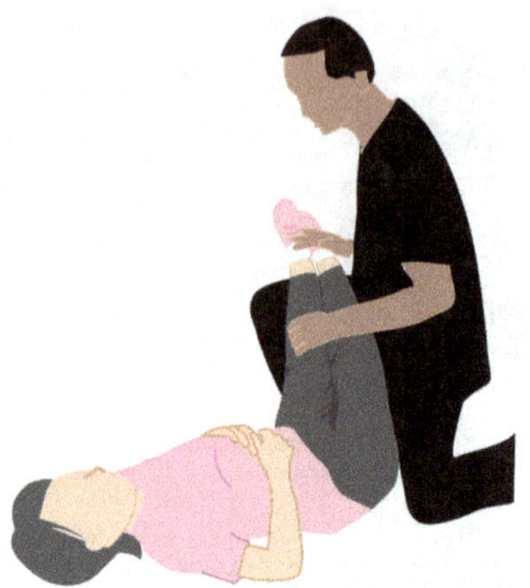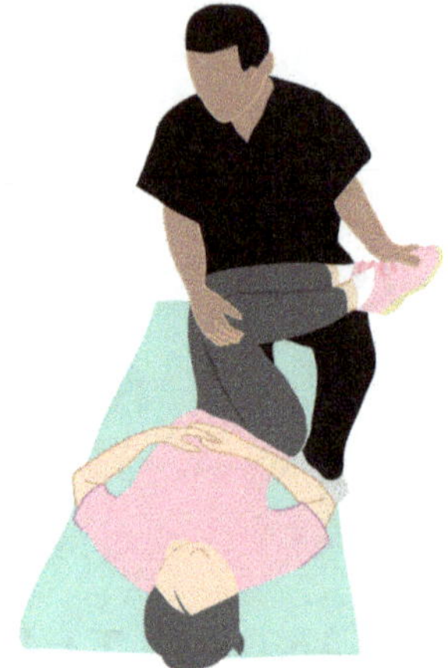

RIGHT AND LEFT ROTATION

Muscles involved: On the opposite side: multiphids, rotators and external oblique. On the same side: internal oblique. In the leg, the opposite pyriform is stretched, the sacropelvic, sartorio, psoas major and iliac, femoral biceps, gluteus maximus muscles and posterior fibers of the gluteus medius.

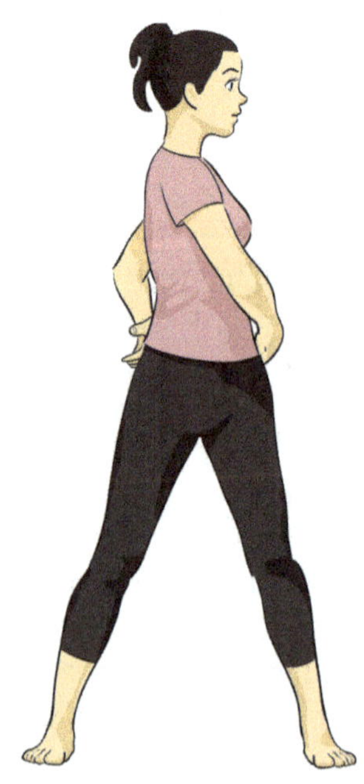

Auto: Starting from the movement of the hara, (1) shift the weight onto the leg of the side turning. (2) You start to rotate your hip to that side by smoothly moving the turn up towards your head. The shoulders and arms naturally accompany this movement.

With a therapist: The patient lies in supine position with their legs bent. The therapist rotates the patient's hip to the most mobile side, bringing the knees to the ground.

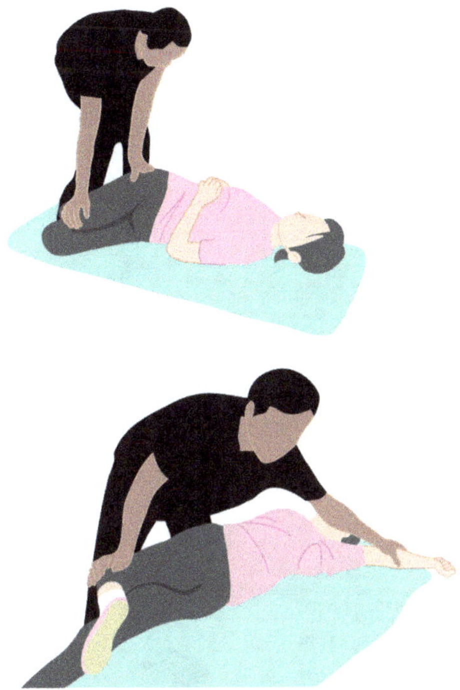

This movement can be performed more acutely by crossing one bent leg over the other straight one and performing an opposite stretch of the other arm.

TRACTION

Muscles involved: This exercise releases the intervertebral joints, especially of the lumbar spinal column.

Auto: This exercise is difficult to do by yourself.

With a therapist: The patient lies in supine position with their legs bent. The therapist places his interlocked hands under both of the patient's popliteal fossa.

He performs traction by dropping the weight of his body backwards.

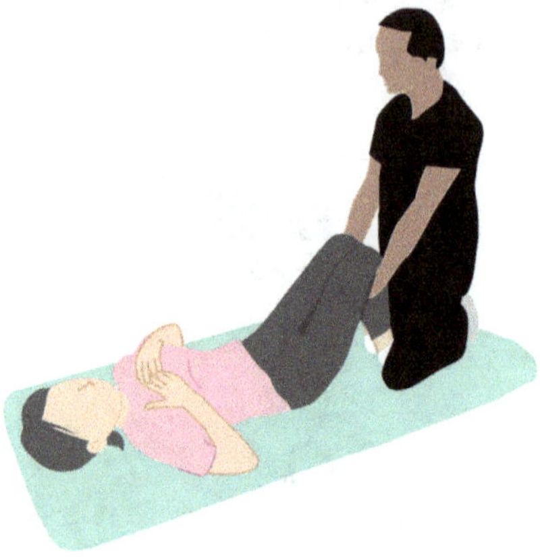

COMPRESSION

Muscles involved: This exercise compresses the intervertebural joints, especially of the lumbar spinal column.

Auto: This exercise is difficult to do by yourself.

With a therapist: Here the patient is in a supine position with their legs straight. The therapist applies pressure to the patient's head with both palms, pushing in the direction of his feet with a gentle movement.

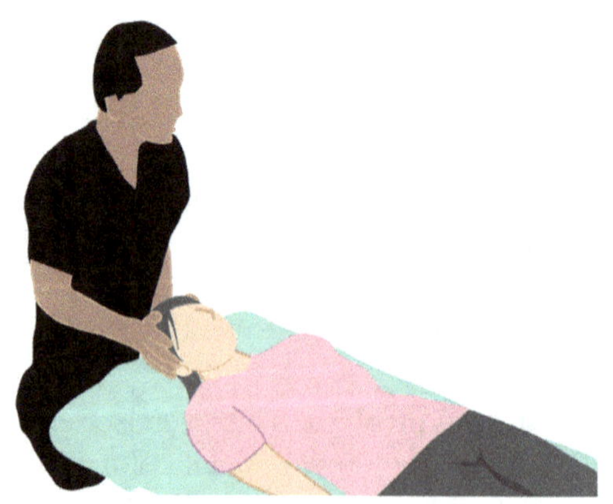

If the patient's body offers some kind of resistance or feels pain, we will work only the traction movement.

It is important for the therapist to know how to convey the best way to move to the patient so as not to harm the body. The patient has most responsibility for recovery. If he understands how he should move his body and does it, recovery will be faster and deeper.

We have explained the movements of the spinal column focusing on work on the lumbar area. We should not forget that the spinal column forms a single part and that what happens in one part is transmitted to the rest. When the lumbar region is affected, sooner or later it will appear in the dorsal or cervical spinal column levels.

Aze Shiatsu Stretching

Prone Decubitus

Hip rotation movement

The hip movement enables the therapist to observe the joint connections from the bottom to the top. Comparing the movement in both the right and left directions.

Generally it is worked with a knee flexed 90º. With a more pronounced flexion, the effect of movement is more concentrated in the lumbar spinal column. With a lesser flexion the movement goes to the dorsal spinal column (interscapular region).

Work is on the sacroiliac joint region on the opposite side to the way the feet are facing.

We stretch the muscles involved with external and internal rotation (the spinal column erector group and internal and external oblique) depending on the leg in question. In addition, the femoral rectum is slightly stretched.

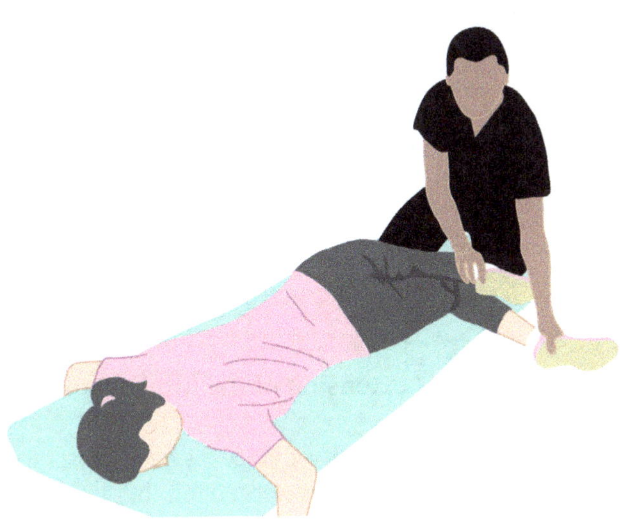

Stretching the sacroiliac joint

Rotating only one hip while keeping the other leg fixed, enables the medial femoral region to be stretched until it reaches the sacroiliac joint. The adductor muscles are stretched and are used to check the condition of the sacroiliac joint; the one on the side of the stretch should open, while the one on the opposite side stays still or closes.

Work is not done on the knee so as to not block the hip.

In addition, it enables us to observe the relationship between the hip and the lumbar area. If there is no imbalance, the stretch reaches the lumbar region that rotates following the natural joint movement.

As in the previous case, the angle of the flexed knee will determine the area where the stretch reaches.

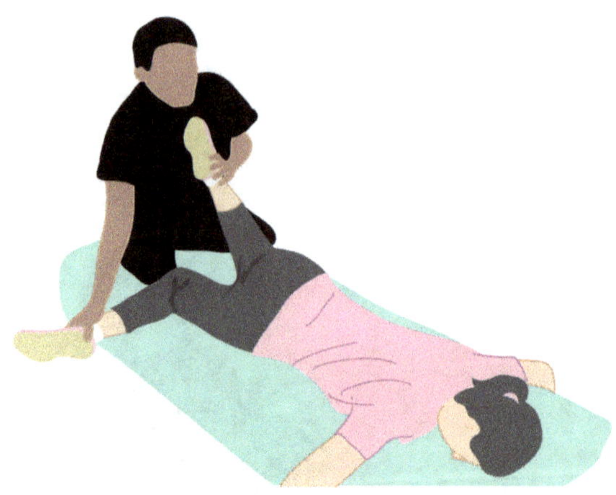

Stretching the quadriceps / extension of the lumbar spinal column

With his hands the therapist brings the patient's heels closer to the gluteus by applying pressure from the toes. Observing the flexibility in both legs.

With this movement two aspects must be taken into account, on one hand, it stretches the anterior femoral region.

On the other, when the anterior part of the legs (sural and femoral regions) are blocked, the hip performs a movement that increases physiological lumbar lordosis.

Care must be taken if the patient has lumbar hernias or hyperlordosis.

Stretching muscles: quadriceps, iliac psoas, sartorium (by its hip flexor action), tensor fasciae latae (by its hip flexor action), anterior tibial, extensor digitorum longus.

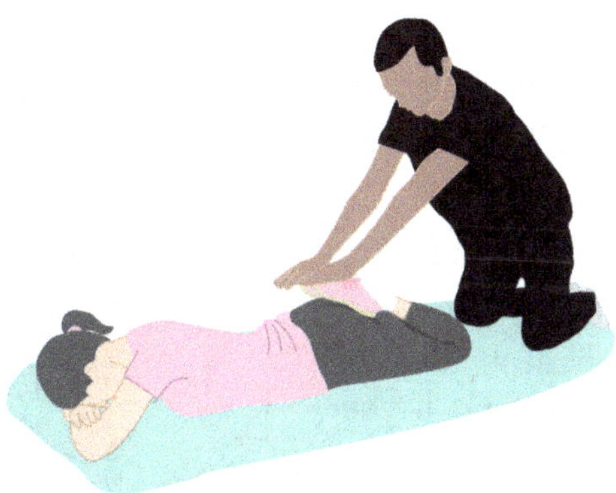

Stretching the calcaneal tendon

In this case, the therapist makes a dorsal foot flexion to stretch the calcaneal tendon. First, perform the movement on the two legs simultaneously. Then repeat with each leg independently. Comparing both legs.

The relationship between the calcaneal tendon and the state of the psoas must be taken into account; when the calcaneal tendon is shortened, the psoas are also affected.

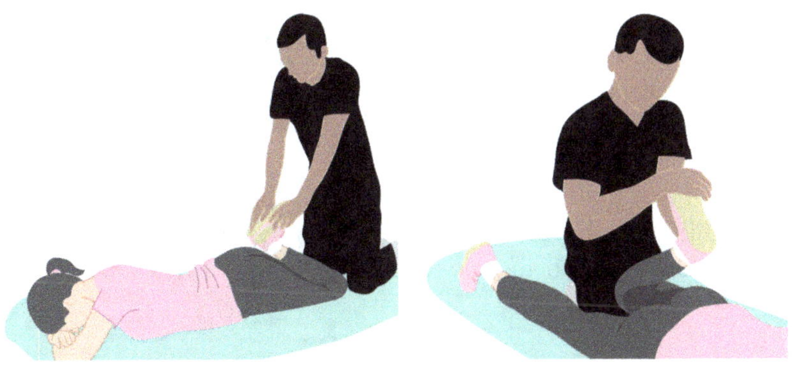

Stretching the soleus muscles (not the calf muscles that perform the knee flexion), plantar fascia, flexor digitorum longus and the flexor hallucis longus, in addition to the calcaneal tendon. Indirectly working on the femoral rectum by touching the heels to the gluteus.

Stretching the tarsal and calcaneal regions

Flexing the sole of the feet from the toes. The stretched line passes through point S41 in the centre of the tarsal region. This movement also works on the back of the foot and the lines that run through it. The angle of the flexed knee will vary depending on the degree of stretching to be performed.

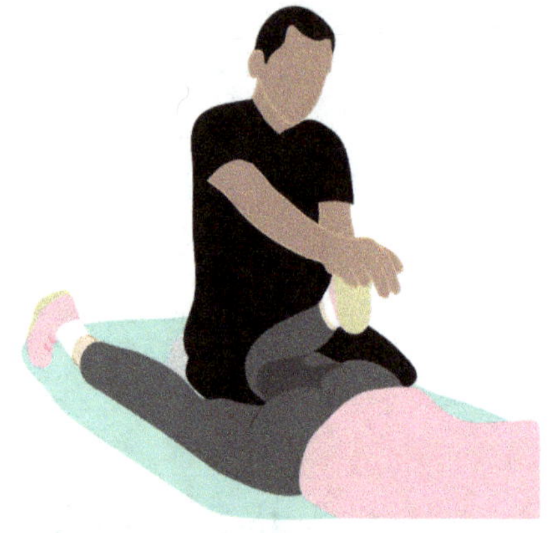

Stretching the muscles: anterior tibial, extensor digitorum longus and extensor hallucis longus muscle.

Stretching the tibial muscles and foot flexors. Eversion

Performing a foot eversion movement (dorsal flexion, abduction and external rotation).

Stretching the medial sural regions (up to point PS6), calcaneal tubercle and internal malleolus.

Stretching muscles: anterior tibial, posterior tibial, flexor digitorum longus, flexor hallucis longus, extensor hallucis longus.

Stretching the soleus muscles (not the calf muscles that perform the knee flexion), plantar fascia, flexor digitorum longus and the flexor hallucis longus, in addition to the calcaneal tendon. Indirectly working on the femoral rectum by touching the heels to the gluteus.

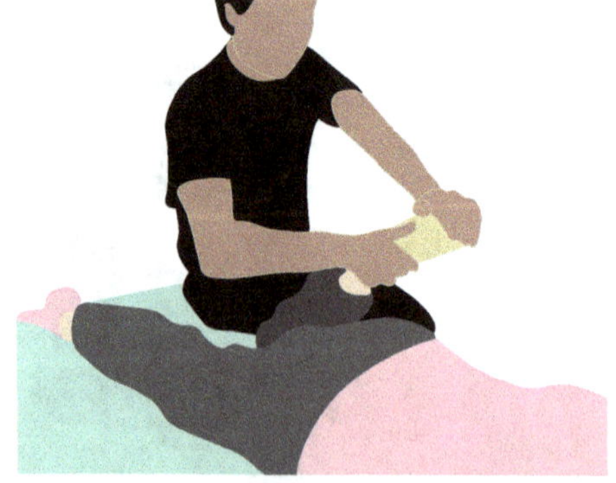

Stretching lateral peroneal muscles. Inversion

Performing a foot inversion movement (plantar flexion, adduction and internal rotation).

Stretching the lateral tibial regions, lateral sural and external malleolus (GB40).

Stretching muscles: peroneus longus, peroneus brevis, anterior tibial, extensor digitorum longus.

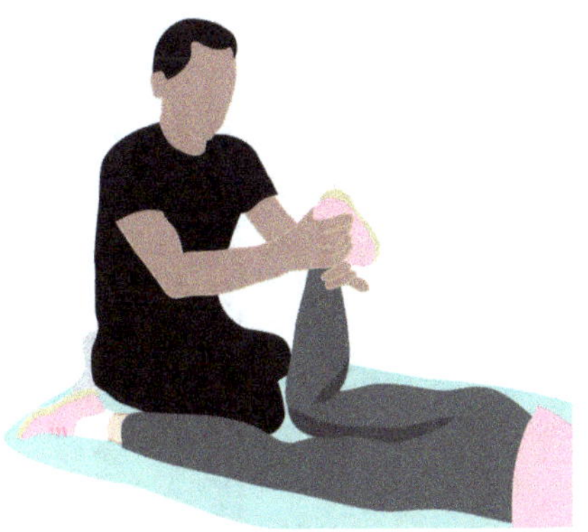

Stretching the soleus muscle and the calcaneal tendon region.

Performing a dorsal flexion and internal ankle rotation. It acts on the lateral, anterior tibial and external malleoli regions.

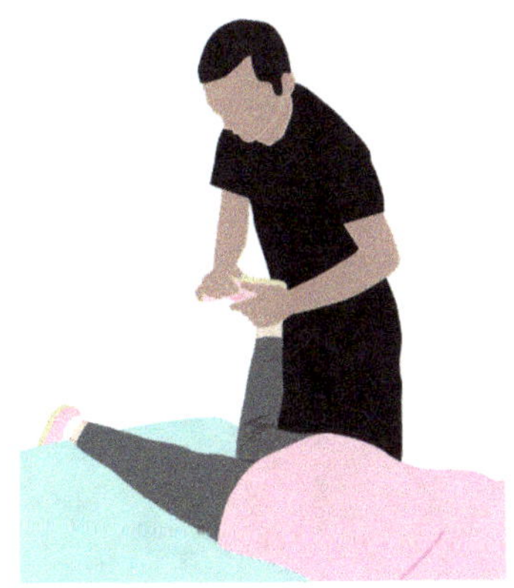
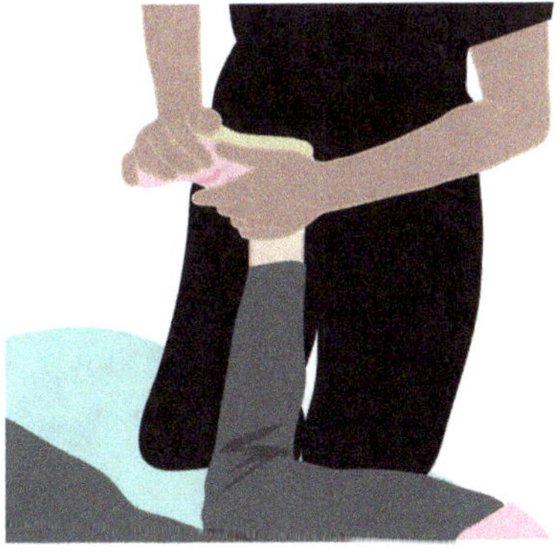

Stretching the soleus muscle and the calcaneal tendon region.

Performing a dorsal flexion and external ankle rotation.. It acts on the sural medial and internal malleoli regions.

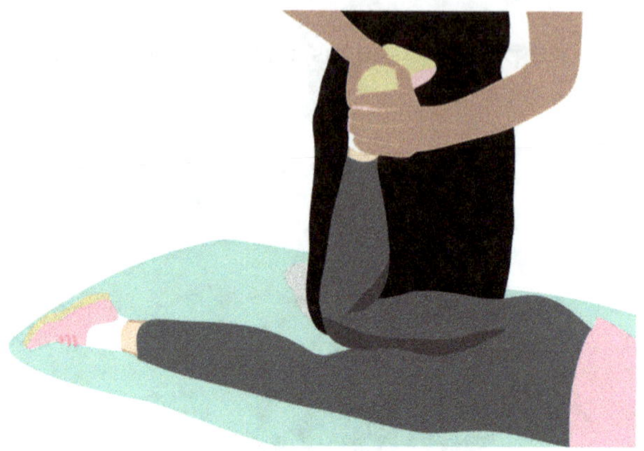

The ankle joint movement

With this movement, the ankle joint and the meridians passing through it are relaxed and stimulated.

You can apply pressure to the centre point of the tarsal region (S41) while performing this exercise.

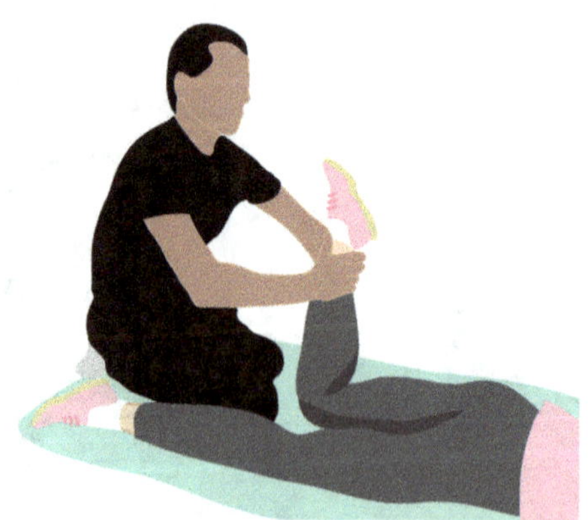

General stretching of the leg

Traction of all leg joints, especially the coxofemoral joint. The patient's leg in anatomical position without rotating the ankle.

Direct the stretch towards the opposite shoulder by connecting all joints from the ankle to the shoulder. Observing the connection of all joints according to the aspa theory.

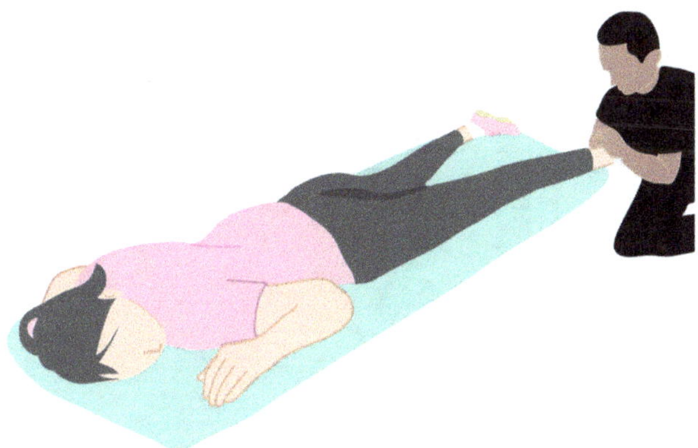

Leg traction and releasing the pyramidal muscle.

Leg traction with the ankle rotated outwards. It goes all the way to the coxofemoral joint. The pyramidal muscle and sciatic nerve are released. Very useful for patients with sciatica and acute lumbalgia. In addition, the *anterior femoral* region is stretched.

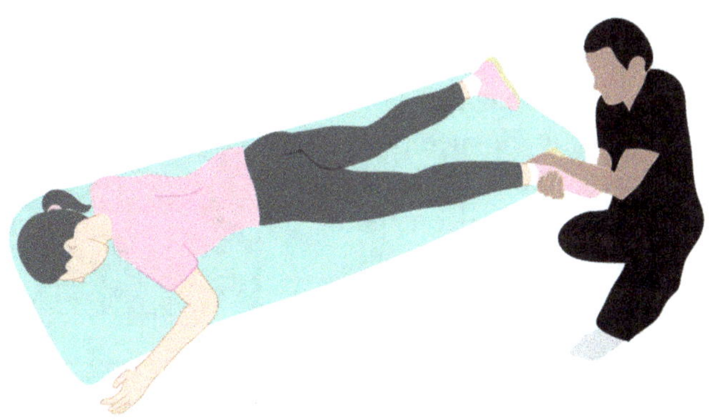

Leg traction and releasing the pyramidal muscle

Leg traction with the ankle rotated inwards. It reaches the coxofemoral and sacroiliac joint, mainly stretching the pyramidal muscle. Useful in chronic lumbalgia to "wake up" ancient contractures. In addition, the *anterior femoral* region is stretched.

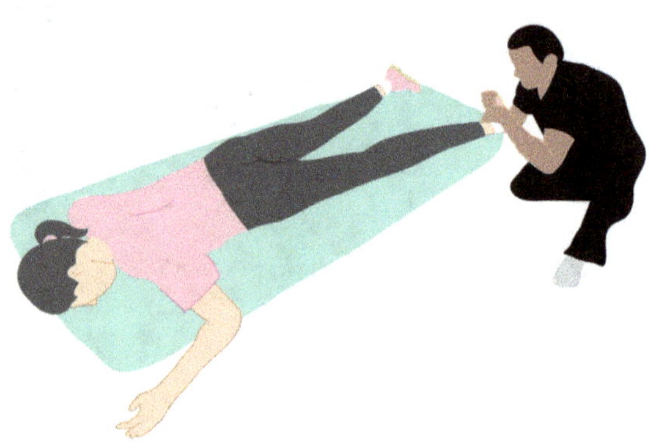

Stretching the sacroiliac region and pyramidal muscle.

Without blocking the sacrum, work is on the sacroiliac joint.
For working on the pyramidal muscle, block the sacrum with one hand and rotate the hip internally from the ankle with the other hand.

Stretching the muscles: pyramidal, internal and external obturator and gluteus. They are the hip stabilizers to maintain their balance.

Be careful if there are knee problems: performing the movement with the palm of the hand on the knee and the elbow on the patient's ankle.

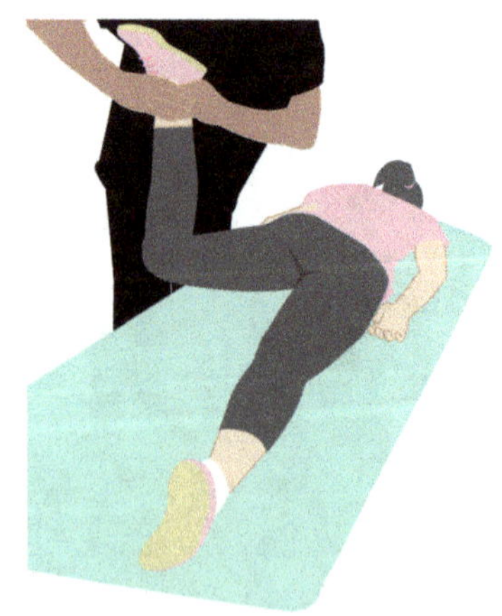

Stretching the psoas

Raise the far leg by placing the hand above the patient's knee. With the other hand the far hip is locked to concentrate the stretch.

Performing a slight abduction of the leg to concentrate the effect of the stretch on the psoas muscle.

This produces a stretch of the anterior femoral region, especially the proximal insertion of the quadriceps.

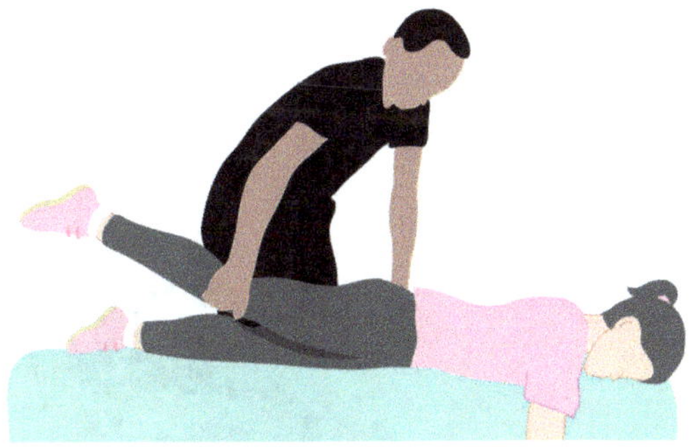

Stretching the anterosuperior iliac spine region

Raise the far leg by placing your hand above the knee. Block the hip with the other hand to concentrate the stretch and avoid hyperextension of the lumbar spinal column.

Work is on the muscle insertions in the anterosuperior and anteroinferior iliac spines.

Performing slight leg aduction to concentrate the stretch on the anterior rectum. This exercise does not work the quadricep muscle bellies that do not pass through the hip joint.

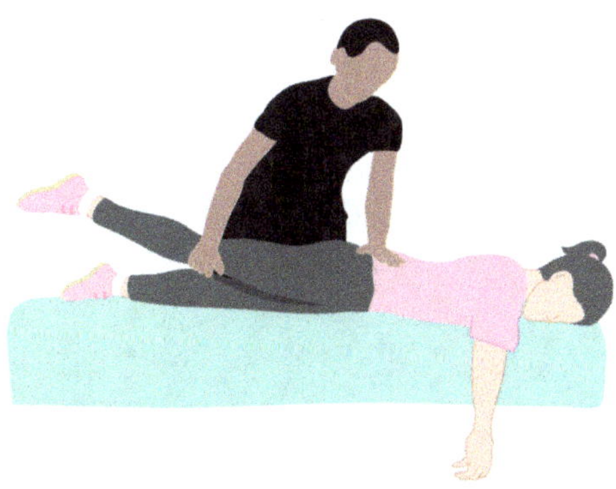

Stretching the anterior femoral region

It is a similar movement to the previous one, but in this case a hyper-flexion of the knee is performed, controlled by the therapist's shoulder, which causes the quadriceps to stretch. Lifting the leg, without causing pain, the stretch reaches the psoas muscle and femoral rectum.

A sharper stretch that works on all the quadricep muscle bellies, especially on muscle insertions in the anterosuperior iliac spine and patellar tendon.

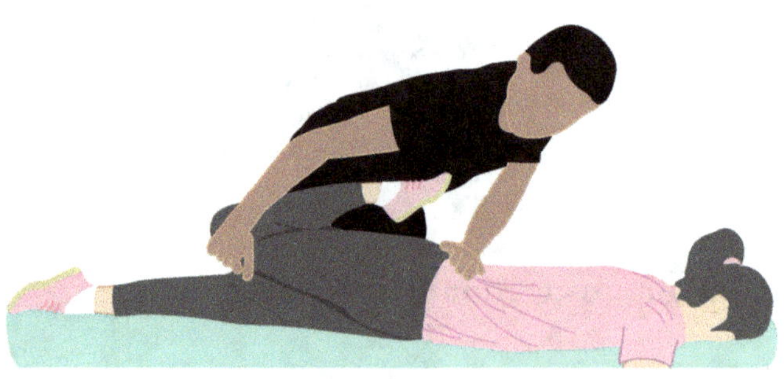

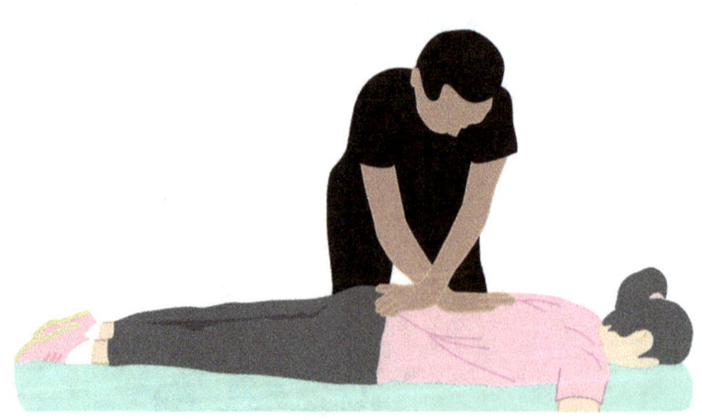

Right iliac crest movement

With crossed hands, one over the superior lumbar area to secure the spinal column and the other pushes the right iliac crest down (mainly using the thenar eminence). The therapist repeats the exercise several times by moving the hand along the iliac crest.

The left iliac ridge region and the lumbar region are stretched: B52 line. At the muscle level, we work on the quadratus lumborum and the thorolumbar aponeurosis.

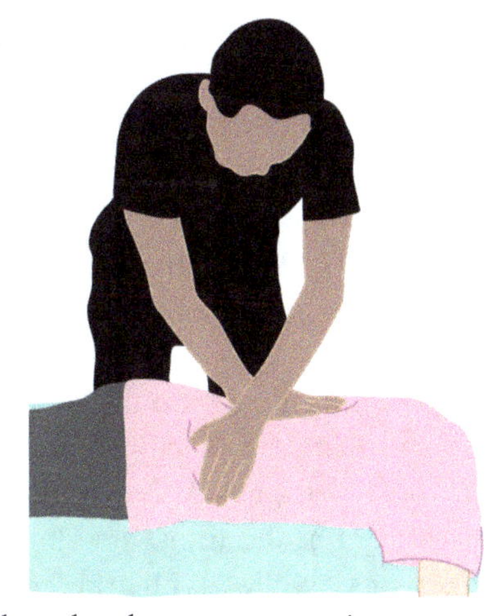

Left iliac crest movement

Repeating the previous exercise on the left side. The hand on the spinal column remains fixed and the other hand moves to the right side to push the iliac crest down (mainly using the hypotenar eminence).

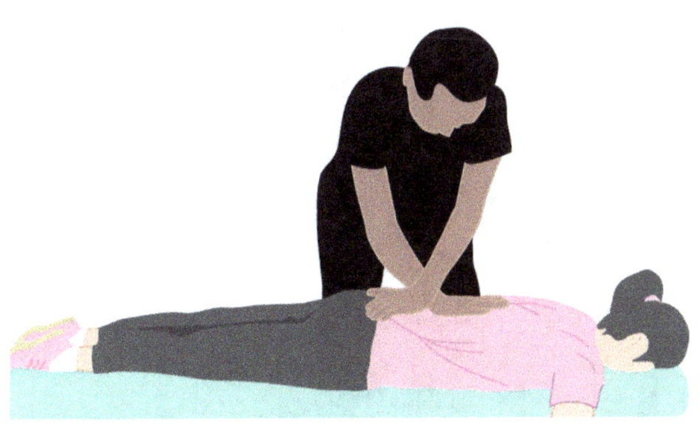

Lumbar vertebrae (rotating) movement

It serves as a diagnostic method of the lumbar region as well as to improve intervertebral mobility, especially of the transverse processes.

Blocking the spinal column from moving by placing one hand on the insertions of the quadratus lumborum in the transverse lumbar processes while with the other hand raise the hip from the antero-superior iliac spine.

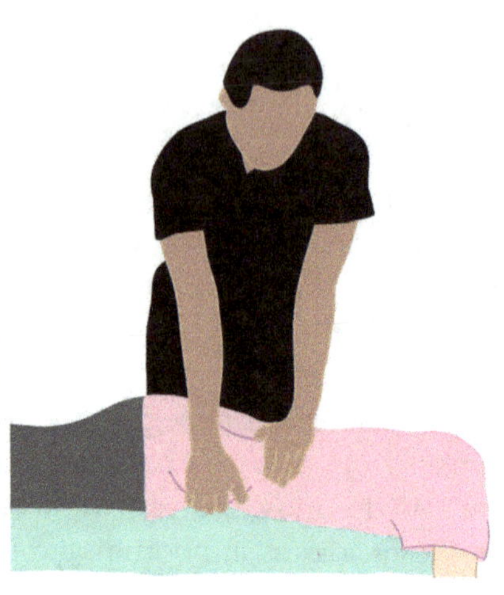

In addition, the *lumbar* regions, B52 *line* and *iliac crest* are mobilized.

Rocking the hip

Releasing and relaxing the fascia lata tensor and the insertion of the femoral rectum into the anterosuperior iliac spine.

Just gently push the hip from the gluteus and let it return to its starting position. Repeat several times rhythmically.

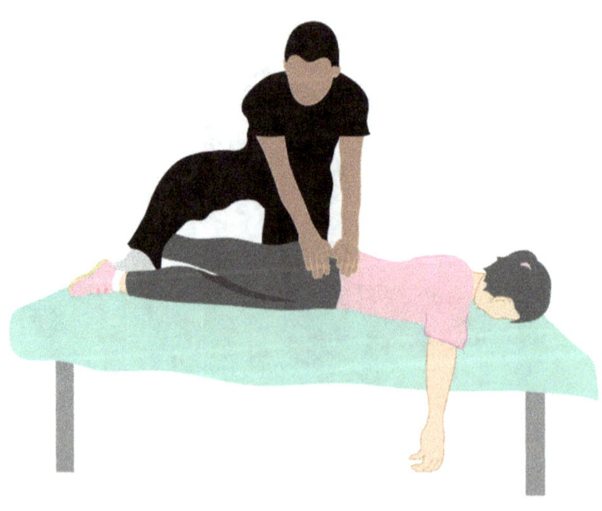

Releasing the hip joint

It acts on the sacroiliac joint ligaments, coxofemoral joint, semitendinous and semimembranous. It also works on the gluteus medius by stretching the posterior fibers and releasing the anterior ones.

When the patient has lumbalgia, he tends to place his leg in this position to mitigate pain. To balance the hip and improve sciatica we must perform the stretch to the less painful side.

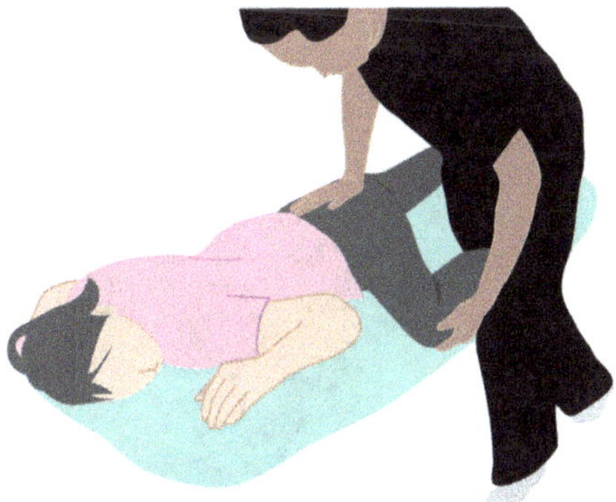

It can be used as a test by performing the exercise on both sides and comparing the results.

Complete the work by applying palm pressures around the coxofemoral joint and following the inferior edge of the iliac crest.

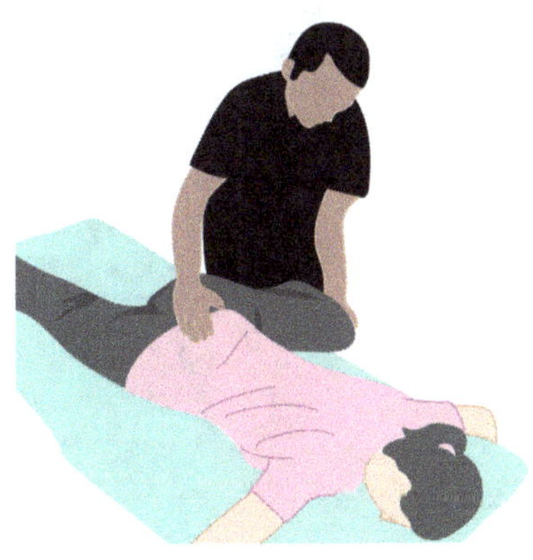

General relaxation of the back

The therapist uses his own body to perform the passive back extension without hurting himself; rocking the hip prevents any possible injury. The exercise can be performed by sitting on the massage bed next to the patient or on your knees on the bed above the patient's body. Relaxing the interscapular and infrascapular and lumbar regions, and stretching the abdominal and chest muscles.

Special care should be taken with people with hyperlordosis or lower back pain.

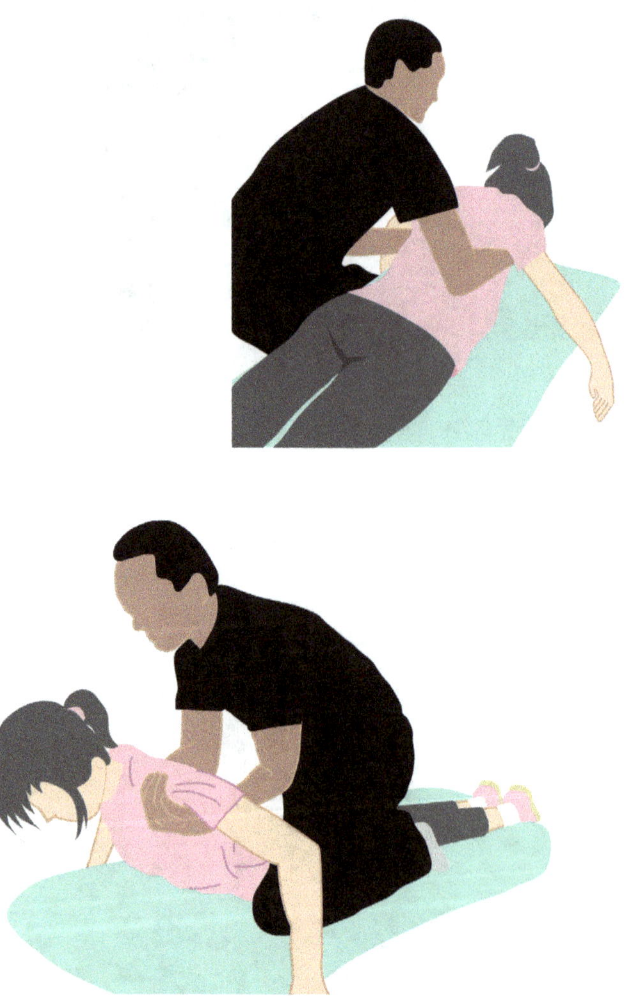

Aze Shiatsu Stretching

Supine Decubitus

Spinal column compression

In the first place, the cervical region is compressed, as it is able to reach the dorsal and even lumbar area.

The intervertebral spaces are shortened. This exercise is for diagnosing possible herniated discs. It can also be done from the heels of the feet.

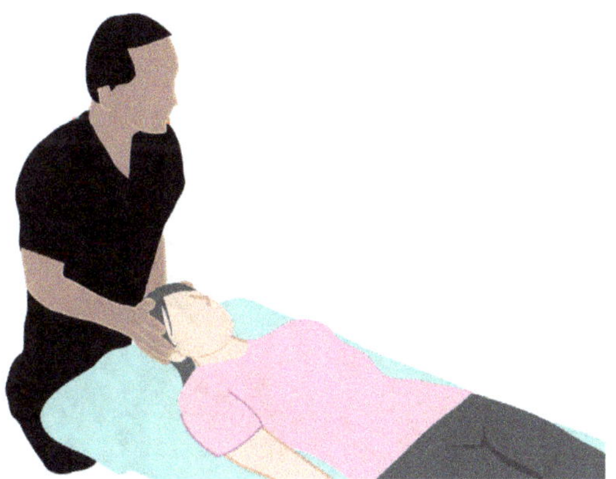

Spinal column traction

Releasing the lumbar intervertebral joints. It is one of the most important exercises for working on the spinal column. It helps to restore circulation in the lower back thereby aiding Shiatsu work. It is also used to diagnose the condition of the lumbar area. If the patient feels pain while performing this exercise, the therapist should think of two possibilities: one, that there is a problem with the disc that must be supervised by a doctor. And two, there is inflammation in the area that needs to be rested before receiving Shiatsu therapy.

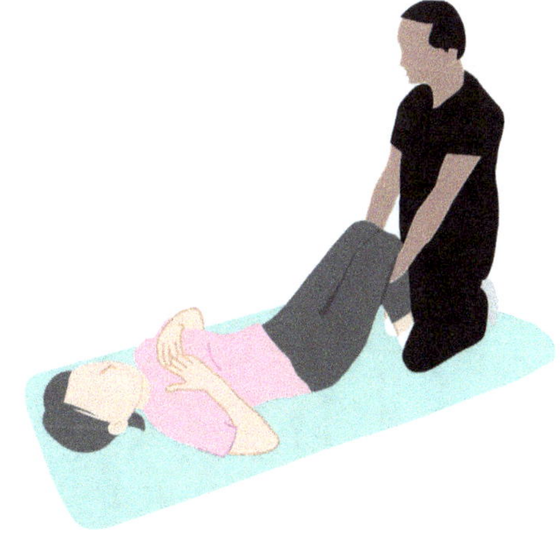

Lumbar spine flexion

It produces a pelvis retroversion, which decreases lumbar lordosis. It produces relief especially in people with lumbar problems.

Stretching the infrascapular and lumbar region in addition to the sacrum.

Stretching muscles: gluteus maximus, hamstring (origin or proximal area), spinal column extensors (lumbar paravertebral group) that rectify lumbar lordosis (longissimus, iliocostal, spinalis, semi-spinalis, multiphid, intertransversals).

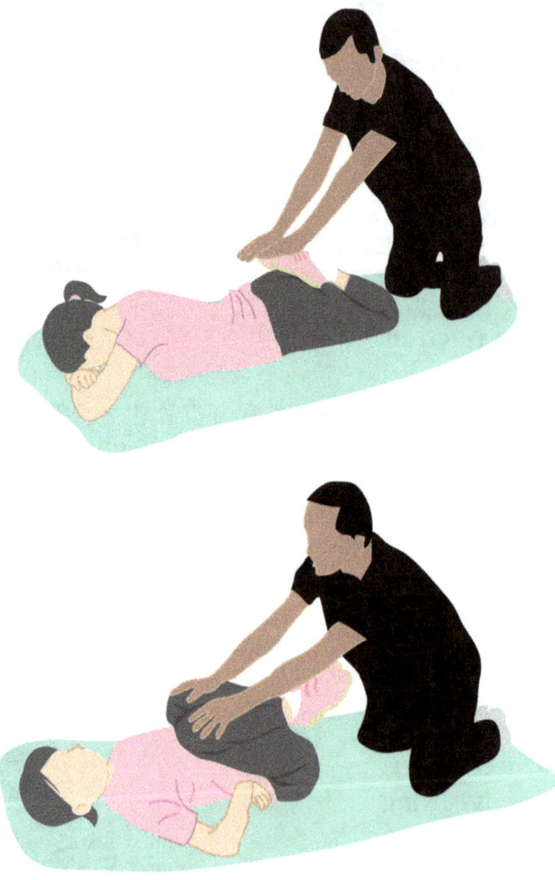

Extension of the spinal column

Spinal column lateralization

The patient's legs rest on the therapist's raised leg; who, with one hand on the knees, pushes and blocks the flexing legs at an angle of 90°.

The infrascapular and lumbar region on the opposite side are stretched, especially the lumbar region: B52 line (Shishitsu).

By lateralizing the lumbar spinal column we stretch the quadratus lumborum, the internal and external oblique on the opposite side.

By rotating internally, these muscles are stretched: adductor magnus, adductor medius and pectineo.

By rotating internally: pyramid, internal and external obturators, all gluteus and sartorious (by its rotating action).

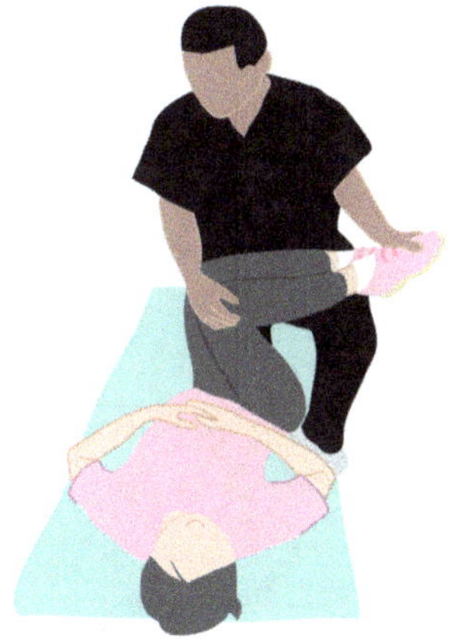

Left leg, internal rotation

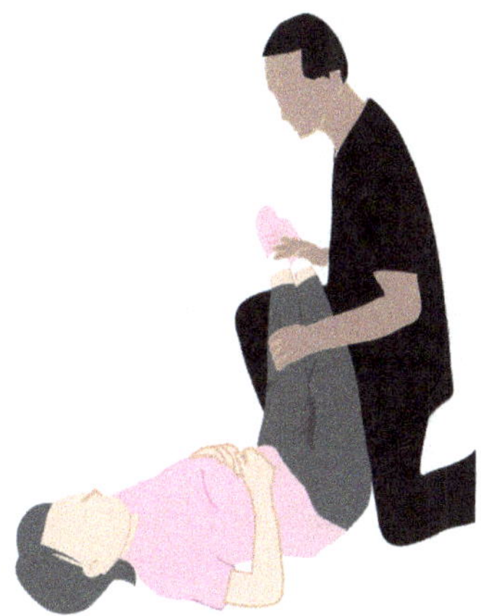

Right leg, external rotation

Hip rotations

Rotations are performed in both directions, right and left.

This is a movement to check the condition of the hip joint. In turn, joint mobility is released.

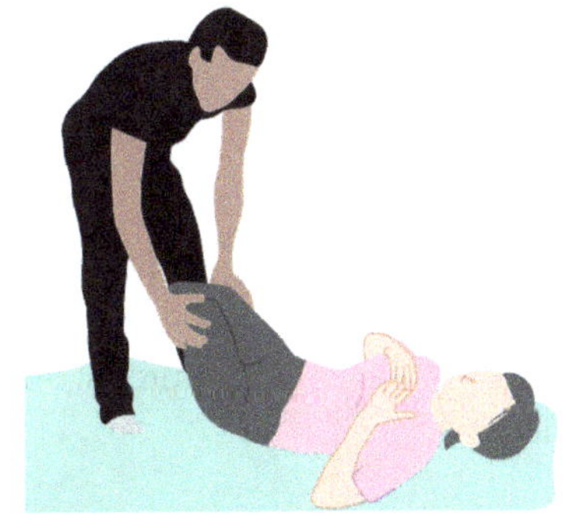

335

Rotation of the spinal column

Notice how the therapist's leg keeps the patient's heels touching his gluteus. This position concentrates the exercise in the lower back. Therefore, work is done on the infrascapular and lumbar region, impacting less on the interscapular region.

Stretching muscles: oblique of the abdomen, part of the anterior rectum of the abdomen, transversal of the abdomen, quadratus lumborum, multifids, intertransversals, fascia lata tensor and iliotibial tract.

Stretching the lateral femoral region

The lumbar area should remain touching the bed to avoid rotating the spinal column. The exercise sequence will be as follows: knee flexion, hip flexion, hip adduction passing the foot to the other side, and finally stretching. One hand controls the head of the femur while the other stretches from the knee.

Stretching is performed on the Gallbladder meridian, especially above point GB31 located approximately in the centre of the region.

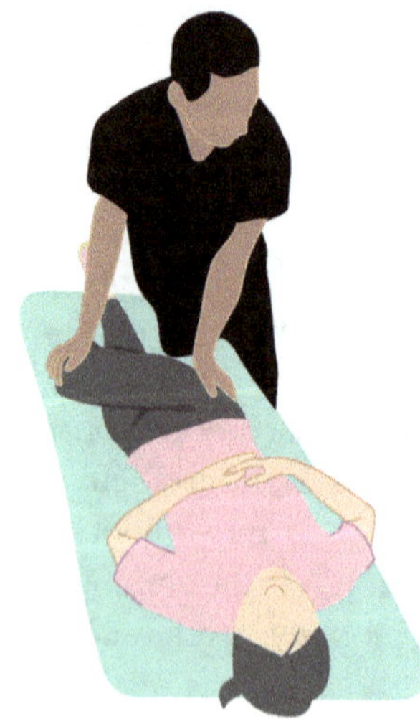

Stretching muscles: fascia lata tensor and iliotibial tract, gluteus (for its flexor action).

The following series of three stretches shows variations of the same exercise over the medial femoral region. One hand rests on the antero-superior iliac spine on the opposite side and the other performs the stretch from the patient's knee. Varying where the hand is placed on the knee influences each of the three lines of the *medial femoral* region.

Stretching the muscles: *adductor magnus, medius and minimus, internal rectum, pectineo and iliac psoas.*

Medial femoral stretch, central line and over the medial inguinal region. The hand on the femorotibial joint. Working on the liver meridian.

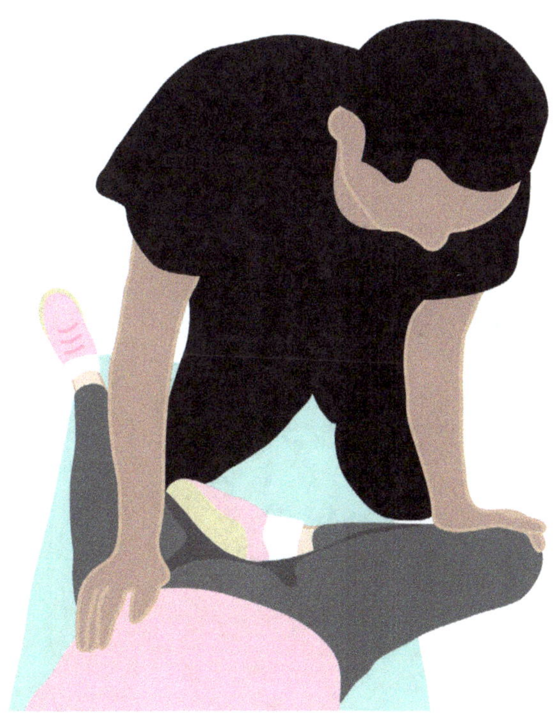

Medial femoral stretch, superior line and superior inguinal region.

Hand on the medial condyle of the femur. Working on the Spleen-Pancreatic meridian.

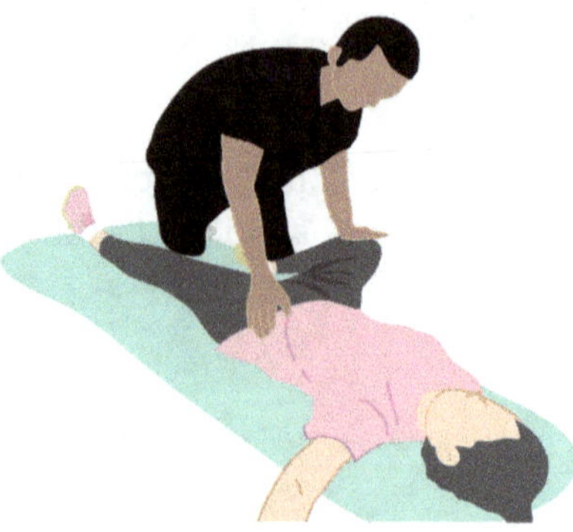

Medial femoral stretch, inferior line and inferior inguinal region.

Hand on the medial condyle of the tibia. Working on the kidney meridian.

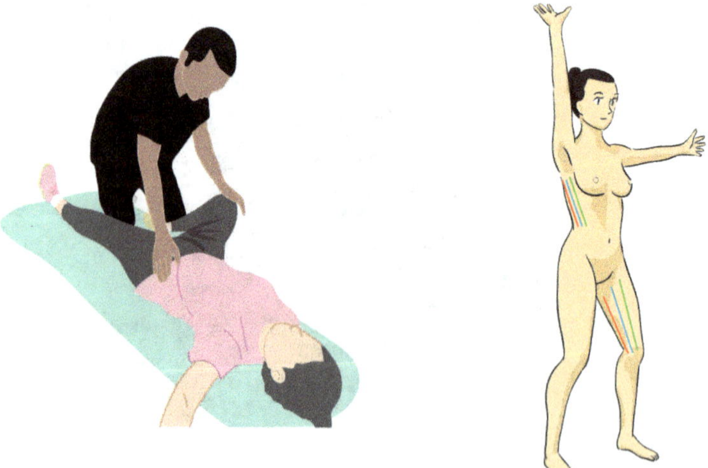

The medial femoral region is a Kyo area that is reflective in the lateral costal area on the other side according to the aspa theory. The three lines intersect and appear in reverse order.

The next series of three stretches is used for working the muscles and Shiatsu regions of the back of the leg. Depending on the degree of hip flexion, the exercises will be concentrated in one or the other of those regions. In any case, these exercises work along the path of the bladder meridian that runs through this area.

Stretching the posterior sural region

Without raising the patient's leg, work is done on the calcaneal tendon. Rising it one palm from the bed, work is carried out on the posterior sural region.

Stretching muscles: sural triceps (especially from the gastrocneum as the knee remains extended), calcaneal tendon, flexor digitorum longus, flexor hallucis and posterior tibial muscles.

The first image, with the leg flat on the bed, shows the work on the calcaneal tendon. The second, with a slightly lifted leg, works on the *posterior sural* region.

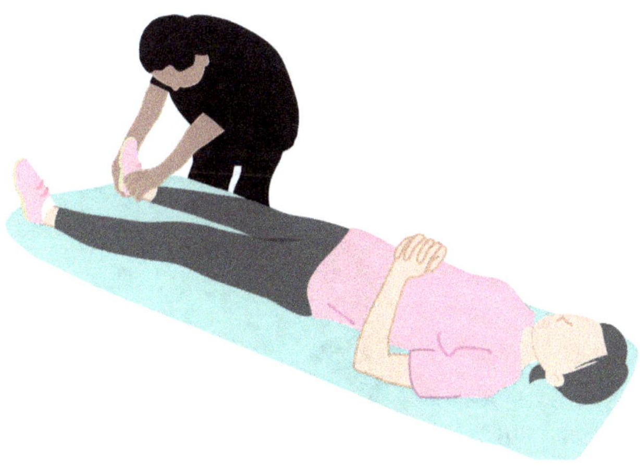

Stretching the posterior femoral region

Raising the extended leg increases the range of the leg's stretch. The *posterior femoral* region and the hamstring musculature are now reached.

Stretching muscles: sural triceps (calves and soleus), flexor digitorum longus, flexor hallucis, posterior tibial and hamstring muscles.

The first image shows the work on the popliteal fossa region.
The second, performing dorsal flexion of the ankle from the feet, works on the hamstring muscles and the posterior femoral region, in addition to the flexors digitorum and the plantar fascia.

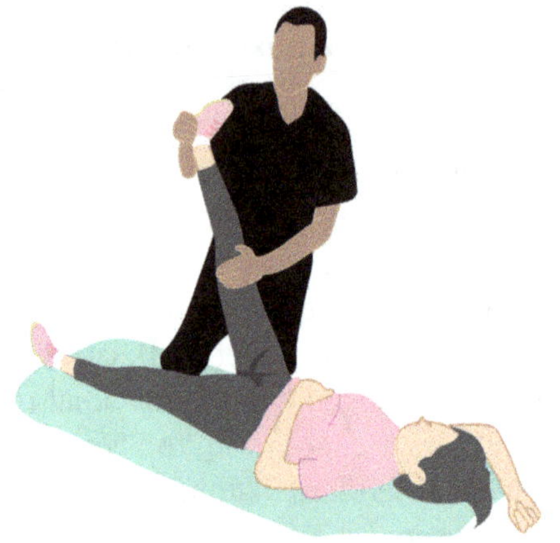

Hip traction, one leg

Different areas are worked on depending on the degree the hip opens.

If the degree of openness is minimal, exercise affects the top of the sacroiliac joint and the quadratus lumborum (lumbar region: B52 line, Shishitsu).

If the degree is maximum, work is done on the sacroiliac joint on the same side.

In whichever case, traction can be combined with applying pressure on the popliteal fossa region, with the three middle fingers of both hands.

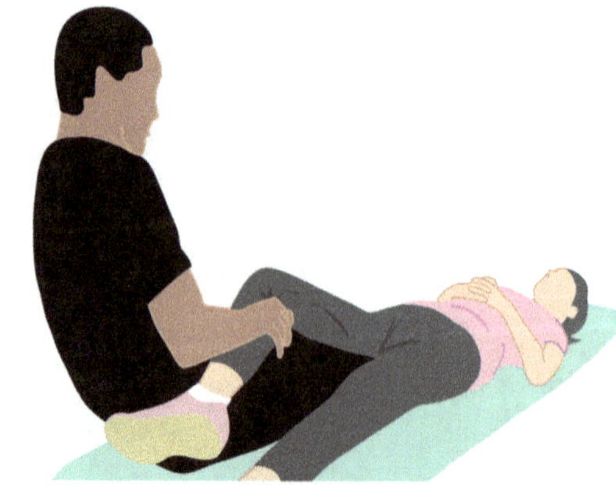

Hip traction from the knee

Depending on the patient's mobility, and their reaction to the exercise, traction will be performed over different areas. If the patient has sufficient mobility, when raising the hip, work is done on the quadriceps and muscle insertions in the anterosuperior iliac spine. If the patient has little mobility, the hip remains on the bed and we work on the insertion of the gluteus medius and sacroiliac joint ligaments. Used for lower back pain, and work along the edge of
the iliac crest.

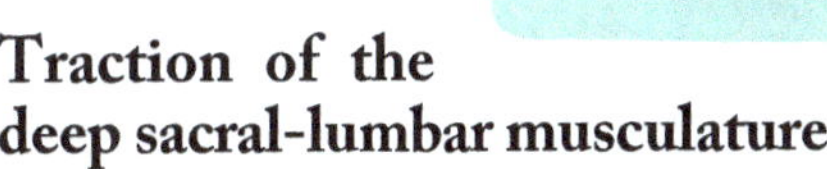

Traction of the
deep sacral-lumbar musculature

This movement works on the sacroiliac joint and on the deep musculature of the last lumbar vertebrae (multifids, rotators and thorolumbar aponeurosis).

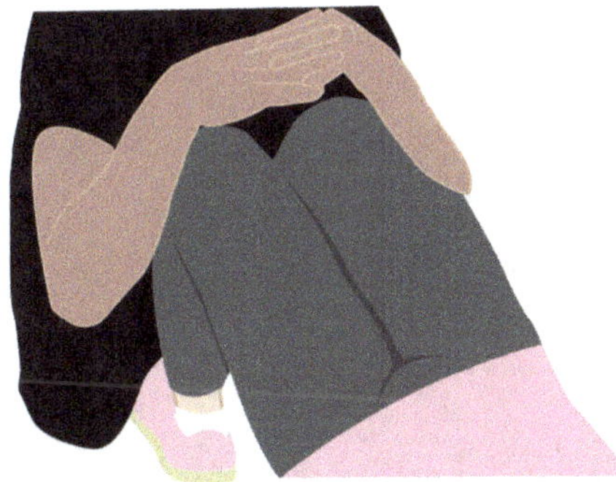

Stretching the anterior femoral area

It acts on the quadriceps, even reaching the psoas. Caution should be exercised depending on the patient's flexibility. Also, in people with hyperlordosis or lumbar problems.

Stretching muscles: quadriceps and iliac psoas.

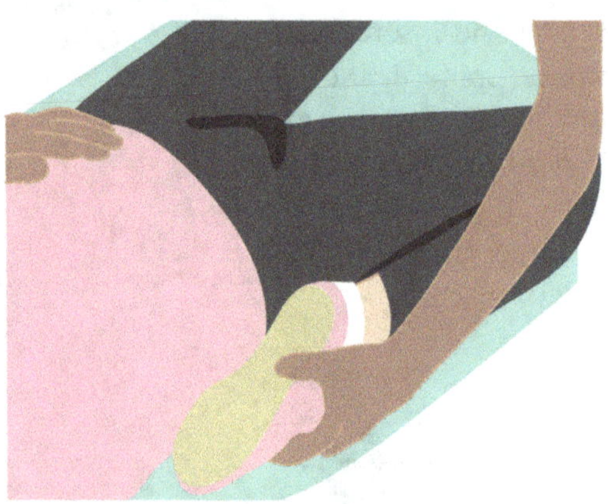

Combined stretching of the inguinal region and the origin of the hamstring area

Knee and hip flexion works on the origin of the hamstrings. Keeping the opposite knee on the bed accentuates the stretch of the inguinal region on that side. If the patient raises the knee when performing the opposite flexion, we can understand that there is shortening of the hamstring musculature.

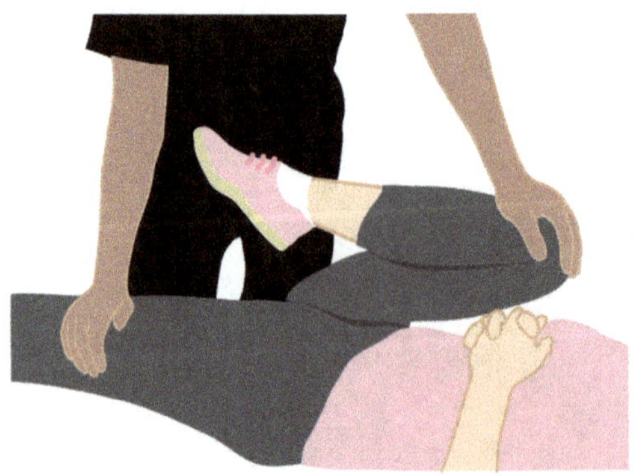

Hip movement in both directions

Making full and rhythmic hip turns in both directions. It mobilizes the hip joint as a warm-up and helps locate possible areas of tension. Allowing you to observe the condition of the large joints of the leg: hip, knee and ankle.

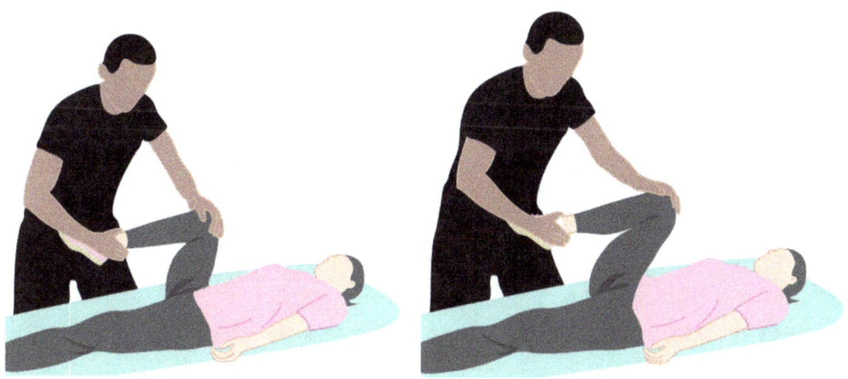

Stretching after hip movement

This exercise complements the previous work. Making wide hip turns inwards, covering the patient's entire mobility range. In places where you feel the movement is difficult, perform a stretch with knee bent and to the maximum with the hip.

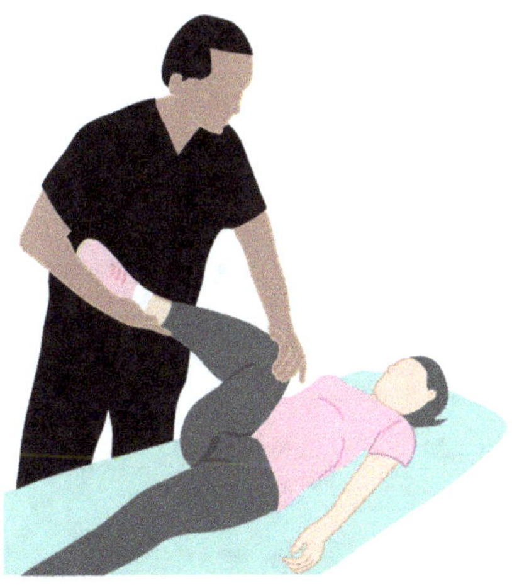

Now perform the exercise by turning the hip outwards.

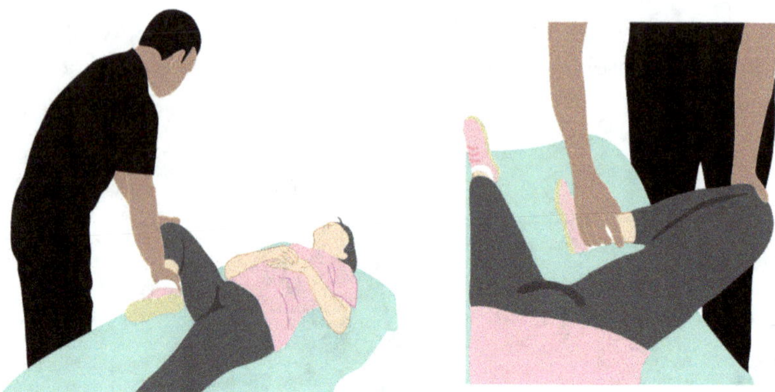

General stretching the leg

The main goal of this movement is to release all joints of the leg, especially the coxofemoral joint, lumbar region, and even the dorsal region.

The therapist should observe how all the joints connect. The movement should reach the hip joint and should be directed towards the opposite shoulder in the aspa form.

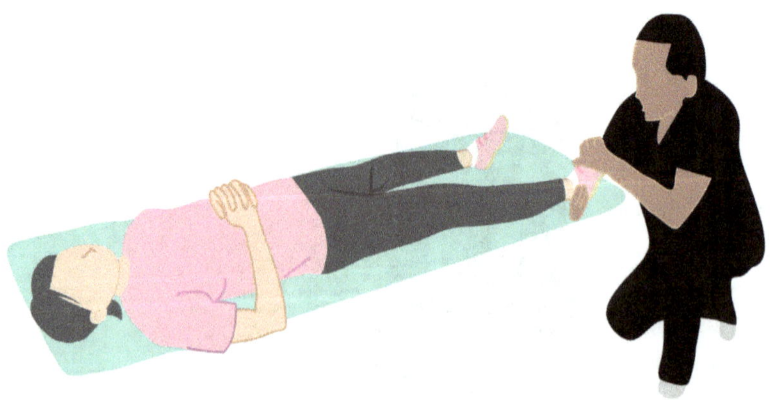

Hip traction and the release of the pyramidal muscle

The patient's leg should be in abduction and the ankle rotated outwards. The ankle must be locked well so that the stretch reaches the head of the femur and the complete distension of the entire posterior muscles occurs. Stretching the *posterior femoral and posterior sural* regions, as well as the *medial sural and inguinal* region. The hamstrings, adductors, gluteus maximus and gluteus minimus are therefore stretched.

Release of the pyramidal muscle and other lateral rotator muscles of the hip: femoral quadrant, internal obdurator, external obdurator, gemellus superior and gemellus inferior.

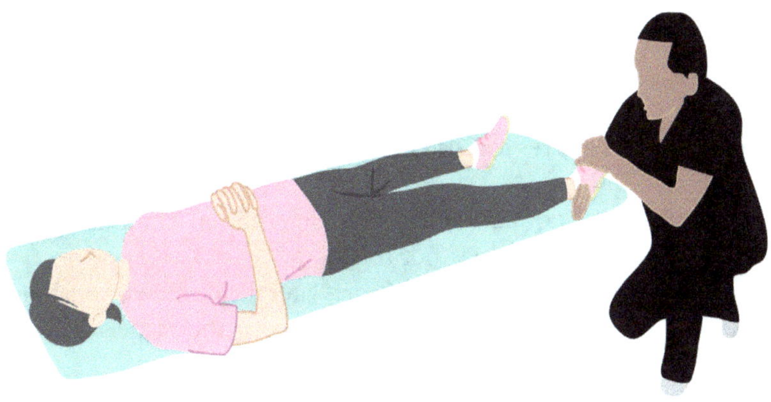

Hip traction and pyramidal stretch

Stretching the lateral area of the leg: *lateral femoral and lateral of the tibia* (anterior tibial muscle) regions. The patient's leg should be in slight abduction and the ankle rotated inwards. As in the previous case, a good ankle-level lock ensures a full stretch of the leg's lateral muscles, as well as the *femoral biceps, gluteus maximus, gluteus medius, sartorious and iliac psoas.* Stretching the *lateral femoral region, lateral of the tibia* (including point S36-Sanri) and *lateral fibula.*

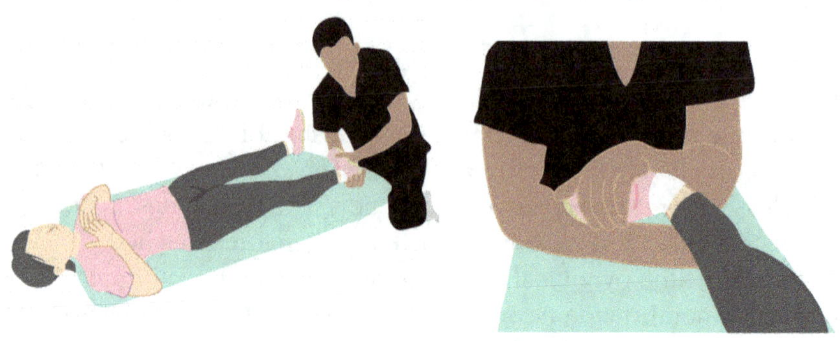

Stretching the pyramidal muscle and the rest of the lateral hip rotators.

Stretching the lateral region of the tibia

Perform plantar flexion and internal ankle rotation. The other hand must control the knee so it does not rotate.

We work the lateral regions of the tibia, lateral calcaneus, tarsal and B60 region. It is necessary to consider how it affects the ankle's external ligaments.

Muscle stretch: anterior tibial, extensor digitorum longus and extensor hallucis longus muscle.

Stretching the stomach meridian.

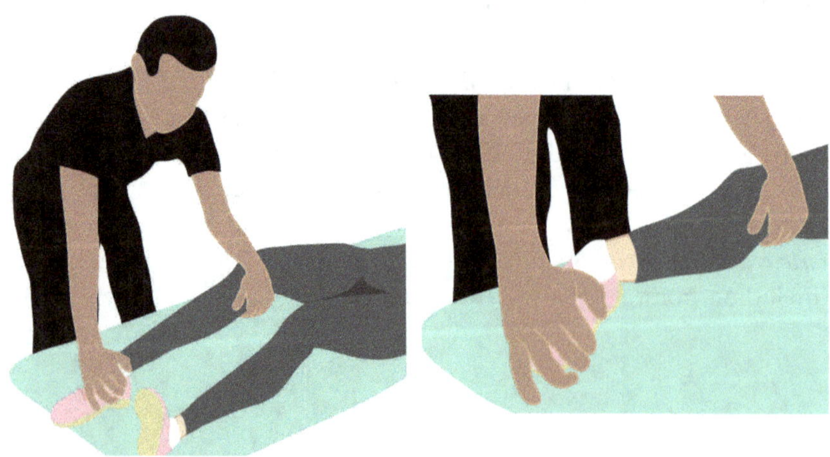

Stretching the medial sural region

Performing dorsal flexion and lateral ankle rotation. Block the knee from moving with the other hand. Work is done on the medial sural region (only the lower half), the medial calcaneal region and the K3 region. Also on the ankle's deltoid ligament (medial side).

Stretching the Spleen-Pancreas meridian (up to SP6).

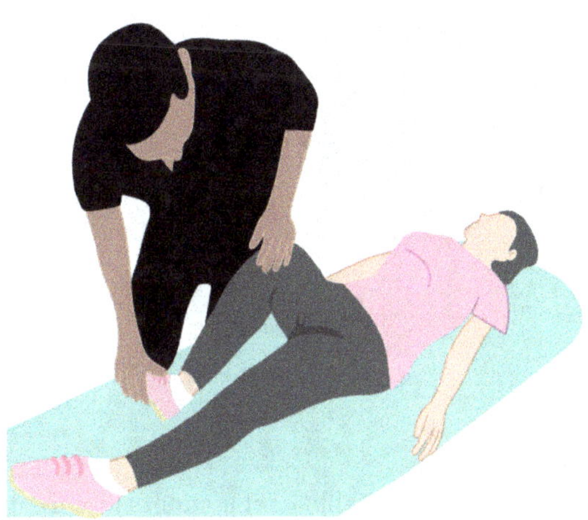

Hip joint release

Maximum external hip rotation and maximum knee flexion. You have to reach the limit of both movements to start stretching. The gluteus medius muscle is worked.

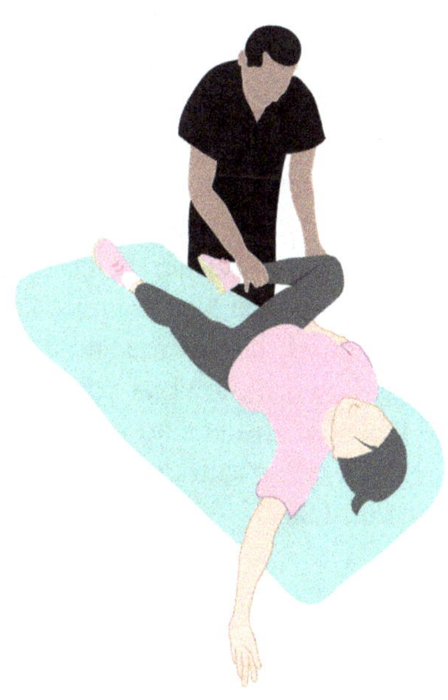

Hip joint movement

This movement is used to check how the coxofemoral joint functions. Exercise is applied from the therapist's hara projecting the weight of his body onto the patient's knee; his whole body acts in this movement.
Small circles should be made concentrated on the joint.

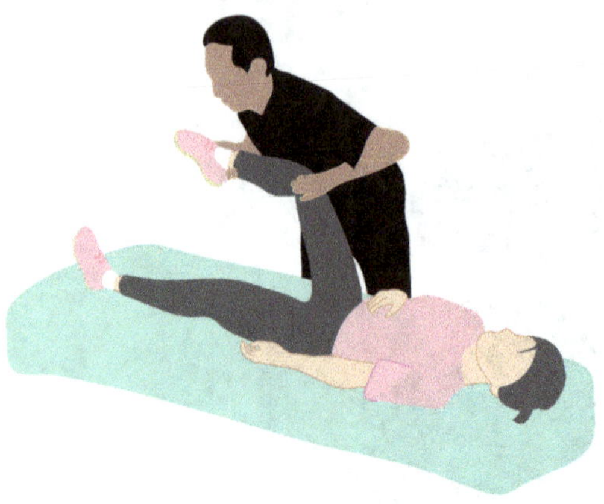

Knee stretch

This exercise works the knee joint and ligaments by the rotational movement of the ankle. To do this, the knee must be blocked by pressing with one hand in the direction of the bed, while the other performs the ankle rotations from the heel in both directions. First, perform the exercise with internal ankle rotations. This works on the fibular collateral ligament.Then, repeat the exercise with external ankle rotations. Work is now on the tibial collateral ligament and pes anserinus (insertions of the sartorius, internal rectum and semitendinous muscles).

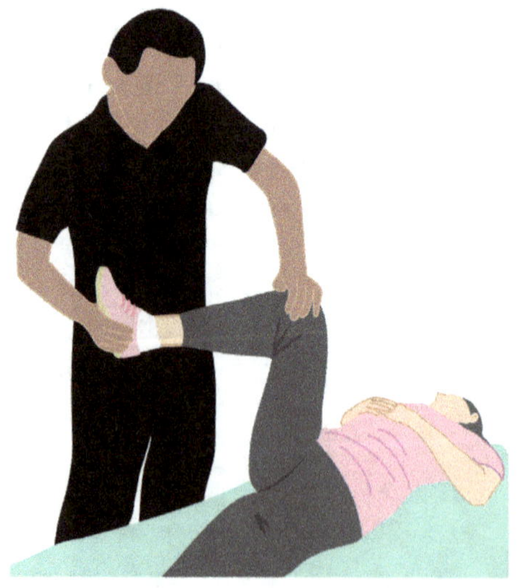

Both exercises move the knee meniscus; therefore it is important to check the condition of the joint at that level.

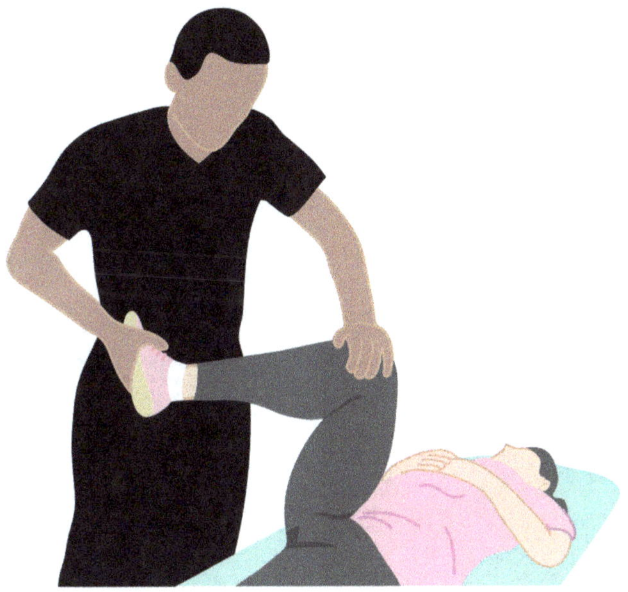

Hip joint movement (medial rotation)

Locking the knee and making the movement from the ankle to move the head of the femur. The therapist should use the rotation of his body (from his hara) to perform the movement.

Attention should be paid to the knee joint, especially in people with knee problems.

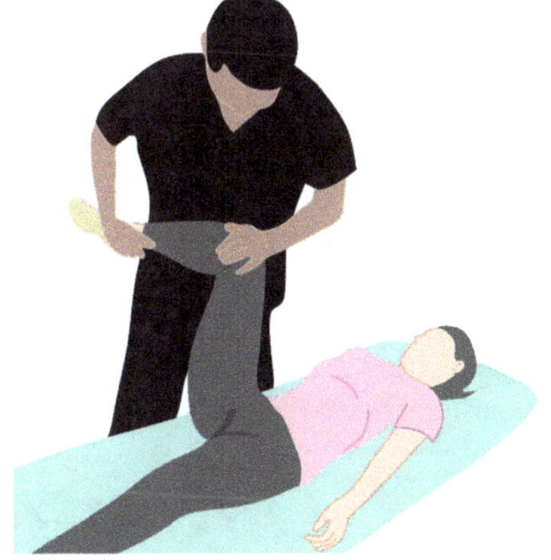

Hip joint movement (lateral rotation)

This exercise performs the opposite movement to the previous one.
As in the previous case, attention should be paid to the knee joint, especially in people with knee problems.

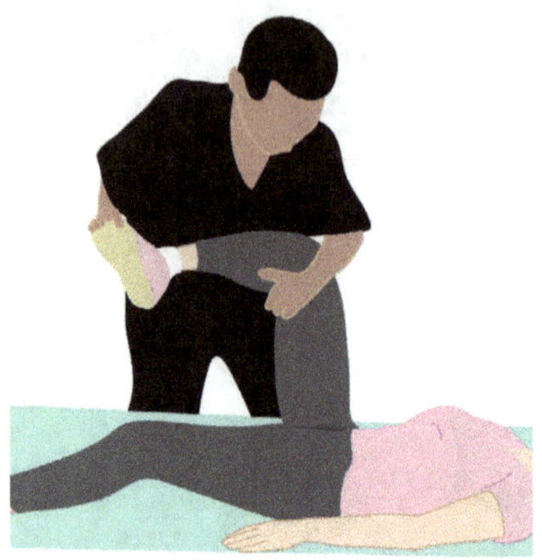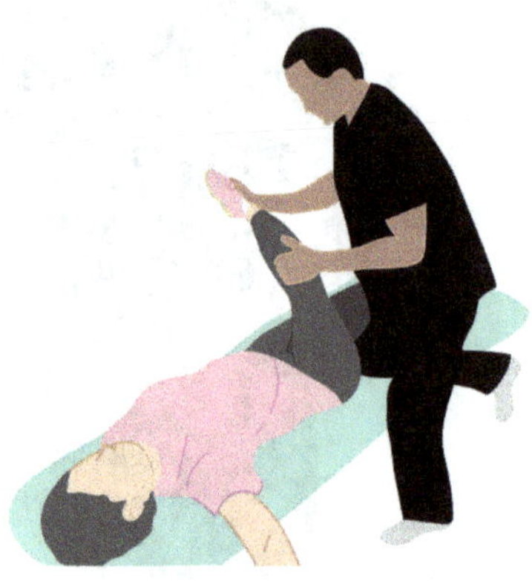

Connected stretch in Aspa 1

This stretch connects the joint, tendon, muscle and energy structures in Aspa from the knee to the shoulder.

The therapist should start by placing one hand on the patient's bent knee and then the other on the shoulder very gently. 60% of the stretch is concentrated on the hand on the knee. The direction of this stretch is very important: the circular movement of the patient's hip must be respected. That's why we don't stretch the knee in the direction of the patient's feet, but toward the centre of the body.

Stretching the lateral, infrascapular and lumbar femoral, interscapular regions.

Connected stretch in Aspa 2

If the patient's arm is stretched, the stretch also affects the axillary area, the ribs, and the latissimus dorsi and deltoid muscles.
In this case the therapist causes a much sharper stretch by transmitting the weight of his body through his knee. When stretching the arm too, the stretch is maximum, so it should be done gently and carefully.
Stretching the *lateral, infrascapular and lumbar femorals, interscapular, intercostal, axillar and medial brachial.*

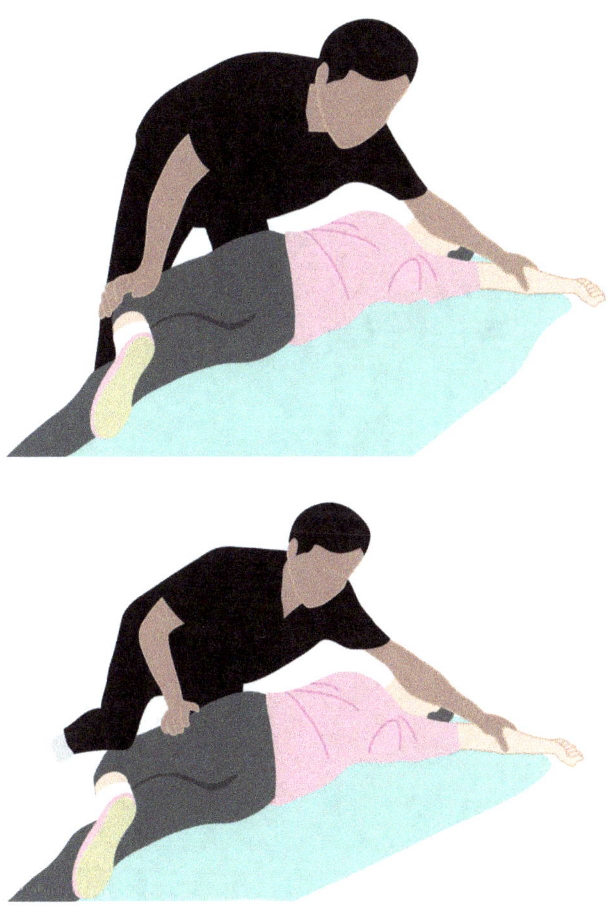

Glosary
of
Japanese
Terms

Below is a number of Japanese terms used in Shiatsu teaching. They describe important aspects to understand Shiatsu therapy and its roots, what its purpose is, and how it works.

1. 手当て **TEATE:** TREATMENT
   手　　TE means **hand**.
   当て　ATE means **put.**
   Literally: Touch with your hands.

2. 病気 **BYOUKI:** ILLNESS
   病　BYOU means **suffering.**
   気　KI means **energy.**
   Literally: Suffering of the Ki.

3. 指圧 **SHIATSU**
   指　SHI means **fingers.**
   圧　ATSU means **pressure.**
   Literally: Finger pressure.

4. 腰　**KOSHI:** CENTRE OF THE BODY / LUMBAR AREA
   月　TSUKI means **body.**
   要　KANAME means the **most important.**
   Literally: The most important part of the body.

5. 肝腎要　**KAN-JIN-KANAME:** THE MOST IMPORTANT THING FOR TREATMENT
   肝　KAN means **liver**.
   腎　JIN means **kidneys.**
   要　KANAME means most important.
   Literally: The liver and kidneys are the most important. The most important areas for any treatment are the Liver and Kidney meridians.

6. めんけん　**MENKEN:** REACTION
   Treatment is a stimulation. Even if the treatment is right, the body

reacts when stimulated. It usually lasts two days and then the patient gets better.

7. **上虚下実　JYO-KYO-KA-JITSU:** A TYPE OF TREATMENT

上　JYO means **up.**

虚　KYO means **empty.**

下　KA means **down.**

実　JITSU means **fullness.**

Literally: Up, empty; down, full. Imagining the human body, we split it in two, placing the navel in the part above. The body is completely relaxed under the navel, full of energy as if it had roots.

8. **頭寒足熱　ZU-KAN-SOKU-NETSU:** A TYPE OF TREATMENT

頭　ZU (ATAMA) means **head.**

寒　KAN means **cold.**

足　SOKU (ASHI) means **feet.**

熱　NETSU means **hot.**

Literally: Cold head, hot feet. This Japanese phrase teaches us a course of action to maintain health; meaning that by keeping the lower body warm, especially the feet, and improving the circulation, more oxygen and food get to the cells, helping them to detoxify and improve possible organic imbalances. On the contrary, the upper body is always cold and relaxed, plus it has no stress. Although people currently live in the modern city, the body is accustomed to the opposite situation.

9. **八方目　HAPPOUMOKU**

八方　HAPPOU means the **eight directions.**

目　MOKU means **eyes.**

Literally: Look in all eight directions. Through the eyes with a glance, trying to cover eight different directions feeling the patient's KI.

10. 目測　　**MOKUSOKU**

目　　MOKU means **eyes.**

測　　SOKU means **measure.**

Literally: Measure with the eyes. When working with the patient we have to measure where the painful points are with the eyes.

11. 気を配る　**KI WO KUBARU:** EMPATHIZING WITH THE OTHER

気　　KI means **energy.**

配る　KUBARU means to **share out.**

Literally: Sharing out energy/Ki. It means having empathy for someone else and helping them.

12. 手おくれ　**TEOKURE:** NON-EFFECTIVE TREATMENT

手　　　TE means **hand.**

おくれ　OKURE means **too late**.

Literally: Apply the hand too late. Treatment that, although appropriate, is applied too late and is worse for the delay.

13. 虚実補瀉　**KYOJITSU-HOSYA**

HO. Lay the hand to complement emptiness.

SYA. Apply pressure to remove excess energy.

Literally: If the body is in KYO (empty), you have to complement it. If it is in JITSU (full), you need to remove it.

14. 無心　**MUSHIN:** INTUITIVELY

無　　MU means **nothing.**

心　　SHIN (KOKORO) means **heart.**

Literally: Without thinking, getting carried away by the knowledge learned. There is a lot of information you have to receive during training for a technique or struggle, free from thoughts and emotions.

15. 長生き　**NAGAIKI:** LONG LIFE

長い　　NAGAI means long.

生きる　IKIRU means to live.

Literally: Long breathing/long life.

This phrase can have two senses:

  1. Living for a long time.

  2. Deep breathing.

So NAGA IKI means: "To live many years you have to breathe deeply and slowly".

16.   足首   **ASHIKUBI (ANKLE)**   手首   **TEKUBI (WRIST)**

足首   ASHI means **feet.**

足   TE means **hand.**

首   KUBI means **neck.**

Literally: There are three very important areas for treatment called 'the neck': the neck itself, the wrist and ankle. Special action points are located for general Shiatsu treatment.

17.   於血   **OKETSU**

於   O means **toxin.**

血   KETSU means **blood**.

Literally: Ancient blood. Ki (energy) and Ketsu (blood) have to circulate constantly. If they become clogged and do not circulate properly it is said that there is stagnation of Ki or Ketsu. This area is called Oketsu (dirty blood).

18.   診断即治療   **SHINDAN-SOKUCHIRYOU**

Literally: Diagnosis and therapy are done at the same time. When the therapist applies Shiatsu pressure to the patient's body, he receives information, through the hands and fingers, of the state of the skin, muscles and body temperature. Therefore, the professional therapist can determine the necessary treatment to perform.

19.   全身治療   **ZENSHIN-CHIRYOU**

Literally: Treatment of all body parts as a whole. The best method to get to the cause is to take care of the whole body first and then the areas that have pathological symptoms.

20. 按腹　　**ANPUKU:** TREATMENT FROM THE HARA

Literally: Diagnosis and treatment of the abdominal area.

Many distal joint and muscular ailments can be alleviated and improved by working the abdominal area, without working the area involved directly. Also, working the abdomen improves the functioning of the organs and bladder, providing elasticity and increased blood supply.

21. 腹黒い　　**HARAGUROI:** PERSON WITH BAD INTENTIONS

腹　　HARA means **abdomen**.

黒い　KUROI means **black.**

Literally: black Hara (abdomen). Malevolent person.

22. 腹を見せる　**HARA WO MISERU**

信頼する　　**SHINRAI SURU**

Literally: Teach the Hara area (trust).

As in the case of animals, which show their belly when they feel confident, people who are comfortable with the pressure expose the Hara area.

23. 背を向ける　**SE WO MUKERU**

背　　　　SE means **back.**

を向ける　　WO MUKERU means **giving someone**.

Literally: Turning your back on someone. Quit, stop doing, stop helping.

24. 守破離　　**SHU HA RI**

守　SHU means **keeping, obeying, respecting traditional wisdom**, and learning fundamental techniques. We must imitate the master's teachings without hesitation until we reach perfection. 破　HA means **break up**. Model your own style. Adapt the technique respecting the teachings of the teacher.

離　RI means **to separate**. When all movements are natural, Shiatsu becomes one, it merges with the spirit. Shiatsu-shi is ready to create its own style.

Japanese numbers

1 ICHI
2 NI
3 SAN
4 SHI (YON)
5 GO
6 ROKU
7 NANA (SHICHI)
8 HACHI
9 KYU
10 JYU
11 JYU ICHI
12 JYU NI
13 JYU SAN
14 JYU SHI
15 JYU GO
16 JYU ROKU
17 JYU SHICHI
18 JYU HACHI
19 JYU KU
20 NI JYU

Acknowledgments

Putting this book together took about a year and a half. The main purpose for doing so has been to improve the location and perform more detailed work on Shiatsu Aze. To build the "column" I started with a few pages and gradually the result came about.

I want to thank all my team who have made it possible for this project to see the light of day.

SHIGERU ONODA
Founder of Aze Shiatsu
Shiatsupractor

Illustrators:

María Torres Dos Ramos, Raquel García Fernández, Tatio Viana, Carmen Toro de Federico, Daigo Ohnuma.

Editing and reviewing texts and images:

Raúl Gómez Villa, Luz María García, Manuel Tirado, César Fernández, Julio Ortiz, Antonio Alonso Casas, Carmen Yagüe, Osamu Suzuki, Chikako Kanai, Mateo García, Kita Naoko y Masumi Mihara.

Supervising anatomical terminology:

Dr. Hiroshi Ishizuka (Director of the Japan Shiatsu College).

Photographs:

Claudia Costanzo, Loukia Stathatou.

Models:

Nuria Colorado, Osamu Suzuki.

Bibliography

参考文献

ATLAS GRÁFICO DE ACUPUNTURA SEIRIN, Seirin, edición Könemann, 2000.

HIRATSUKA KOUICHI, ¿Qué es la Osteopatía?, edición Goma-Shobou, 2003.

JAPAN SHIATSU COLLEGE SHIATSU RIRON KOUGIROKU, Teoría del Shiatsu, J.S.C. 1979. KAN POU GAIRON KEI KETSU HEN, Introducción de la medicina del kanpou y puntos tsubos, edición KK Ishiyakus-Shuppan, 1980.

KAWANA RITSUKO, Tsubo no kenkou Hyakka, edición Shufu to Seikatsusha. 2002.

NAMIKOSHI TORU, Tratado completo de terapia Shiatsu, edición Edaf, Madrid, 1992.

ONODA SHIGERU, Libro completo de Shiatsu, edición Gaia, Madrid,1998.

— Curso básico de Shiatsu, edición Gaia, Madrid,2002.

— Introducción a la práctica del Shiatsu, edición Dilema, 2003.

— Autoshiatsu, edición Edaf, Madrid, 2002.

— Tratamiento de la Lumbalgia mediante Shiatsu, edición Gaia, 2001.

— Atsu he no kodawari. Qué es la presión? Edición Taniguchi-Shoten, Japón 2008.